BIOCHEMISTRY OF CATECHOLAMINES

The Biochemical Method

By

Toshiharu NAGATSU

UNIVERSITY PARK PRESS
Baltimore · London · Tokyo

UNIVERSITY PARK PRESS
Baltimore · London · Tokyo

Library of Congress Cataloging in Publication Data

Nagatsu, Toshiharu.
  Biochemistry of catecholamines.

  Bibliography: p.
  1. Catecholamines. 2. Catecholamines—Analysis.
I. Title.   [DNLM: 1. Air pollution—Collected
works. 2. Ecology—Collected works.   WA754 E17 1973]
QP801.C33N3   599'.01'4   73-10351
ISBN 0-8391-0093-0

Originally published by
UNIVERSITY OF TOKYO PRESS

BIOCHEMISTRY OF CATECHOLAMINES

FOREWORD

Since 1965, when I initiated the study of enzyme inhibitors produced by microorganisms, Dr. Nagatsu, the author and the discoverer of tyrosine hydroxylase, has collaborated with me in the study of new inhibitors of enzymes involved in biosynthesis and metabolism of catecholamines. This work was of great assistance in microorganism-produced enzyme inhibitor research. As a result of his collaborative work, new and interesting inhibitors of tyrosine hydroxylase and dopamine-β-hydroxylase, showing expected hypotensive effect, were discovered. From these studies I began to recognize the importance of the biochemistry of catecholamines. At the same time, I realized the importance of catecholamines in the control of human and animal behavior.

As recent as 15 years ago, the biochemical base of hypertension, psychoses, and neurological diseases was practically unknown; however, at present, this situation has changed markedly. For example, we now know that L-DOPA is a specific drug for parkinsonism, and also various neuroreptics that block dopaminergic neurones are now successfully used for treatment of schizophrenia. The mechanism of the pharmacological effects of these compounds can be determined from the biochemistry and the pharmacology of the related catecholamines. These catecholamines studies cover the mechanisms of various diseases and may, in addition, cover human behavior, feelings and emotions. Moreover, new, useful compounds are now being developed on the basis of catecholamine biochemistry.

At the present time, biochemistry and biology are progressing in two directions. The first concerns the mechanism of life, construction of cells and their heredity; these studies have been generally classified as molecular biology. Studies in molecular biology have given us abundant basic knowledge on the genetics and the biosyntheses of living compounds. The second area involves the rapidly progressing biochemistry of human behavior and disease. These studies provide a rational approach to exact diagnosis, and to achieving effective treatment of diseases. The extraordinary progress in this area is an important contribution to human welfare.

The purpose of this book is to present and discuss recent advances in research on the function, biochemistry, and pharmacology of catechol-

v

amines. In addition, detailed experimental methods showing how important results were obtained are also presented. Dr. Nagatsu has studied the
enzymology involved in biosyntheses and metabolisms of catecholamines
in their relation to pharmacology and disease. This book will be useful for
experts in the biochemistry of catecholamines, and will also be valuable for
researchers and students in medical sciences in general.

We are most grateful to Dr. Nagatsu for his contributions to this difficult
and complex field, and we are even more grateful for his efforts in compil-
ing and writing this book, which I believe will be an important and useful
contribution to scientific literature.

July 1973

Hamao UMEZAWA, *Director*
Institute of Microbial Chemistry

PREFACE

Catecholamines are unique among various hormones in that not only their metabolic pathway but also the enzymes related to their biosynthesis and metabolism have been almost completely elucidated. These biochemical findings of catecholamines are valuable in understanding the physiological, pathological and pharmacological functions of catecholamines. The biochemical and enzymological techniques developed in catecholamine research are also useful in biological and medical investigation of the sympathetic autonomic nervous system which may be closely related to the pathogenesis of various diseases, such as hypertension and mental or nervous diseases.

This book is intended to present biochemical facts about catecholamines and detailes of investigative techniques, especially in the field of enzymology, that have been developed over the last 20 years. It is an enlargement of a previous review: Nagatsu, T.: Biosynthesis and metabolism of catecholamines (in Japanese). *J. Jap. Biochem. Soc.*, **37**, 697 (1965). After the publication of the review in Japanese, I received many requests for an English translation. I also received many inquiries on the details of enzyme assays such as those of tyrosine hydroxylase and dopamine-β-hydroxylase. I decided to expand the review and add details of techniques in catecholamine biochemistry, especially enzymology. Although many modifications of the assay techniques are possible, experiment examples, such as the preparation of an incubation mixture for an enzyme assay, have been included. Specific descriptions of assays that may be useful in the laboratory are given but readers can modify them to fit their own experimental plans.

I hope that this book can be of some help to reseachers in the clinical and basic aspects of various fields of medicine and biology.

Publication of this book was delayed because of an interruption caused my spending a sabbatical year at the Roche Institute of Molecular Biology (Nutley, New Jersey, U. S. A.) in 1972.

References up to 1971 were included in the first draft and as many important reports appeared in 1972, some of them have been included in the Supplement.

vii

Several interesting reports have appeared after the preparation of the second draft.

As described in the text, catecholamine biosynthesis and metabolism in the sympathetic nervous system and the adrenal medulla were found to be regulated both by feedback regulation at the tyrosine-hydroxylase stage and by the changes in the levels of the enzymes such as tyrosine hydroxylase and dopamine-β-hydroxylase probably due to the changes in protein synthesis of the enzymes. The increased levels of tyrosine hydroxylase and dopamine-β-hydroxylase after chronically increased sympathetic nerve activity (Mueller, R. A., Thoenen, K. and Axelrod, J.: Adrenal tyrosine hydroxylase: compensatory increase in activity after chemical sympathectomy. *Science*, **163**, 468 (1969); Viveros, O. H., Arqueros, L., Connett, R. J. and Kirshner, N.: Mechanism of secretion from the adrenal medulla. IV. The fate of storage vesicles following insulin and reserpine administration. *Mol. Pharmacol.*, **5**, 69 (1969)) as well as the decreased levels of tyrosine hydroxylase and aromatic L-amino acid decarboxylase after the administration of L-DOPA were discovered (Dairman, W. and Udenfriend, S.: Decrease in adrenal tyrosine hydroxylase and increase in norepinephrine synthesis in rats given L-DOPA. *Science*, **171**, 1022 (1971); Dairman, W., Christenson, J. G. and Udenfriend, S.: Decrease in liver aromatic L-amino acid decarboxylase produced by chronic administration of L-DOPA. *Proc. Natl. Acad. Sci. U. S. A.*, **68**, 2117 (1971)). These advances in the regulation mechanism of catecholamine biosynthesis and metabolism have been summarized in a recent review (Cotton, M. de V., Udenfriend, S. and Spector, S. *eds*: Regulation of catecholamine metabolism in the sympathetic nervous system. *Pharmacol. Rev.*, **24**, 161–449, Williams and Wilkins Co., Baltimore (1972)).

Blood vessels have very dense sympathetic nerve innervations and are therefore rich in norepinephrine and the enzymes of its biosynthesis and metabolism. They should be important sources of norepinephrine in blood and urine (Spector, S., Tarver, J. and Berkowitz, B.: Effects of drugs and physiological factors in the disposition of catecholamines in blood vessels. *Pharmacol. Rev.*, **24**, 191 (1972)).

The radioimmunoassay for dopamine-β-hydroxylase (Rush, R. A. and Geffen, L. B.: Radioimmunoassay and clearance of circulating dopamine-β-hydroxylase, *Circ. Res.*, **31**, 444 (1972)) has been used in the determination of enzyme in blood, and it is possible to use it to measure enzyme protein including the active and inactive forms.

Mass fragmentographic assaying of catecholamines using a mass spectrometer as a detector for the gas chromatography was carried out by Costa *et al.* (Costa, E., Green, A. R., Koslow, S. H., Lefevre, H. F., Revuelta, A. V. and Wang, C.: Dopamine and norepinephrine in noradrenergic axons: A study *in vivo* of their precursor product relationship by mass fragmentography and radiochemistry. *Pharmacol. Rev.*, **24,** 167 (1972). Koslow, S. H., Cattabeni, F. and Costa, E.: Norepinephrine and dopamine: assay by mass fragmentography in the picomole range. *Science*, **176,** 177 (1972)) and should be quite useful as a highly specific and sensitive assay for tissue catecholamines. A simple and sensitive fluorometric method for the assay of norepinephrine, epinephrine and dopamine in urine by means of thin-layer chromatography has been reported (Takahashi, R. and Gjessing, L. R.: A fluorometric method combined with thin-layer chromatography for the determination of norepinephrine, epinephrine and dopamine in human urine. *Clin. Chim. Acta*, **36,** 369 (1972)). To increase the specificity of a catecholamine assay, complete separation of the catecholamines, either by gas chromatography or thin-layer chromatography, is preferable. A simplified enzymatic radioassay for dopamine and norepinephrine had been established in Axelrod's Laboratory by Coyle, J. T., Jr. and Henry, D. (Catecholamines in fetal and newborn rat brain. *J. Neurochem.*, in press, 1973). This method used catechol-*O*-methyltransferase and radioactive *S*-adenosylmethionine for labeling the dopamine and norepinephrine, then differentiates both amines by periodate oxidation. It appears to be simple and highly sensitive for the assay of tissue catecholamines.

Several important reviews have also appeared in the period 1971–1972. They have been included in the Review bibliography.

February 1973

Toshiharu NAGATSU, *Professor*
Aichi-Gakuin University

ACKNOWLEDGEMENTS

I wish to thank Professor Hamao Umezawa (Director, Institute of Microbial Chemistry, Tokyo, Japan) for his kind encouragement and arrangement for the publication of this book and for his foreword, and Dr. Sidney Udenfriend (Director, Roche Institute of Molecular Biology, Nutley, New Jersey, U. S. A.) for his kind encouragement and advice since my work with him as a NIH international postdoctoral fellow at the National Institutes of Health (Bethesda, Maryland, U. S. A.) from 1962 to 1964.

My thanks are also due to Professor Kunio Yagi (Institute of Biochemistry, Nagoya University, Nagoya, Japan) for introducing me to catecholamine biochemistry starting with the fluorescence assay of catecholamines, and to Professor Keisuke Fujita (President, Fujita-Gakuen University School of Medicine, Toyoake, Aichi, Japan) who had helped me in establishing a biochemistry laboratory in Aichi-Gakuin University School of Dentistry.

I am grateful to Dr. Julius Axelrod (National Institute of Mental Health, Bethesda, Maryland, U. S. A.) for his personal information on dopamine-β-hydroxylase assay, to Professor Miki Akino (Department of Biology, Faculty of Science, Tokyo Metropolitan University, Tokyo, Japan) for his critical reading of and advive concerning the section on phenylalanine hydroxylase, to Professor Kerry T. Yasunobu (Department of Biochemistry and Biophysics, University of Hawaii, Honolulu, Hawaii, U. S. A.) for reviewing the description of his purification procedure of monoamine oxidase, and to Dr. Donald E. Wolf and Mrs. Idamarie Eggers (Merck Sharp and Dohme Research Laboratories, Rahway, New Jersey, U. S. A.) for their careful review of the Appendix (Chemical Properties of Catecholamines).

I deeply acknowledge the help of my colleagues in the Department of Biochemistry, School of Dentistry, Aichi-Gakuin University, especially the capable assistance of Miss Yuko Nishikawa and Miss Yumiko Shibahara in the preparation of this book.

Finally, I wish to acknowledge deeply the invaluable help from my wife, Dr. Ikuko Nagatsu, in every respect for the preparation of this book.

The Author

CONTENTS

BIOCHEMISTRY OF CATECHOLAMINES

Introduction

Biogenic amines which possess a 3,4-dihydroxyphenyl (catechol) nucleus, are generally called catecholamines (catechol amines) and are derivatives of 3,4-dihydroxyphenylethylamine. Three catecholamines, epinephrine (adrenalin), norepinephrine (noradrenalin) and dopamine (hydroxy-tyramine), are present in animals and plants (Fig. 1). They are located in the biosynthetic pathway in the following order, dopamine → norepine-phrine → epinephrine, but each has its own biological activity. Epinephrine is a typical hormone which is secreted from the adrenal medulla. It is transported to various target organs by the bloodstream, taken up by the organs, and serves to regulate metabolism in the target organs. Nor-epinephrine is also secreted from the adrenal medulla but only in small amounts. It is generally contained in the sympathetic nerves, discharged from the nerve endings as a chemical transmitter, and acts in the area in which it is discharged probably by binding with a "receptor" in the target organs. Norepinephrine is, therefore, called a "local hormone" or a "tissue hormone." Norepinephrine and dopamine are also contained in the brain, and are supposed to be chemical transmitters. The physiological role of dopamine is not yet as clear as those of epinephrine and norepinephrine, but recent findings showing a high concentration of dopamine in the extrapyramidal system of the brain strongly suggest its physiological im-portance in the brain. Catecholamines produce many important physio-logical effects in the brain, the cardiovascular system, and other organs.

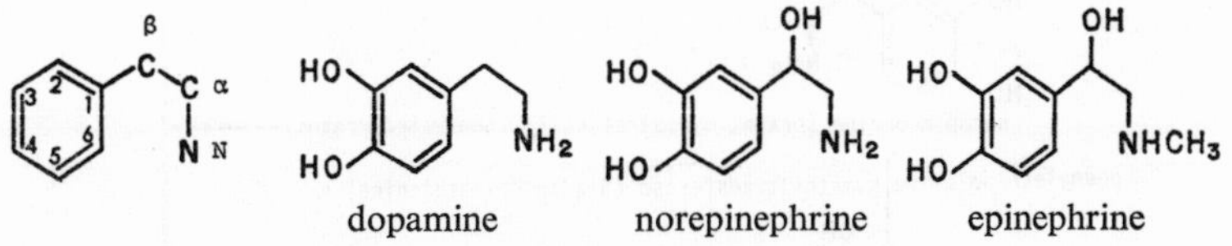

Fig. 1. Structures of catecholamines.

Recent studies have stressed their pathological importance in nervous diseases, including parkinsonism and psychoses, such as mental depression, in heart diseases, and in hypertention.

The first catecholamine to be discovered was epinephrine (adrenalin),

3

which is the predominant hormone in the adrenal medulla (Abel and Crawford, 1897; Takamine, 1901; Aldrich, 1901). Epinephrine was synthesized in 1904 (Stolz). Simultaneously, the second catecholamine to be discovered, norepinephrine (noradrenalin), which lacks the *N*-methyl group found in epinephrine, was also synthesized (Stolz, 1904). The discovery of norepinephrine in the animals, however, was not made until 40 years later (Euler, 1946a). It was discovered in sympathetically innervated organs and sympathetic nerves (Euler, 1946a) as well as in urine and the adrenal medulla (Holtz, Credner and Kroneberg, 1947). The third catecholamine to be discovered, dopamine, which lacks the hydroxy group at the β-carbon site of the norepinephrine side chain was found in animals at about the same period (Holtz, Credner and Strübing, 1942; Goodall, 1950a, b).

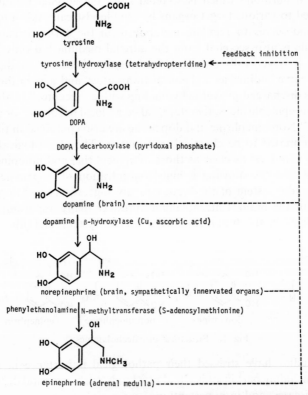

Fig. 2. The main biosynthetic pathway of catecholamines and its regulation (Udenfriend, 1966b).

On the other hand, studies on the biosynthesis and metabolism of cate-cholamines and on the related enzymes began around 1930. DOPA decar-boxylase which decarboxylates DOPA to dopamine was first discovered among the biosynthetic enzymes (Holtz, 1939). As a result, the following main metabolic pathway of catecholamines was proposed: tyrosine → DOPA → dopamine → norepinephrine → epinephrine (Blaschko, 1939). This hypothetical pathway was later proved by isotope experiments (Udenfriend and Wyngaarden, 1956). By 1964, all the enzymes of the bio-synthesis of catecholamines had been discovered and the biosynthetic pathway and the mechanism of biosynthetic regulation were elucidated (Udenfriend, 1966a, b) (Fig. 2).

In regard to the enzymatic degradation of catecholamines, the oxidative deamination by monoamine oxidase was discovered first (Blaschko and Schlossmann, 1936; Blaschko, Richter and Schlossmann, 1937a, b). An-other important step in the study of the metabolism of catecholamines

COMT : catechol-O-methyltransferase
MAO : monoamine oxidase

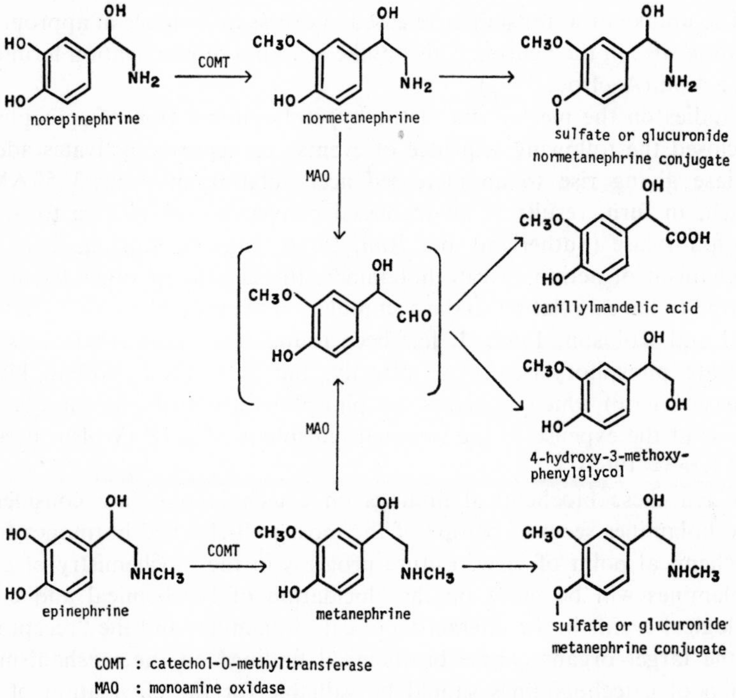

Fig. 3. The main metabolic pathway of catecholamines (Axelrod, 1959).

was the discovery of *O*-methylated catecholamine metabolites, i.e., 4-hydroxy-3-methoxymandelic acid (vanillylmandelic acid) (Armstrong, Shaw and Wall, 1956; Armstrong, McMillan and Shaw, 1957), metanephrine (3-methoxyepinephrine) and normetanephrine (3-methoxynorepinephrine) (Axelrod, 1957), as the major metabolites of catecholamines. Catechol-*O*-methyltransferase proved to be the enzyme responsible for the *O*-methylation of catecholamines (Axelrod, 1957). These findings led to the complete elucidation of the metabolic pathway of catecholamines (Fig. 3).

Catecholamines were found to be stored in subcellular granules in the adrenal medulla (Blaschko and Welch, 1953; Hillarp, Lagerstedt and Nilson, 1953) as well as in the sympathetic nerves (Euler and Hillarp, 1956; Euler, 1958; Schümann, 1956, 1958b; Potter and Axelrod, 1963b). Opinions differ as to whether the transmitter, norepinephrine, is directly transferred to the receptor from the granules or whether it first passes through an intermediate station. This postulated storage area is referred to as the extragranular pool from which the release may even occur in several steps (Euler, 1966a).

The uptake of a transmitter released in excess takes place at appropriate binding sites in the neuron. This uptake is a kind of inactivation terminating action (Axelrod, 1965).

Studies on the mechanism of the hyperglycemic action of epinephrine disclosed the following sequence of events: epinephrine activates adenyl cyclase giving rise to an increased accumulation of cyclic-3′,5′-AMP, which, in turn, results in an increased conversion of inactive to active phosphorylase (Sutherland and Rall, 1960) (Fig. 4). Starting from this mechanism of action of catecholamines, the actions of other hormones proved to have a relation to the accumulation of cyclic-3′,5′-AMP (Sutherland and Robison, 1966). It has been found that cyclic AMP does not activate phosphorylase kinase directly, but activates a protein kinase (kinase kinase) which catalyzes the phosphorylation of phosphorylase *b* kinase at the expense of the terminal phosphate of ATP (Walsh, Perkins and Krebs, 1968).

When these biochemical findings on catecholamines are considered, catecholamines seem to be one of the most well-clarified hormones from biochemical point of view. Future progress in the biochemistry of catecholamines will be made on the elucidation of biochemical and enzymological events in the interaction of catecholamines and the "receptors" in the target organs. These biochemical findings on the mechanism of action of catecholamines should be valuable for the elucidation of the general mechanism of action of the hormones, "the chemical messengers."

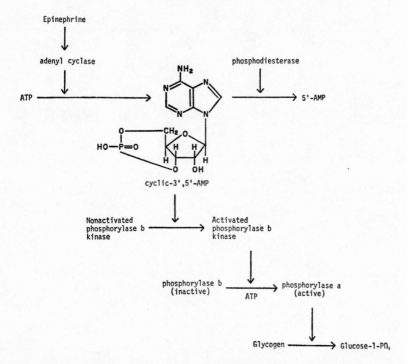

Fig. 4. The hyperglycemic action mechanism of epinephrine (Sutherland and Rall, 1960).

Chapter I

Biosynthesis of Catecholamines

I. 1.　Main Biosynthetic Pathway of Catecholamines

Based on the similarity of structure of catecholamines and tyrosine and
phenylalanine, theories on the biosynthesis of catecholamines from tyrosine
were established (Halle, 1906). The first experimental evidence on the
formation of catecholamines from DOPA was achieved in 1938 (Imaizumi,
1938). DOPA decarboxylase, which is responsible for the formation of
dopamine, was discovered in 1939 (Holtz, 1939). As a result, the following
biosynthetic pathway was derived; tyrosine → DOPA → dopamine → norepinephrine → epinephrine (Blaschko, 1939). In 1947, it was shown that
radioactive phenylalanine administered to rats was incorporated into epinephrine in the adrenal medulla (Gurin and Delluva, 1947). A series of isotopic experiments showed that phenylalanine-C^{14}, tyrosine-C^{14} and DOPA-
C^{14} could be incorporated into epinephrine in the adrenal medulla, but
neither tyramine-C^{14} nor phenethylamine-C^{14} proved to be precursors of
adrenal epinephrine (Udenfriend, Cooper, Clark and Baer, 1953; Udenfriend and Wyngaarden, 1956). Dopamine-C^{14} was also shown to convert
to epinephrine in the adrenal medulla (Leeper and Udenfriend, 1956).
Norepinephrine-C^{14} was shown to be directly converted to epinephrine
(Masuoka, Schott, Akawie and Clark, 1956). These *in vivo* experiments
supported the following biosynthetic pathway: phenylalanine → tyrosine
→ DOPA → dopamine → norepinephrine → epinephrine (Fig. 2, p. 4).
It was subsequently found that perfusion of the intact, isolated calf adrenal
with a well-oxygenated artificial medium containing C^{14}-labeled tyrosine
resulted in the formation of labeled dopamine, norepinephrine and epinephrine (Rosenfeld, Leeper and Udenfriend, 1958). They also reported that
the hydroxylation step essential for the conversion of tyrosine to DOPA
appears to be the rate-limiting reaction in the over-all sequence. The presence of dopamine in the adrenal gland also supports the main biosynthetic
pathway (Goodall, 1950a, b, 1951; Shepherd and West, 1953).

The results *in vivo* described above were also confirmed by *in vitro* experiments showing the formation of dopamine and norepinephrine from
DOPA-C^{14} in the homogenate of bovine adrenal medulla (Demis, Blaschko
and Welch, 1955, 1956).

It was shown that the turnover rate of epinephrine in the adrenal medulla was very slow (a half-life of nine days in the rat) (Udenfriend, Cooper, Clark and Baer, 1953). The rate of turnover of norepinephrine in the adrenal gland was similar to that of epinephrine (Udenfriend and Wyngaarden, 1956). These results suggest that a very slow rate-limiting step in the biosynthesis of catecholamines is present before the synthesis of norepinephrine. Tyrosine hydroxylase which forms DOPA from tyrosine is now thought to be the rate-limiting step (Levitt, Spector, Sjoerdsma and Udenfriend, 1965).

This main biosynthetic pathway of catecholamines was confirmed in other organs besides the adrenal gland. In the brain, norepinephrine was concentrated in the hypothalamus (Vogt, 1954). Dopamine was also discovered in the brain (Carlsson, Lindqvist, Magnusson and Waldeck, 1958). In mammalian brain, practically all of the dopamine was localized in the extrapyramidal system such as corpus striatum (Carlsson, 1959a, b). In human brain also, dopamine was localized in the extrapyramidal system (Sano, Gamo, Kakimoto, Taniguchi, Takesada and Nishinuma, 1959). Dopamine was found also in the splenic nerve (Schümann, 1956) and was localized in the cytoplasma, whereas the norepinephrine was localized in granular elements of the nerves (Schümann, 1958b).

The incubation of the sympathetic ganglia and nerves with radioactive tyrosine and DOPA resulted in the formation of radioactive dopamine and norepinephrine; epinephrine was also thought to have been formed, but it was not certain (Goodall and Kirshner, 1957). In contrast to the chromaffin cells of the suprarenal medulla, the biosynthesis of catecholamines in the mammalian sympathetic nervous tissue proceeds mainly up to norepinephrine. By administering tyrosine-C^{14} or DOPA-H^3 to guinea pigs it was possible to achieve sufficient labeling of the dopamine and norepinephrine in the brain to permit measurement of their turnover rate (Udenfriend and Zaltzman-Nirenberg, 1963). The half-life of norepinephrine was about 4 hr, suggesting a rate of synthesis of at least 0.03 to 0.04 $\mu g/g$ per hr or 2.4 $\mu g/day$ for the whole guinea pig brain. The half-life of dopamine was about 2.5 hr, and the calculated rate of synthesis was 0.11 $\mu g/g$ per hr or 7.9 $\mu g/$ day for the whole brain.

The heart, which is a sympathetically innervated organ, can synthesize norepinephrine from tyrosine. This was proved from the evidence that the isolated, perfused guinea pig heart converted tyrosine-C^{14} to norepinephrine-C^{14} (Spector, Sjoerdsma, Zaltzman-Nirenberg, Levitt and Udenfriend, 1963). The calculated rate for the formation of norepinephrine was 0.03 to 0.05 $\mu g/g$ per hr and the estimate on the rate of synthesis of norepinephrine in intact mammalian heart was 0.03 to 0.2 μg/g per hr. These results showed that the heart itself is capable of synthesizing norepinephrine from the dietary precursor tyrosine at a rate which is consistent with estimated rates of formation *in vivo* (Spector, Sjoerdsma, Zaltzman-Nirenberg, Levitt and Udenfriend, 1963).

By 1964, all the enzymes relating to the biosynthesis of catecholamines had been discovered. The dietary precursor of catecholamines is mainly tyrosine, but dietary phenylalanine can be converted to tyrosine in the liver. The enzyme which converts phenylalanine to tyrosine, i.e., phenylalanine hydroxylase, was first discovered in the liver (Udenfriend and Cooper, 1952a). It was purified and separated into two proteins (Mitoma, 1956; Kaufman, 1957); phenylalanine hydroxylase, a component which requires a reduced pteridine cofactor, and dihydropteridine reductase, a component which requires NADPH (Kaufman, 1962a, 1966a). The enzyme, tyrosine hydroxylase, which catalyzes the conversion of tyrosine to DOPA, was discovered in the adrenal medulla, brain, and sympathetically innervated tissues (Nagatsu, Levitt and Udenfriend, 1964a, b). Before the discovery of tyrosine hydroxylase, tyrosinase was assumed to be the enzyme which converts tyrosine to DOPA, however, tyrosinase appears to work only in the formation of melanin in mammalian tissues. Tyrosine hydroxylase also requires a reduced pteridine as a cofactor (Nagatsu, Levitt and Udenfriend, 1964b), and it can hydroxylate phenylalanine to tyrosine (Ikeda, Levitt and Udenfriend, 1965). Therefore, the conversion of phenylalanine to tyrosine also can occur in the brain, adrenal medulla, and various sympathetically innervated tissues. Dopa decarboxylase, which decarboxylates DOPA to dopamine, was discovered in 1938 (Holtz, Heise and Lüdtke, 1938; Holtz, 1939). It was purified and found to require pyridoxal phosphate as a cofactor, and to decarboxylate various aromatic L-amino acids. Consequently, the name, aromatic L-amino acid decarboxylase was proposed for the enzyme (Lovenberg, Weissbach and Udenfriend, 1962). The side chain hydroxylation of dopamine to norepinephrine is catalyzed by dopamine-β-hydroxylase. The enzyme was isolated from the adrenal medulla and characterized (Levin, Levenberg and Kaufman, 1960). This enzyme is a copper protein and requires ascorbic acid as a cofactor (Friedman and Kaufman, 1965; Goldstein, Lauber and McKereghan, 1965). The final step for the formation of epinephrine from norepinephrine in the adrenal medulla was found to be catalyzed by phenylethanolamine-*N*-methyltransferase (Kirshner and Goodall 1957b; Axelrod, 1962b). The donor of the methyl group of epinephrine is *S*-adenosylmethionine. It is noted that among five enzymes related to the biosynthesis of epinephrine,

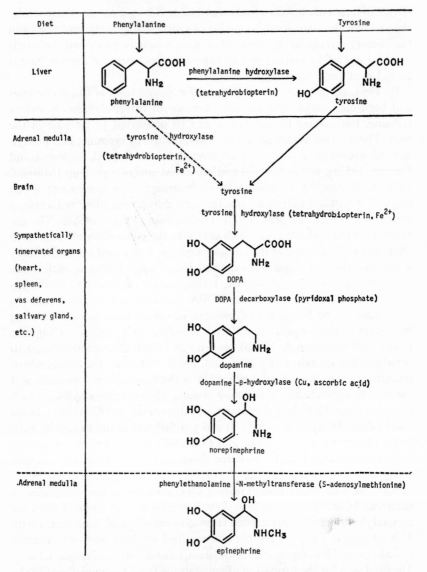

Fig. 5. The tissue distribution of enzymes and cofactors related to the biosynthesis of catecholamines.

three enzymes, i.e., phenylalanine hydroxylase, tyrosine hydroxylase, and dopamine-β-hydroxylase, belong to monooxygenases (Hayaishi, 1964). As the cofactors of these biosynthetic enzymes, reduced pteridine (phenyl-alanine hydroxylase and tyrosine hydroxylase), pyridoxal phosphate (DO-PA decarboxylase), and ascorbic acid (dopamine-β-hydroxylase) are required.

Figure 5 shows what is presently known about the tissue distribution of enzymes related to the biosynthesis of catecholamines. Dietary tyrosine is the precursor of catecholamine biosynthesis. Dietary phenylalanine is converted to tyrosine by phenylalanine hydroxylase in the liver, and the formed tyrosine can also be the precursor. Phenylalanine hydroxylase is exclusively localized in the liver. In contrast, tyrosine hydroxylase is exclusively localized in catecholamine-containing organs. Tyrosine hydroxylase can also hydroxylate phenylalanine to tyrosin. Therefore, phenyl-alanine can be converted to tyrosine at the site of catecholamine biosynthesis. This reaction may be negligibly low in normal animals. However, in the phenylketonuric patient who hereditarily lacks liver phenylalanine hydroxylase, the formation of tyrosine from phenylalanine for catechol-amine biosynthesis by tyrosine hydroxylase in sympathetically innervated organs could be of significance.

In some parts of the brain, such as the extrapyramidal system, dopamine is supposed to be the end product of the catecholamine biosynthesis. In other parts of the brain and in all the sympathetically innervated organs, norepinephrine is the end product. In the adrenal medulla, norepinephrine is further N-methylated to epinephrine, which is the main catecholamine.

The biosynthesis of catecholamines from tyrosine proceeds very rapidly, and the intermediates, such as DOPA and dopamine whose tissue concentrations are very low, do not accumulate.

In the following sections, each enzyme in the biosynthesis of catechol-amines will be described.

I. 2. Phenylalanine Hydroxylase*

L-Phenylalanine, tetrahydropteridine: oxygen oxidoreductase (4-hydroxylating) [EC 1. 14. 3. 1]. Trivial name: Phenylalanine 4-hydroxylase, Phenylalanine hydroxylase.

Phenylalanine hydroxylase is an oxygenase which catalyzes the hydroxylation of phenylalanine to tyrosine and requires tetrahydrobiopterin as a cofactor (Kaufman, 1966 a, b). This enzyme was first discovered in the

---

* I wish to thank Dr. Miki Akino (Department of Biology, Faculty of Science, Tokyo Metropolitan University, Tokyo) for his careful review of this chapter and for his valuable suggestions.

soluble fraction of rat liver (Udenfriend and Cooper, 1952a) and, subsequently, it was reported that the system consists of two protein fractions and requires reduced NAD (Mitoma, 1956). Two enzymes of the phenylalanine hydroxylation system were separately purified from sheep liver and rat liver, respectively, and NADPH was demonstrated as the cofactor in the following reaction (Kaufman, 1957):

$$NADPH + H^+ + O_2 + phenylalanine \longrightarrow NADP^+ + H_2O + tyrosine$$

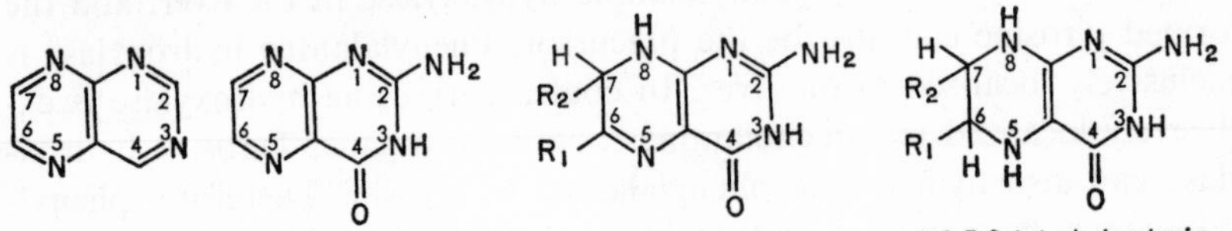

| | pteridine | pterin (2-amino-3,4-dihydro-4-oxopteridine) | 7,8-dihydropterin | 5,6,7,8-tetrahydropterin |

	Pterin derivatives	R_1-	R_2-
Folic acid	N-[p-{[(2-amino-4-hydroxy-6-pteridinyl)-methyl]amino} benzoyl]glutamic acid	$HOOC-(CH_2)_2-CH-NH-CO-\bigcirc-NH-CH_2-$ $\qquad\qquad\qquad\quad\;$ COOH	H-
6,7-Dimethyl-pterin	2-amino-4-hydroxy-6,7-dimethylpteridine	H_3C-	H_3C-
7-Methyl-pterin	2-amino-4-hydroxy-7-methylpteridine	H-	H_3C-
6-Methyl-pterin	2-amino-4-hydroxy-6-methylpteridine	H_3C-	H-
Sepiapterin	2-amino-4-hydroxy-6-lactyl-7,8-dihydropteridine	$H_3C-\overset{H}{\underset{OH}{C}}-\overset{O}{C}-$	H-
Neopterin	2-amino-4-hydroxy-6-(D-erythro-1',2',3'-trihydroxy-propyl)pteridine	$HO-\overset{H}{\underset{H}{C}}-\overset{H}{\underset{O}{C}}-\overset{H}{\underset{O}{C}}-$	H-
Biopterin	2-amino-4-hydroxy-6-(L-erythro-1',2'-dihydroxypropyl)pteridine	$H_3C-\overset{H}{\underset{O}{C}}-\overset{H}{\underset{O}{C}}-$	H-

Fig. 6. Nomenclature and structure of pterins.

It was then reported that in addition to NADPH another cofactor which appeared to be different from any of the known vitamins and coenzymes was involved in the reaction (Kaufman, 1958b). It was found that tetrahydrofolic acid (Kaufman, 1958a) and tetrahydropterins (2-amino-4-hydroxy-5,6,7,8-tetrahydropteridines), such as 6,7-dimethyl-5,6,7,8-tetrahydropterin and 6-methyl-5,6,7,8-tetrahydropterin, can replace the natural cofactor (Kaufman, 1959, 1961, 1962b). The nomenclature and structure of pterins are shown in Fig. 6. A substance showing cofactor activity in the phenylalanine hydroxylation system was isolated from rat liver and identified as dihydrobiopterin (2-amino-4-hydroxy-6-(L-*erythro*-1′,2′-dihydroxypropyl)-7,8-dihydropteridine) (Fig. 7), and the following mechanism (Fig. 8) of the reaction was proposed (Kaufman, 1963a):

$$\text{tetrahydropterin} + \text{phenylalanine} + O_2 \xrightarrow{\substack{\text{phenylalanine hydroxylase} \\ \text{(rat liver enzyme)}}}$$

$$\text{dihydropterin (quinoid form)} + \text{tyrosine} + H_2O$$

$$\text{dihydropterin (quinoid form)} + \text{NADPH} + H^+ \xrightarrow{\substack{\text{dihydropteridine reductase} \\ \text{(sheep liver enzyme)}}}$$

$$\text{tetrahydropterin} + \text{NADP}^+$$

Fig. 7. Structure of 7,8-dihydrobiopterin.

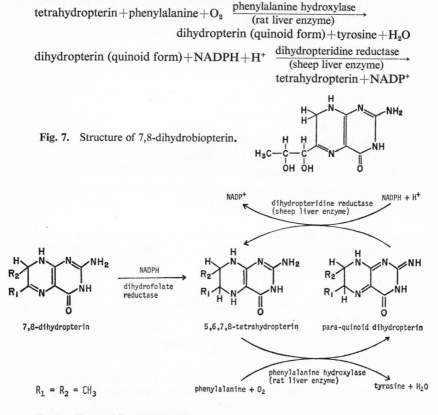

Fig. 8. The pteridine (6,7-dimethylpterin) transformations during the enzymatic conversion of phenylalanine to tyrosine (Kaufman, 1963b, 1964).

Sum: phenylalanine$+O_2+$NADPH$+H^+ \longrightarrow$ tyrosine$+H_2O+$NADP$^+$

Many reviews on phenylalanine hydroxylase have been published by Kaufman (1962b, 1963b, 1964, 1966a, b, 1970).

I. 2. 1. TISSUE DISTRIBUTION

Phenylalanine hydroxylase is localized in the soluble fraction of the liver (Udenfrined and Cooper, 1952a), and rat liver has shown high activity. Activity is also present in rabbit liver (Kaufman, 1957), human liver (Kaufman, 1969) and monkey liver (Cotton, 1971). The postulated relations of gene-enzyme-disease was first unequivocally demonstrated, and the enzyme is lacking in the liver of phenylketonuric patients (Jervis, 1953). Phenylalanine hydroxylase was discovered in insect tissue (fat body of silkworm) (Akino, 1965, personal communication), and was also found in spinach leaves (Nair and Vining, 1965) and in some bacteria such as Pseudomonas (Guroff and Ito, 1963), and rat kidney and pancreas (Friedman, Lloyd and Kaufman, 1972).

I. 2. 2. ASSAY METHOD

See section III. 1.

I. 2. 3. PURIFICATION

Eighty-five to ninety percent pure phenylalanine hydroxylase was purified from rat liver (rat liver enzyme) (Kaufman, 1962c; Kaufman and Fisher, 1970). Dihydropteridine reductase (sheep liver enzyme) which is necessary to regenerate tetrahydrobiopterin from quinoid dihydrobiopterin was purified from sheep liver (Kaufman, 1962c).

A. *Purification of phenylalanine hydroxylase (rat liver enzyme)*

The purification procedure established by Kaufman and Fisher (1970) is shown in the chart below.

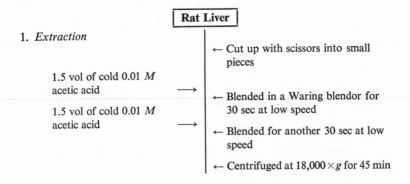

	Rat Liver	
1. *Extraction*		← Cut up with scissors into small pieces
1.5 vol of cold 0.01 *M* acetic acid $\longrightarrow$		← Blended in a Waring blendor for 30 sec at low speed
1.5 vol of cold 0.01 *M* acetic acid $\longrightarrow$		← Blended for another 30 sec at low speed
		← Centrifuged at 18,000$\times g$ for 45 min

Supernatant

2. *Ethanol fractionation*

Ethanol ($-30°$--$-40°$C)
to 0–10% at $-2°$C   ⟶ | ← Centrifuged at 4,000 ×g for 15 min
to 10–21% at $-4°$C   ⟶ | ← Centrifuged at 4,000 ×g for 15 min

Second Precipitate

¼ of the original vol
of 0.033 M potassium
phosphate buffer, pH 7.4 ⟶

| **Ethanol Fraction** |

3. *First $(NH_4)_2SO_4$ fractionation*

20.3 g of $(NH_4)_2SO_4$ to each
100 ml of solution   ⟶ | ← Centrifuged at 18,000 ×g for 20 min

Supernatant

5.60 g of $(NH_4)_2SO_4$ to each
100 ml of original solution ⟶ | ← Centrifuged at 18,000 ×g for 20 min

Precipitate

¼ of the original vol of
0.033 M Tris buffer, pH 6.8⟶

| **First $(NH_4)_2SO_4$ Fraction** |

4. *Calcium phosphate gel treatment*

10 ml of cold 0.1 M
L-phenylalanine and then
100 ml of cold water to
each 100 ml of solution   ⟶

73 ml (0.35 vol) of calcium
phosphate gel (20 mg/ml) ⟶ | ← Addition for 15 min during stirring
    | ← Stirring for another 10 min
    | ← Centrifuged

Gel Precipitate

Elution with 210 ml of 0.02 M
potassium phosphate buffer,
pH 6.8   ⟶ | ← Centrifuged

Gel Precipitate

Elution with 160 ml of 0.1 M
potassium phosphate buffer,
pH 6.8 $\longrightarrow$ | ← Centrifuged

The Active Gel Eluate
(0.1 M supernatant)

5. *Second (NH₄)₂SO₄ fractionation*

18.2 g of (NH₄)₂SO₄ to
each 100 ml of eluate $\longrightarrow$ | ← Centrifuged at 18,000 × g for 20 min

Supernatant

7.35 g of (NH₄)₂SO₄ to each
100 ml of starting solution $\longrightarrow$ | ← Centrifuged at 18,000 × g for 20 min

Precipitate

¼ of the original vol of
0.01 M Tris buffer, pH 7.0 $\longrightarrow$

| **Second (NH₄)₂SO₄ Fraction** |

Sephadex G-25 (1.5 × 23 cm) Column
(equilibrated with 0.005 M Tris buffer, pH 7.0)

0.005 M Tris buffer, pH 7.0 $\longrightarrow$ | ← Collected 5-ml fractions

| **Desalted Second (NH₄)₂SO₄ Fraction** |

6. *DEAE-cellulose column*
chromatography

Enzyme Fraction Containing 1.5 g of Protein

DEAE-Cellulose Column (1.9 × 40 cm)
(equilibrated with 0.005 M Tris buffer, pH 7.0)

Gradient elution (the first
bottle containing 300 ml of
0.01 M Tris buffer, pH 7.0,
the second containing 300 ml
of 0.01 M Tris buffer, pH 7.0,
and 0.22 M KCl, connected
in series) $\longrightarrow$

| ← Collected 6 ml fractions in the collecting tubes containing 0.3 ml of 3 M KCl (final KCl concentration in each tube, 0.15 M)

Active Fractions
(between 300 and 540 ml of eluant)

| ← Concentrated by ultrafiltration

> **DEAE-Cellulose Eluate**

7. *Sephadex G-200 gel filtration* |

Enzyme Solution
containing 200–400 mg protein

|

Sephadex G-200 Column (2.5 × 60 cm)
which had been equilibrated with 0.01 M Tris buffer, pH 7.0,
0.01 M KCl, and pretreated with crude side-fractions from DEAE-
cellulose step

| ← Eluted with 0.01 M Tris buffer, pH 7.0, 0.1 M KCl

Active Fractions
(between 150 and 200 ml of eluant)

The enzyme was purified about 400-fold with a yield of about 5 % and the specific activity of the most purified fraction was 0.5–0.6 μmoles of tyrosine formed/min/mg protein. The enzyme was determined to be 85–90 % pure by polyacrylamide gel electrophoresis with and without sodium dodecyl sulfate and by sucrose gradient centrifugation and could be stored at −80°C up to one year with a 30% loss in acticity. Two active forms of phenylalamine hydroxylase, corresponding to approximate molecular weights of 210,000 and 110,000 (Kaufman and Fisher, 1970), could be separated either by chromatography on Sephadex G-200 or by sucrose density centrifugation.

B. *Purification of dihydropteridine reductase (sheep liver enzyme)* (Kaufman, 1962c, 1967)
For the assay of phenylalanine hydroxylase, the addition of dihydropteridine reductase and a tetrahydropteridine cofactor, such as 6,7-dimethyltetrahydropterin, is necessary. Dihydropteridine reductase was purified from sheep liver (Kaufman, 1962c, 1967) and the purification procedure described by Kaufman is shown in the chart below.

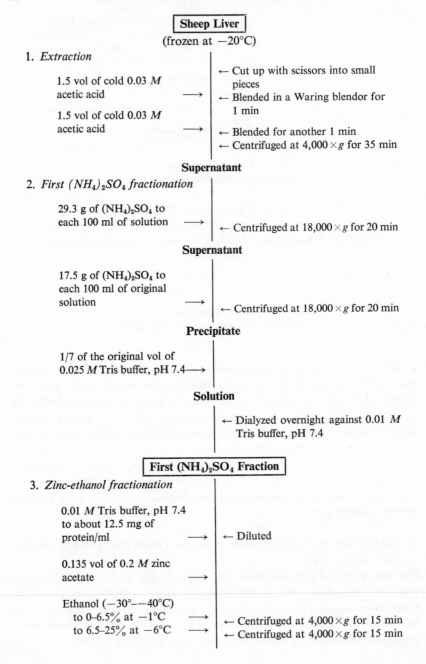

Sheep Liver

(frozen at $-20°C$)

1. *Extraction*

    1.5 vol of cold 0.03 *M*
acetic acid   ⟶

    ← Cut up with scissors into small
    pieces
    ← Blended in a Waring blendor for
    1 min

    1.5 vol of cold 0.03 *M*
acetic acid   ⟶

    ← Blended for another 1 min
    ← Centrifuged at $4,000 \times g$ for 35 min

Supernatant

2. *First $(NH_4)_2SO_4$ fractionation*

    29.3 g of $(NH_4)_2SO_4$ to
each 100 ml of solution   ⟶

    ← Centrifuged at $18,000 \times g$ for 20 min

Supernatant

    17.5 g of $(NH_4)_2SO_4$ to
each 100 ml of original
solution   ⟶

    ← Centrifuged at $18,000 \times g$ for 20 min

Precipitate

    1/7 of the original vol of
0.025 *M* Tris buffer, pH 7.4⟶

Solution

    ← Dialyzed overnight against 0.01 *M*
    Tris buffer, pH 7.4

First $(NH_4)_2SO_4$ Fraction

3. *Zinc-ethanol fractionation*

    0.01 *M* Tris buffer, pH 7.4
to about 12.5 mg of
protein/ml   ⟶   ← Diluted

    0.135 vol of 0.2 *M* zinc
acetate   ⟶

    Ethanol $(-30°--40°C)$
to 0–6.5% at $-1°C$ ⟶   ← Centrifuged at $4,000 \times g$ for 15 min
to 6.5–25% at $-6°C$ ⟶   ← Centrifuged at $4,000 \times g$ for 15 min

Second Precipitate

1/8 of the original diluted
vol of 0.033 M potassium
phosphate buffer, pH 6.8 ⟶ | ← Centrifuged

Supernatant

| ← Dialyzed overnight against 0.033 M
potassium phosphate buffer, pH 6.8

| **Zinc-Ethanol Fraction** |

4. *Second alkaline* $(NH_4)_2SO_4$
fractionation

0.033 M potassium phosphate
buffer, pH 6.8, to a protein
concentration of about
10 mg/ml   ⟶ | ← Diluted

14 g of $(NH_4)_2SO_4$ to each
100 ml of diluted solution ⟶

1 N NH$_4$OH to pH 8.2 ⟶

Another 23.8 g of $(NH_4)_2SO_4$
to each 100 ml of pH 8.2
solution   ⟶ | ← Centrifuged at 18,000 × g for 20 min

Supernatant

18.3 g of $(NH_4)_2SO_4$
to each 100 ml   ⟶ | ← Centrifuged at 18,000 × g for 20 min

Precipitate

0.01 M Tris buffer, pH 7.4 ⟶ | ← Dialyzed overnight against 0.01 M
Tris buffer, pH 7.4

| **Second $(NH_4)_2SO_4$ Fraction** |

5. *Calcium phosphate gel treatment*

0.01 M Tris buffer, pH 7.4,
to a protein concentration
of about 10 mg/ml   ⟶

About 0.3 vol of calcium
phosphate gel (dry weight
=20 to 22 mg/ml)   ⟶ | ← Centrifuged

Gel Precipitate

Elution with potassium
phosphate buffer, pH 6.8,
equal to the starting vol
after dilution $0.008\ M \longrightarrow$
                      $0.1\ M \longrightarrow$ ← Centrifuged
                                            ← Centrifuged

| **The Active Gel Eluate (0.1 M)** |

6. *Alumina Cγ treatment*

                                    ← Dialyzed against a large excess of
    0.1 N acetic acid   0.01 M Tris buffer, pH 7.4
    to pH 5.4 $\longrightarrow$

    0.06–0.08 vol of
    alumina Cγ gel (12 mg/ml) $\longrightarrow$ ← Centrifuged

    Elution with potassium
    phosphate buffer, pH 6.8,
    equal to the starting vol
    after dilution $0.008\ M \longrightarrow$
                       $0.1\ M \longrightarrow$ ← Centrifuged
                                           ← Centrifuged

| **The Active Gel Eluate (0.1 M)** |

7. *Third $(NH_4)_2SO_4$ fractionation*
   (Kaufman, 1967)

    14 g of $(NH_4)_2SO_4$ to each
    100 ml of gel eluate $\longrightarrow$ ← With continuous mechanical
                                            stirring
    1 N NH$_4$OH to pH 8.0 $\longrightarrow$

    28.7 g of $(NH_4)_2SO_4$ to each
    100 ml of starting material $\longrightarrow$ ← Centrifuged at $16,000 \times g$ for 15 min

Supernatant   **Precipitate**

                       10% of the starting
20.3 g of $(NH_4)_2SO_4$ volume of 0.02 M
to each 100 ml of   phosphate buffer,
starting material$\longrightarrow$ pH 6.8 $\longrightarrow$

10% of the starting   ←Centrifuged at
volume of 0.02 M $16,000 \times g$ for   Dialyzed against a
phosphate buffer,   15 min   large excess of 0.01 M
pH 6.8 $\longrightarrow$ potassium phosphate,
                        $\longleftarrow$ ←pH 6.8

| **Second Fraction** | | **First Fraction** |

90% of the dihydropteridine   low specific activity,
reductase, high specific   almost completely free
activity   of dihydrofolate reductase

The purification after alumina C_γ stage was between 80- and 100-fold with a yield of 13 % and the enzyme was stable for months when stored at $-20°C$. Dihydropteridine reductase and dihydrofolate reductase were purified simultaneously up to the alumina C_γ stage and could not be separated, but dihydrofolate reductase relatively free of dihydrofolate reductase could be obtained after the third ammonium sulfate fractionation (Kaufman, 1967a; Akino, personal communication).

I. 2. 4. PROPERTIES

The properties of 85 to 90 % pure phenylalanine hydroxylase purified from rat liver were described by Kaufman and Fisher (1970). Two major active forms were separated by Sephadex G-200 chromatography, and their molecular weights were estimated to be approximately 110,000 and 210,000. Each phenylalanine hydroxylase was shown to be capable of existing as a monomer (51,000 to 55,000 molecular weight), dimer (110,000 molecular weight) and tetramer (210,000 molecular weight). Polyacrylamide electrophoresis on gels of varying acrylamide concentrations revealed that the enzyme exists as two isoenzymes, each having a molecular weight of 110,000. The dimer of each isoenzyme will dissociate to the monomer by dilution of the enzyme or by increasing the temperature from 0° to 30°C. From these results, it was concluded that phenylalanine hydroxylase exists in multiple forms (Kaufman and Fischer, 1970).

Phenylalanine hydroxylase was proved to be an oxygenase by the O^{18}_2 experiment (Kaufman, Bridgers, Eisenberg and Friedman, 1962) and 7,8-dihydrobiopterin, which had been isolated from rat liver (Kaufman, 1963a) (Fig. 7), was proved to be converted to an active form of 5,6,7,8-tetrahydrobiopterin by dihydrofolate reductase (Matsubara, Katoh, Akino and Kaufman, 1966; Kaufman, 1967a,b; Nagai (Matsubara), 1968).

$$\text{NADPH} + \text{H}^+ + 7,8\text{-dihydrobiopterin} \xrightarrow{\text{dihydrofolyte reductase}} \text{NADP}^+ + 5, 6, 7, 8\text{-tetra-} \\ \text{hydrobiopterin}$$

In this reaction phenylalanine is converted to tyrosine by molecular oxygen, and the tetrahydropterin is converted to a "oxidized pterin." The structure of the primary oxidation product formed from tetrahydropteridines during the phenylalanine hydroxylase-catalyzed oxidation was examined and it was shown that the oxidized pteridine intermediate is at the oxidation level of a dihydropteridine and that it does not have a double bond at the sixth carbon position of the pteridine ring (Kaufman, 1961).

Thus, the intermediate cannot be either the 7,8- or 5,8-dihydropteridine. It was found that during the reduction of the intermediate with NADP-H[3], no tritium was incorporated into a stable position on the pteridine ring and when a tetrahydropteridine labeled with tritium on the pyrazine ring was oxidized, very little tritium was lost. These results are not consistent with a 5, 6-dihydro structure for the primary oxidation product, and they strongly support a quinoid structure (Kaufman, 1964). Based on these results, the reaction mechanism for phenylalanine hydroxylase shown in Fig. 8 was proposed.

Besides tetrahydrobiopterin, various tetrahydropterins, such as 6,7-dimethyltetrahydropterin (DMPH$_4$), 7-methyltetrahydropterin, and 6-methyltetrahydropterin, can function as cofactors (Kaufman, 1962b). Tetrahydroneopterin   (2-amino-4-hydroxy-6-(L-erythro-1',2',3'-trihydroxypropyl) tetrahydropteridine) was also shown to work as a cofactor (Akino, personal communication). Sepiapterin (2-amino-4-hydroxy-6-lactyl-dihydropteridine) was proved to be converted to dihydrobiopterin by sepiapterin reductase, which was purified from rat liver (Matsubara, Katoh, Akino and Kaufman, 1966), and the product from sepiapterin was identified as 7,8-dihydrobiopterin (Nagai (Matsubara), 1968).

From the reaction sequence of phenylalanine hydroxylase (Kaufman, 1959),

$$\text{phenylalanine} + XH_4 + O_2 \longrightarrow \text{tyrosine} + XH_2 + H_2O$$

$$XH_2 + NADPH + H^+ \longrightarrow XH_4 + NADP^+$$

where XH_4 = tetrahydropteridine and
      XH_2 = dihydropteridine,

the ratio, NADPH oxidized/tyrosine formed, should be 1.0. This was proved with the natural cofactor, tetrahydrobiopterin, (Kaufman, 1963a), 6-methyltetrahydropterin or 6, 7-dimethyltetrahydropterin (Kaufman, 1959; Storm and Kaufman, 1968). However, with 7-methyltetrahydropterin as a cofactor, the ratio, NADPH oxidized/tyrosine formed, was about 3.0. This extra electron consumption was strictly phenylalanine dependent (Strom and Kaufman, 1968), and molecular oxygen was the most likely acceptor for the extra electrons being consumed and could be reduced to H_2O_2. This was proved from the findings that the extra XH_4 oxidized was accompanied by extra O_2 consumption and that the ratio, NADPH oxidized/tyrosine formed, was 5 where the hydroxylase system was coupled to peroxidase (Kaufman, Storm and Fisher, 1970).

$$\text{phenylalanine} + 3XH_4 + 3O_2 \longrightarrow \text{tyrosine} + 3XH_2 + 2H_2O_2 + H_2O$$

$$2H_2O_2 + 2XH_4 \longrightarrow 2XH_2 + 4H_2O$$

Sum: $\quad \text{phenylalanine} + 5XH_4 + 3O_2 \longrightarrow \text{tyrosine} + 5XH_2 + 5H_2O$

Based on these results, the following mechanism of the enzyme—catalyzed reaction was proposed (Storm and Kaufman, 1968; Kaufman, Storm and Fisher, 1970):

$$E + XH_4 + RH \longrightarrow E(XH_4, O_2, RH)$$

$$E(XH_4, O_2, RH) \longrightarrow E(XH_2, O_2^=, 2H^+, RH)$$

$$E(XH_2, O_2^=, 2H^+, RH) \overset{a}{\underset{b}{\diagdown}} \begin{array}{l} E + XH_2 + RH + H_2O_2 \\ E + XH_2 + ROH + H_2O \end{array}$$

where RH = amino acid substrate.

In this mechanism the ratio of XH_4 oxidized to tyrosine formed is determined by the relative rates of reaction a and b, and these rates are dependent on the structures of both the substrate and the pteridine.

With 7-methyltetrahydropterin as a cofactor, increasing the enzyme concentration or salt concentration, and reducing the temperature of the reaction were found to lower the ratio, NADPH oxidized/tyrosine formed, to nearly 1.0. These results suggested that there are at least two forms of the enzyme, probably monomer and polymer, that have different catalytic efficiencies: one form catalyzes an oxidation of the 7-methyltetrahydropterin that is only loosely coupled to the hydroxylation reaction, whereas the other catalyzes a tightly coupled reaction (Kaufman, Storm and Fisher, 1970; Fisher and Kaufman, 1970). This hypothesis agrees with the recent finding on the existence of multiple forms of phenylalanine hydroxylase (Kaufman and Fisher, 1970).

A protein, phenylalanine hydroxylase stimulator (PHS), which stimulates highly purified rat liver phenylalanine hydroxylase has been discovered in partially purified sepiapterin reductase (Kaufman, 1970). It showed marked stimulation with its natural cofactor, tetrahydrobiopterin, slight stimulation with 6-methyltetrahydropterin, but no stimulation with 6,7-dimethyltetrahydropterin. Excess phenylalanine inhibited phenylalanine hydroxylase in the presence of PHS and tetrahydrobiopterin. From kinetic data, PHS appears to affect a reversible association-dissociation of the hydroxylase (Kaufman, 1970).

Dihydropteridine reductase activity can be measured in a system containing H_2O_2 and peroxidase. It was found that in this assay system dihydropteridine reductase purified from rat, rabbit, sheep, cow or cat liver can utilize either NADH or NADPH (Nielsen, Simonsen and Lind, 1969). However, when dihydropteridine reductase was coupled with phenylalanine hydroxylase, NADPH was a predominant cofactor (Kaufman, 1957).

Aged rat liver phenylalanine hydroxylase was reactivated by the addition of Fe^{2+} and cystein, and α,α'-dipyridyl inhibited the activity. These results suggest involvement of the Fe^{++} ion in the enzyme reaction (Kaufman, 1962b). Phenylalanine hydroxylase of Pseudomonas (ATCC 11299a) was activated by preincubating the enzyme with Hg^{++}, Cd^{++}, Cu^+, Cu^{++}, or Fe^{++}, but the metals changed neither the K_m value towards an oxygen, substrate or pteridine cofactor nor the molecular weight of the enzyme (Guroff and Rhoads, 1967; Guroff, 1970). It has been found that pure rat liver phenylalanine hydroxylase (Kaufman and Fisher, 1970) contains 1 to 2 moles of iron per mole of enzyme (assuming 100,000 molecular weight) and that the iron is essential for the hydroxylase activity (Fisher, Kirkwood and Kaufman, 1972).

The purified enzyme is relatively specific for L-phenylalanine. The α-alanine side chain is essential as a substrate, but some replacements in the benzene ring are allowable. The following compounds showed some activity: β-2-thienylalanine, 2-fluorophenylalanine, 3-fluorophenylalanine, and 4-fluorophenylalanine. The following compounds were almost completely inactive: D-phenylalanine, m-tyrosine, o-tyrosine, glycyl-DL-phenylalanine, acetaminocinnamic acid, phenylglycine, β-phenylserine, phenylamine, β-phenyllactate, α-phenyl-α-alanine, benzylmalonate, phenylpyruvate and 1-phenyl-2-acetaminobutanone-3 (Kaufman, 1962c).

When p-deuterophenylalanine was incubated with bacterial phenylalanine hydroxylase, the migration of deuterium from the p-position to the m-position was discovered (Fig. 9) (Guroff, Reifsnyder and Daly, 1966). m-Tritiotyrosine was produced from p-tritiophenylalanine with bacterial and liver phenylalanine hydroxylase (Guroff, Levitt, Daly and Udenfriend, 1966), and from p-chlorophenylalanine or p-bromophenylalanine, the main product was either m-chlorophenylalanine or m-bromophenylalanine. However, no fluorinated tyrosine was detected after the action of either bacterial or liver phenylalanine hydroxylase on p-fluorophenylalanine (Guroff, Kondo and Daly, 1966). Three products were produced from p-methylphenylalanine; m-methyltyrosine, p-methyl-m-hydroxyphenylalanine (p-methyl-m-tyrosine), and p-hydroxymethylphenylalanine. The production of m-methyltyrosine is due to the hydroxylation-induced migration of alkyl groups. The appearance of p-methyl-m-hydroxyphenylalanine suggests the migration of a hydroxy group. The formation of p-hydroxymethylphenylalanine demonstrates an unexpected side-chain hydroxylation by a pteridine-requiring enzyme normally involved in aromatic hydroxylation. The phenomenon of hydroxylation-induced intramolecular migration has been designated "NIH shift," since the phenomenon was discovered by scientists (Guroff, Daly, Jerina, Renson, Witkop and Udenfriend, 1967) at the National Institutes of Health (NIH, Bethesda, Maryland, U.S.A.).

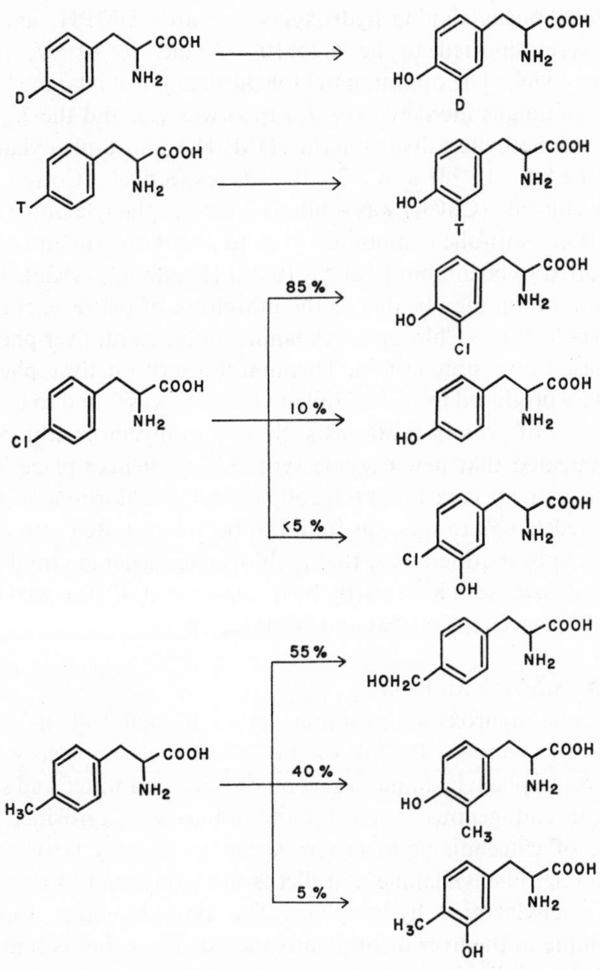

Fig. 9. Action of phenylalanine hydroxylase on 4-substituted phenylalanine (NIH shift; Guroff, Daly, Jerina, Renson, Witkop and Udenfriend, 1967).

Tryptophan is hydroxylated to 5-hydroxytryptophan with phenylalanine hydroxylase, but this reaction may have little physiological significance on the formation of serotonin *in vivo* (Renson, Weissbach and Udenfriend, 1962).

Reported K_m values of a rat liver phenylalanine hydroxylase system towards NADPH, 6,7-dimethyltetrahydropterin (DMPH$_4$), tetrahydrobiopterin and L-phenylalanine were $1 \times 10^{-4}M$, $5.7 \times 10^{-5}M$, $6.5 \times 10^{-6}M$, and $1 \times 10^{-3}M$, respectively (Kaufman, 1963b, 1969). K_m values of the human liver phenylalanine hydroxylase towards DMPH$_4$ and L-phenylalanine were reported to be $5.7 \times 10^{-5}M$ and $1 \times 10^{-3}M$, respectively (Kaufman, 1969). The optimum pH for purified phenylalanine hydroxylase in the Cynomolgus monkey (*Macaca irus*) was 7.6, and the K_m values towards 6,7-dimethyltetrahydropterin (DMPH$_4$) and L-phenylalanine were found to be $8.5 \times 10^{-5}M$ and $5.7 \times 10^{-4}M$, respectively (Cotton, 1971).

Cupric chloride (CuCl$_2$) was inhibitory for the phenylalanine hydroxylation reaction. Antifolic compounds such as amethopterin and aminopterin were reported to be inhibitory at $5 \times 10^{-4}M$ (Kaufman, 1962c). The mechanism of inhibition may be due to the inhibition of the regeneration of the pteridine cofactor. *p*-Chlorophenylalanine inhibited rat liver phenylalanine hydroxylase irreversibly *in vivo*. This inhibition of rat liver phenylalanine hydroxylase produced by *p*-chlorophenylalanine was found to be prolonged by inhibitors of protein synthesis such as puromycin or ethionine. These results indicated that new enzyme synthesis must take place in the liver before the activity is restored (Guroff, 1969a). *p*-Chlorophenylalanine-C[14] administered *in vivo* to rats was found to be incorporated into the enzyme protein. It appears, therefore, that *p*-chlorophenylalanine inhibits phenylalanine hydroxylase at least partly by its incorporation into enzyme protein near or at the active site (Gál and Millard, 1971).

I. 2. 5. PHYSIOLOGICAL ROLE

Phenylalanine hydroxylase reaction serves a dual role in mammalian metabolism (Kaufman, 1962b). First of all, it is a compulsory step in the combustion of phenylalanine to carbon dioxide and water and secondly, it provides an endogenous source for the amino acid, tyrosine. The direct precursor of catecholamines *in vivo* seems to be only tyrosine, and not phenylalanine. Phenylalanine in a diet is first converted to tyrosine in the liver by phenylalanine hydroxylase. The tyrosine either formed from phenylalanine in the liver or originally included in a diet is transported to the adrenal medulla, brain, and sympathetically innervated tissues, where it is converted to DOPA and then to catecholamines first by tyrosine hydroxylase (Nagatsu, Levitt and Udenfriend, 1964a, b) and then by the subsequent biosynthetic enzymes. Dietary phenylalanine can be converted to tyrosine in sympathetically innervated organs by tyrosine hydroxylase (Ikeda, Levitt and Udenfriend, 1965) (see I. 3.). However, it may not be a direct precursor of catecholamines. In the case of phenylketonuria in which phenylalanine hydroxylase activity is not found in the liver, the hydroxylation reaction of phenylalanine to tyrosine by tyrosine hydroxylase in sympathetically innervated tissues may be of physiological significance. In fact, the formation of tyrosine from phenylalanine was proved *in vivo* to take place in phenylketonuria, although the rate was only 5% in a normal man (Udenfriend and Bessman, 1953). This hydroxylation in phenylketonuria may be due to tyrosine hydroxylase in sympathetically innervated tissues. When phenylalanine was administered to a rat, it accumulated in the liver. Fifteen minutes after administration tyrosine increased due to the hydroxylation of phenylalanine by phenylalanine hydroxylase in the liver. Tyrosine in the brain started to increase 30 min after administration. These results suggest that tyrosine formed from phenylalanine in the liver is transported into the brain via blood (Carver, 1965).

The biosynthesis of catecholamines in the brain needs special attention because of the presence of the blood-brain barrier towards catecholamines. In general, catecholamines cannot pass through the blood-brain barrier (Weil-Malherbe, Axelrod and Tomchick, 1959; Weil-Malherbe, Whitby and Axelrod, 1961). This means that catecholamines in the brain are not transported by means of the blood, but are synthesized in the brain tissue. The precursor amino acids, such as phenylalanine, tyrosine and DOPA can penetrate the blood-brain barrier into the brain. DOPA is not detectable in the blood, therefore, either phenylalanine or tyrosine can be a precursor of catecholamines in the brain; both are capable of passing through the blood-brain barrier. The uptake of L-tyrosine by the brain, *in vivo*, is rapid and stereo-selective. Circulating L-tyrosine rapidly attains equilibrium in the brain (Chirigos, Greengard and Udenfriend, 1960). Phenylalanine is taken up by the brain, but the picture is complex because of the enzymatic production of tyrosine in the liver; phenylalanine inhibits tyrosine uptake by brain. This fact may be significant for the understanding of phenylketonuria (Guroff and Udenfriend, 1962; Udenfriend, 1963).

The activity of the phenylalanine-hydroxylating system in the liver of newborn rats in the absence of an added cofactor and dihydropteridine reductase (sheep liver enzyme) was significantly lower (50–70%) than the average activities of adult males and females. This relative defect in hydroxylating ability can be traced to the lower levels of the pteridine cofactor and probably dihydropteridine reductase in the livers of newborn rats. The cofactor reached adult levels within the first day of life. The conversion *in vivo* of phenylalanine to tyrosine in newborn rats was about the same as that in adult male and female rats (Brenneman and Kaufman, 1965).

I. 3.   Tyrosine Hydroxylase (TH)

L-Tyrosine, tetrahydropteridine: oxygen oxidoreductase (3-hydroxylating) [EC 1. 14. 3. a]. Trivial name: Tyrosine 3-hydroxylase, Tyrosine hydroxylase.

Tyrosine hydroxylase is an oxygenase which catalyzes the conversion of L-tyrosine to L-DOPA, the initial step of norepinephrine biosynthesis, and requires a tetrahydropteridine as a cofactor (Nagatsu, Levitt and Udenfriend, 1964a,b; Udenfriend, 1966c). It is a distinct enzyme from tyrosinase. Prior to the discovery of tyrosine hydroxylase tyrosinase was thought to work in the formation of DOPA in catecholamine biosynthesis, but no evidence for this could be obtained from sympathetically innervated tissues of animals. Tyrosine hydroxylase was found to be the rate-limiting step in the biosynthesis of catecholamines (Levitt, Spector, Sjoerdsma and Udenfriend, 1965). Reviews concerning this enzyme were published by Udenfriend (1966a, b, c).

I. 3. 1.   TISSUE DISTRIBUTION

The tissue distribution of tyrosine hydroxylase coincided with that of catecholamines suggesting that the physiological role of the enzyme is the biosynthesis of catecholamines. The following organs were reported to have the enzyme activity: adrenal medulla, brain, spleen, heart (Nagatsu, Levitt and Udenfriend, 1964b), salivary glands (Sedvall and Kopin, 1967), splenic nerve (Stjärne, 1966b), and vas deferens (Austin, Livett and Chubb, 1967). Intracranial distribution was as follows (in the decreasing order): caudate nucleus, hypothalamus, thalamus, midbrain, medulla oblongata, cerebral cortex and cerebellum (Creveling, Barchas, Nagatsu, Levitt and Udenfriend, 1972). This distribution agrees with that of dopamine or norepinephrine in the brain. Tyrosine hydroxylase was purified from human catecholamine-secreting tumors, such as pheochromocytoma (Nagatsu, T., Yamamoto and Nagatsu, I., 1970) and is thought to be an intraneuronal enzyme. It was shown that denervation resulted in the disappearance of tyrosine hydroxylase activity in the heart (Pool, Covell, Levitt, Gibb and Braunwald, 1967), salivary glands (Sedvall and Kopin, 1967), and kidney (Nagatsu, Rust and DeQuattro, 1969).

Some contradictory results on the subcellular distribution of tyrosine hydroxylase have also been reported. In an early report (Nagatsu, Levitt and Udenfriend, 1964a), enzyme activity in the adrenal medulla, brain, and heart, assayed without the addition of a tetrahydropteridine cofactor, was mainly found in association with particles forming sediments at $15,000 \times g$ to $20,000 \times g$. However, activity was also found in the soluble fractions of these organs when a tetrahydropteridine cofactor was added. The particulate enzyme of bovine adrenal medulla homogenate was difficult to solubilize from either the particles or the acetone powder by treatment with sonic oscillation, repeated freezing and thawing, butanol, various detergents, lipase, or DNase. However, incubation of either the acetone powder or the particles with trypsin resulted in solubilization of the enzyme activity (Petrack, Sheppy and Fetzer, 1968). The soluble enzyme could be obtained also by chymotrypsin digestion (Shiman, Akino and Kaufman, 1971). When the bovine caudate nucleus homogenate was fractionated, most of the tyrosine hydroxylase activity was found in particles forming sediments at $15,000 \times g$ to $20,000 \times g$, and a small part was found in the soluble fraction. The particle-bound enzyme appears to be localized in nerve ending fractions (synaptosomes) and probably in synaptic vesicles (Nagatsu, T. and Nagatsu, I., 1970). The association of tyrosine hydroxylase with the synaptic vesicles in the bovine caudate nucleus was also confirmed with five other enzymes serving as biochemical markers and coordinated by means of electron microscopy (Fahn, Rodman and Côté, 1969).

On the other hand, there are some reports indicating that tyrosine hydroxylase is exclusively localized in the soluble fraction of the adrenal medulla (Laduron and Belpaire, 1968c; Musacchio, 1968) and in the splenic nerve (Stjärne and Lishajko, 1967). Recent finding on the aggregation of tyrosine hydroxylase suggested that bovine adrenal tyrosine hydroxylase is a soluble enzyme. It appears that tyrosine hydroxylase forms aggregates and adsorbs particulate fractions under certain conditions during homogenization (Musacchio, Wurzburger and D'Angelo, 1971; Wurzburger and Musacchio, 1971). Whether the enzyme is particle-bound or not, enzyme activity appears to be inhibited *in vivo* by the end product, catecholamine. Therefore, the localization of tyrosine hydroxylase and that of the newly synthesized catecholamine should be the same, or at least very close in the cell.

I. 3. 2. ASSAY METHOD
See section III. 2.

I. 3. 3. PURIFICATION

Tyrosine hydroxylase is difficult to purify, because it easily aggregates and becomes insoluble during purification. Only partial purification of the natural form of the enzyme was possible from the soluble fraction of beef adrenal medulla (Nagatsu, Levitt and Udenfriend, 1964b; Brenneman and Kaufman, 1964; Nagatsu, T., Yamamoto and Nagatsu, I., 1970). A large part of the enzyme was particle-bound in beef adrenal medulla, and the particulate enzyme was solubilized by incubation with trypsin (Petrack, Sheppy and Fetzer, 1968) or with chymotrypsin (Shiman, Akino and Kaufman, 1971). The enzyme in the particles of bovine caudate nucleus was also solubilized with trypsin (Nagatsu, T., Sudo and Nagatsu, I., 1971). However, the proteinase-treated enzymes appear to be fragments of the matural enzyme, and the relationship between the proteinase-treated enzyme and the native enzyme is not clear yet.

A. *Partial purification from the soluble fraction of bovine adrenal medulla*
   (Nagatsu, Levitt and Udenfriend, 1964b; Nagatsu, T., Yamamoto and
   Nagatsu, I., 1970)

The complete procedure was carried out at 0–4°C. Buffers were all prepared by dilution of $1M$ potassium phosphate buffer, pH 7.5, to the desired concentration. Dialysis was performed overnight against at least a 40-fold excess of the same buffer which was changed twice. Precipitates were collected by centrifugation for 20 min at $15,000 \times g$.

Fractionation with $(NH_4)_2SO_4$. Tissues were homogenized twice with 2 volumes of $0.1M$ buffer in an Ultra Turrax homogenizer for 1 min. The homogenate was centrifuged at $100,000 \times g$ for 60 min and the supernatant was carefully removed. To each 100 ml of the supernatant, 67 ml of saturated $(NH_4)_2SO_4$ solution (adjusted to pH 7.5 with NH_4OH) was added dropwise with constant mixing (40% saturation). The suspension was then stirred for 20 min and centrifuged. The precipitate was dissolved in 5 mM buffer (100 ml per 100 g starting material) and dialyzed against 5 mM buffer. To each 100 ml of the dialyzed solution, 33 ml of saturated $(NH_4)_2SO_4$ solution was added (25% saturation) and after 20 min of mixing, the solution was centrifuged. To the supernatant, 19 ml of saturated $(NH_4)_2SO_4$ solution was added (35% saturation) and after a further 20 min of mixing, the solution was again centrifuged and the supernatant discarded. The precipitate was dissolved in 5 mM buffer (75 ml per 100 g of the starting material).

Charcoal treatment. To each 20 ml of the solution 0.5 g of charcoal was added. The suspension was stirred for 30 min and the charcoal was removed by centrifugation. The solution was dialyzed against 5 mM buffer and then centrifuged.

Hydroxyapatite column. Hydroxyapatite (1 g for 100 mg protein) and powdered cellulose (1:2, w/w) were mixed well, equilibrated with 5 mM buffer and packed in a column. After application of the enzyme solution into the column, gradient elution was performed with 50 ml increments of phosphate buffer of increasing concentration (5, 25, 50, 70, 100 and 400 mM). Peaks of the enzyme activity from the bovine adrenal medulla appeared at 50 mM. Specific activity in the 50 mM fraction was increased about 4-fold by the hydroxyapatite. Since there was a gain in units of enzyme activity during the procedure, especially at the $(NH_4)_2SO_4$ step, the actual degree of purification was unknown. An example of the purification procedure for human pheochromocytoma is shown in Table I. At the $(NH_4)_2SO_4$ step, the enzyme could be stored as a precipitate for a month at $-20°C$ with only a slight loss of activity, but after hydroxyapatite chromatography it became unstable and activity was gradually lost, even at $-20°C$. Storage at $-80°C$ allowed longer retention of activity.

TABLE I. Purification of Tyrosine Hydroxylase from the Pheochromocytoma Tissue.

Purification step	Protein (mg)	Total activity[a] (nmoles/min)	Specific activity[a] (nmoles/min/mg protein)
Homogenate[b]	1160	121	0.10
High-speed centrifugation supernatant	857	117	0.14
$(NH_4)_2SO_4$ fractionation	64.6	360	5.6
Charcoal treatment	43.9	255	5.6
Hydroxyapatite column	4.4	88	20.0

[a] at 30°C.
[b] 9.3 g of pheochromocytoma tissue.

B. *Partial purification from the particulate fraction of bovine adrenal medulla using trypsin digestion* (Petrack, Sheppy and Fetzer, 1968)

It was reported that approximately 90% of the total tyrosine hydroxylase activity of bovine adrenal medulla homogenates is localized in the particuatle fraction of the homogenate. An acetone powder prepared from the particulate fraction was found to retain all of the activity, nevertheless, it could not be extracted from the acetone powder with water, salt solutions or buffers of varying pH and ionic strength. It was not possible to solubilize the enzyme from either the particles or the acetone powder by treatment with butanol, sonic oscillation, repeated freezing and thawing, various detergents, lipase, or DNase, although most of these procedures did not inactivate the enzyme. It was found that incubation of either the acetone powder or the particles with trypsin resulted in solubilization of the activity. Based on these findings, the following procedure for the purification of tyrosine hydroxylase of bovine adrenal medulla particles was established (Petrack, Sheppy and Fetzer, 1968).

Preparation of adrenal medulla particles. Bovine adrenal glands were obtained packed in ice. The glands were trimmed of fat, and the medulla was separated and stored frozen at $-70°C$ until they were ready to be used. No significant loss in activity was found even after several months of storage. For a typical preparation, 47 g of medulla was homogenized with 200 ml of 0.25 M sucrose for three 1 min intervals in a Virtis homogenizer operated at top speed. The volume was adjusted to 470 ml with 0.25 M sucrose, and the homogenate was filtered through four layers of cheese cloth. The filtered homogenate (420 ml) was centrifuged for 1.5 hr at 78,000 × g and the supernatant was discarded. The particulate fraction was washed by suspension in 0.1 M phosphate buffer, pH 6.5 (final volume, 420 ml). The washed particles were again precipitated by centrifugation for 1.5 hr at 78,000 × g. The residue was resuspended in 0.02 M phosphate buffer, pH 6.5, and the volume was adjusted to 180 ml.

Solubilization by trypsin digestion. To 180 ml of the residue suspension 1.8 ml of trypsin solution containing 5 mg per ml was added. The suspension was incubated for 1 hr at 30°C with continuous stirring. Tryptic activity was terminated by the addition of 1.8 ml of trypsin inhibitor containing 10 mg per ml. The trypsin suspension was stored overnight at $-70°C$. The next morning, the suspension was thawed and centrifuged for 2 hr at 105,000 × g. The clear, pale yellow supernatant was collected.

Fractionation with $(NH_4)_2SO_4$. $(NH_4)_2SO_4$ (25.5 g) was slowly added to 145 ml of trypsin supernatant to give approximately 25% saturation and stirring was continued for a total time of 1 hr. The precipitate was removed by centrifugation at 27,000 × g for 1 hr and discarded. $(NH_4)_2SO_4$ (20.6 g) was added to the clear supernatant to give approximately 45% saturation, and stirring was continued for a total of 1 hr. The precipitate was collected by centrifugation at 27,000 × g for 1 hr, suspended in a minimum volume of 0.02 M phosphate buffer, pH 6.5, and dialyzed overnight against the same buffer. The dialyzed solution was adjusted to 6.0 ml and centrifuged for 30 min at 144,000 × g to yield the partially purified enzyme. The purified enzyme did not lose any activity for at least two months when stored at $-70°C$.

C. *Purification from the particulate fraction of bovine adrenal medulla using chymotrypsin digestion* (Shiman, Akino and Kaufman, 1971)

Shiman, Akino and Kaufman (1971) solubilized tyrosine hydroxylase from the particulate fraction of bovine adrenal medulla using chymotrypsin digestion. The enzyme was purified by ammonium sulfate fractionation and Sephadex G-150 or substituted Sepharose 4B chromatography (Sepharose 4B to which 3-iodo-L-tyrosine is attached through its amino group). The procedure using Sephadex G-150 is described below in a form of a flow sheet.

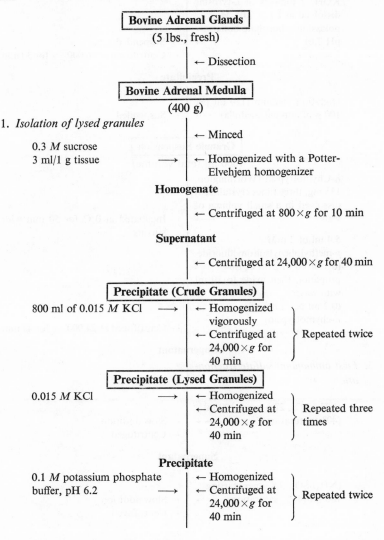

| Bovine Adrenal Glands |
| (5 lbs., fresh) |

← Dissection

| Bovine Adrenal Medulla |
| (400 g) |

1. *Isolation of lysed granules*

← Minced

0.3 *M* sucrose
3 ml/1 g tissue   ⟶   ← Homogenized with a Potter-
Elvehjem homogenizer

Homogenate

← Centrifuged at $800 \times g$ for 10 min

Supernatant

← Centrifuged at $24,000 \times g$ for 40 min

| Precipitate (Crude Granules) |

800 ml of 0.015 *M* KCl   ⟶   ← Homogenized
vigorously
← Centrifuged at   } Repeated twice
$24,000 \times g$ for
40 min

| Precipitate (Lysed Granules) |

0.015 *M* KCl   ⟶   ← Homogenized
← Centrifuged at   } Repeated three
$24,000 \times g$ for   times
40 min

Precipitate

0.1 *M* potassium phosphate   ← Homogenized
buffer, pH 6.2   ⟶   ← Centrifuged at   } Repeated twice
$24,000 \times g$ for
40 min

| **Precipitate (Washed, Lysed Granules)** |
(free of endogenous inhibitors)

2. *Chymotrypsin digestion*

300 ml of digestion medium (1 mmole of EDTA, 10 mmoles of cysteine-HCl, 10 mmoles of KOH, 2 mmoles of L-tyrosine dissolved in 1 *l* of 0.05 *M* potassium phosphate buffer, pH 7.6) ⟶	← Suspended ← Centrifuged at 36,000 × *g* for 30 min

Precipitate

Digestion medium (150 ml per 100 g of adrenal medulla) ⟶	← Suspended

| **Granule Suspension** |
(600 ml total volume)

α-Chymotrypsin (Worthington, 135 mg, three times crystallized) dissolved in a small volume of water ⟶	← Incubated at 0°C for 50 min with stirring
5.4 ml of 2 m*M* *p*-methylphenylsulfonylfluoride (dissolved in 2 ml of iso-propanol, then made to 10 ml with water) (0.2 ml per 5 mg of α-chymotrypsin) ⟶	← Centrifuged at 24,000 × *g* for 45 min

Supernatant

3. *First ammonium sulfate fraction-ation*

(NH$_4$)$_2$SO$_4$, 22.6 g per 100 ml (40% saturation) ⟶	← Slow addition ← Centrifuged

Supernatant

(NH$_4$)$_2$SO$_4$, 3.8 g per starting 100 ml (46% saturation) ⟶	← Slow addition ← Centrifuged

Supernatant

(NH$_4$)$_2$SO$_4$, 14.9 g per starting
100 ml (62% saturation)   ⟶   ← Slow addition
                                ← Centrifuged

Precipitate
(46–62% fraction)

6–8 ml of 0.05 M potassium
phosphate, pH 7.6   ⟶

Cloudy Solution

4. *Sephadex G-150 chromatography*

Sephadex G-150 Column
washed with 4 to 8 g of junk protein (for example 0–40% fraction)
and equilibrated with 0.3 M sucrose buffered at pH 7.6 with 0.05
M potassium phosphate (2.5 × 40 cm)

                          ← Eluted with the same buffer,
                            collected 3-ml fractions

Sephadex Eluate

5. *2nd ammonium sulfate fractionation*

(NH$_4$)$_2$SO$_4$, 31.2 g per 100 ml
(53% saturation)   ⟶   ← Slow addition
                           ← Centrifuged

Precipitate   **Supernatant**

A minimum volume
of 0.05 M potassium   (NH$_4$)$_2$SO$_4$, 4.9 g per
phosphate buffer,   starting 100 ml (60%
pH 7.6   ⟶   saturation)   ⟶   ← Slow addition
                                                    ← Centrifuged

                                             Precipitate

                          A minimum volume of
                          0.05 M potassium
                          phosphate buffer, pH 7.6   ⟶

0-53%   **53-60%**
(NH$_4$)$_2$SO$_4$ **(NH$_4$)$_2$SO$_4$**
Fraction   **Fraction**

(Specific activity,   (Specific activity,
42 nmoles/min/mg,   64 nmoles/min/mg,
at 25°C)   at 25°C)

Disc gel electrophoresis of the purified tyrosine hydroxylase showed two major and several minor bands. The enzyme activity was associated with the two major bands. The two bands from the enzyme preparation with a specific activity of 65 nmoles/min/mg were estimated by densitometry to contain at least 40 % of the stained protein (Shiman, Akino and Kaufman, 1971).

I. 3. 4. PROPERTIES

A. Cofactors and requirements

The properties of an enzyme purified from bovine adrenal medulla and requiring a tetrahydropteridine as a cofactor were reported mainly. The order of the cofactor activity from the lowest to the highest was: tetra-hydrofolate, tetrahydroneopterin, 7-methyltetrahydropterin, 6,7-dimethyl-tetrahydropterin, tetrahydropterin, 6-methyltetrahydropterin, and tetra-hydrobiopterin (Brenneman and Kaufman, 1964; Ellenbogen, Taylor and Brundage, 1965; Nagatsu, T., Mizutani, Nagatsu, I., Matsuura and Sugi-moto, 1972). Tetrahydrobiopterin is thought to be the natural cofactor. At high concentrations (10 and 20 mM), tetrahydropteridines inhibited enzyme activity, however, at high concentrations of 6,7-dimethyltetrahy-dropterin the inhibition observed was completely reversed by the addition of Fe^{++} (Ellenbogen, Taylor and Brundage, 1965). It has been recently reported that 6,7-dimethyl-5,6,7,8-tetrahydropterin gives different kinetics from tetrahydrobiopterin, the possible natural cofactor (Shiman, Akino and Kaufman, 1971). Thus, K_m for tyrosine in the presence of tetrahydrobiopterin ($7 \times 10^{-6}M$) was very small, and high tyrosine con-centrations inhibited the DOPA formation. In contrast, tetrahydrobio-pterin did not inhibit enzyme activity at high concentrations. With tetra-hydrobiopterin as cofactor, the rate of hydroxylation of phenylalanine is much faster than with 6,7-dimethyltetrahydropterin, and faster than the rate of tyrosine hydroxylation (Shiman, Akino and Kaufman, 1971). This inhibition by excess tyrosine may be of physiological significance in the biosynthesis of catecholamines, since the enzyme is about 30 % inhibited at only twice the normal tissue concentration of tyrosine (Shiman, Akino and Kaufman, 1971). Since biopterin has been difficult to prepare, nearly all previous studies on tyrosine hydroxylase have been carried out with the commercially available 6,7-dimethyl-5,6,7,8-tetrahydropterin as an artificial cofactor. The above results by Shiman, Akino and Kaufman (1971) indicate that the results with 6,7-dimethyltetrahydropterin must be inter-preted with some caution and that 6-methyltetrahydropterin would be a better analogue than 6,7-dimethyltetrahydropterin.

The reduced pteridine functioned catalytically in the presence of NADPH and the sheep liver enzyme (dihydropteridine reductase). Based on analogy with the phenylalanine-hydroxylating system, the conversion of tyrosine to DOPA may be formulated as shown in the equations where XH_4 stands for tetrahydropteridine and XH_2 for dihydropteridine (Brenneman and Kaufman, 1964).

$$\text{tyrosine} + XH_4 + O_2 \xrightarrow[\text{hydroxylase}]{\text{tyrosine}} DOPA + H_2O + XH_2$$

$$XH_2 + NADPH + H^+ \xrightarrow[\text{enzyme}]{\text{sheep liver}} XH_4 + NADP^+$$

The role of Fe^{++} ion as cofactor of the enzyme was not yet established, however, there are several indications that Fe^{++} not only stabilizes the enzyme but also stimulates the reaction. The degree of stimulation was different with the stage of purification of the enzyme and with the structure of the tetrahydropteridines added as a cofactor. When Fe^{++} was added to a reaction mixture containing beef adrenal enzyme, mercaptoethanol and tetrahydrofolate, marked stimulation was observed. With 6,7-dimethyl-tetrahydropterin as a cofactor, Fe^{++} stimulated the reaction to a lesser extent. Preincubation of the enzyme resulted in appreciable loss of the enzyme activity, but minimum amounts of Fe^{++} added during the preincubation period prevented this loss (Nagatsu, Levitt and Udenfriend, 1964b). Prior incubation of the adrenal enzyme from particle fractions without Fe^{++} in acetate buffer resulted in a considerable loss of activity, however, preliminary incubation of the enzyme in the presence of Fe^{++} not only prevented inactivation, but resulted in activity higher than that without prior incubation. In contrast, prior incubation of the enzyme with Fe^{+++} resulted in almost complete inactivation of the activity (Petrack, Sheppy and Fetzer, 1968). The fact that α,α'-dipyridyl or o-phenanthroline is markedly inhibitory in vitro and in vivo (Taylor, Stubbs and Ellenbogen, 1969) also suggested a Fe^{++} requirement. Fe^{++} stimulated the enzyme reaction specifically. The following metals had no effect: Mg^{++}, Ca^{++}, Mn^{++}; and Ba^{++}, Co^{++}, Cu^{++}, Zn^{++}, and Cd^{++} inhibited the reaction (Nagatsu, T., Sudo and Nagatsu, I., 1971). Shiman, Akino and Kaufman (1971) reported that purified tyrosine hydroxylase is sensitive to H_2O_2 generated during the non-enzymatic oxidation of tetrahydropterin and that the enzyme can be protected by catalase, peroxidase, or Fe^{++} from H_2O_2-mediated inactivation. It is concluded, therefore, that the previous reports that tyrosine hydroxylase is stimulated by Fe^{++} can be explained by the known ability of Fe^{++} to decompose H_2O_2 (Shiman, Akino and Kaufman, 1971). However, Fe^{++} could show more pronounced stimulation than catalase or peroxidase on the enzyme preparations from human adrenals and pheochromocytoma (Nagatsu, T., Mizutani and Nagatsu, I., 1972). The precise mechanism of the action of Fe^{++} in the enzymatic reaction remains to be elucidated.

The requirement of molecular oxygen as a substrate was confirmed by the O^{18}_2 experiment (Daly, Levitt, Guroff and Udenfriend, 1968). The position of O^{18} in the DOPA formed either from tyrosine-4-O^{18} and O^{16}_2 or from nonisotopic tyrosine and O^{18}_2 by tyrosine hydroxylase was determined. The DOPA formed from tyrosine-4-O^{18} contained only small amounts (about 10%) of O^{18} in the 3 position while DOPA formed from nonisotopic tyrosine and O^{18}_2 contained approximately 90% of the label in the 3 position. Hydroxylation of phenylalanine-4-H^3 with tyrosine hydroxylase resulted in migration of the tritium from the p position since the final product, DOPA, contained 42% of the original radioactivity (NIH shift: Guroff, Daly, Jerina, Renson, Witkop and Udenfriend, 1967).

B. Specificity

Tyrosine hydroxylase is almost specific towards L-tyrosine and L-phenylalanine. D-Tyrosine, tyramine, and tryptophan were inactive as substrate (Nagatsu, Levitt and Udenfriend, 1964b) but L-phenylalanine was hydroxylated to DOPA through tyrosine. Thus, the enzyme catalyzes two similar consecutive steps: phenylalanine → tyrosine → DOPA. However, phenylalanine was not directly converted to DOPA. Free tyrosine appeared during phenylalanine hydroxylation and one explanation is that the enzyme-tyrosine complex dissociates before conversion to DOPA (Ikeda, Levitt and Udenfriend, 1965, 1967). Tyrosine formation by tyrosine hydroxylase found in the brain and sympathetic nervous system may explain the small conversion of phenylalanine-C^{14} to tyrosine-C^{14}, which was observed in patients with phenylketonuria (Udenfriend and Bessman, 1953).

The DOPA formed proved to be L-form (Nagatsu, Levitt and Udenfriend, 1964b).

It was reported that L-m-tyrosine can be converted to L-DOPA both by rat liver phenylalanine hydroxylase and by bovine adrenal tyrosine hydroxylase (Tong, D'Iorio and Benoiton, 1971) and that m-tyrosine can be formed from L-phenylalanine by bovine adrenal tyrosine hydroxylase (Tong, D'Iorio and Benoiton, 1971).

C. *Kinetics*

K_m values assayed in the system containing 6,7-dimethyltetrahydropterin (DMPH$_4$) and mercaptoethanol were: O$_2$, $7.4 \times 10^{-5}M$; phenylalanine, $4 \times 10^{-4}M$; tyrosine, $1 \times 10^{-4}M$; and DMPH$_4$, $5 \times 10^{-4}M$ (Ikeda, Fahien and Udenfriend, 1966). K_m values assayed in a system containing particulate bovine adrenal enzyme were tyrosine, $7 \times 10^{-6}M$; and tetrahydrobiopterin, $1.2 \times 10^{-4}M$ (Shiman and Kaufman, 1970). Optimum pH either in acetate buffer or in phosphate buffer was 5.8–6.3. The optimum temperature was 30°C. The reaction was linear for 10–15 min at 30°C (Ayukawa, Takeuchi, Sezaki, Hara, Umezawa and Nagatsu, 1968).

D. *Inhibitors*

Inhibitors of tyrosine hydroxylase have been widely screened, since the enzyme appears to be the rate-limiting step of catecholamine biosynthesis (Udenfriend, Zaltzman-Nirenberg and Nagatsu, 1965; Levitt, Gibb, Daly, Lipton and Udenfriend, 1967; McGeer, E. G. and McGeer, P. L., 1967; Saari, Williams, Britcher, Wolf and Kuehl, 1967).

Typical inhibitors of tyrosine hydroxylase are shown in Table II.

Substrate analogues such as L-α-methyl-p-tyrosine inhibited the enzyme in competition with tyrosine (Nagatsu, Levitt and Udenfriend, 1964b). L-α-Methyl-p-tyrosine inhibited the enzyme *in vivo*, decreased the endogenous level of catecholamines (Spector, Sjoerdsma and Udenfriend, 1965), and caused the decrease in blood pressure and sedation in man (Sjoerdsma, 1967). Phenylalanine was a substrate and inhibited the formation of DOPA from tyrosine (Ikeda, Levitt and Udenfriend, 1967; Nagatsu and Takeuchi, 1967).

Various catechol compounds including DOPA, dopamine, norepinephrine and epinephrine inhibited the enzyme, indicating the possibility of feedback regulation of the catecholamine biosynthesis (Nagatsu, Levitt and Udenfriend, 1964). The inhibition was in competition with a tetrahydropteridine and uncompetitively with tyrosine (Udenfriend, Zaltzman-Nirenberg and Nagatsu, 1965). 3,4-Dihydroxyphenyl-n-propylacetamide (Hassle 22/54) was the most potent catechol inhibitor (Levitt, Gibb, Daly, Lipton and Udenfriend, 1967). It was shown that in normal sympathetically innervated tissues, such as the brain, heart, spleen and adrenal medulla, the

TABLE II.   Tyrosine Hydroxylase Inhibitors.

Groups	Examples of inhibitors	I_{50} (M)
Tyrosine analogues[1,2]	L-α-Methyl-p-tyrosine	2×10^{-5}
	DL-3-I-α-Methyl-p-tyrosine	3×10^{-7}
Catechols[1,2,3]	Norepinephrine	1×10^{-3}
	3,4-Dihydroxyphenyl-n-propylacetamide (Hassle 22/54)	2×10^{-5}
Tryptophan analogues[4,5]	L-α-Methyl-5-hydroxytryptophan	7×10^{-5}
	DL-5-I-Tryptophan	9×10^{-7}
Fe^{++}-chelating agents[1,6]	α,α'-Dipyridyl	1×10^{-4}
	o-Phenanthroline	1×10^{-5}
	2,4,5-Tripyridyl-s-triazine	1×10^{-4}
	Bathophenanthroline	1×10^{-4}
Naphthoquinones	Aquayamycin[7]	3.7×10^{-7}
	Chrothiomycin[8]	1×10^{-8}
		2.5×10^{-6}
		(Fe^{++}: 2.5×10^{-3})
	Deoxyfrenolicin[9]	1×10^{-4}
		1×10^{-4}
		(Fe^{++}: 5×10^{-4})
	Spinochrome A[10]	4×10^{-6}
	Echinochrome A[10]	2×10^{-4}
	Oudenone[11-13]	3×10^{-4}

1) Nagatsu, Levitt and Udenfriend, 1964b.
2) Udenfriend, Zaltzman-Nirenberg and Nagatsu, 1965.
3) Levitt, Gibb, Daly, Lipton and Udenfriend, 1967.
4) Zhelyaskov, Levitt and Udenfriend, 1968.
5) McGeer, E. G., McGeer, P. L. and Peters, 1967.
6) Taylor, Stubbs and Ellenbogen, 1968, 1969.
7) Ayukawa, Takeuchi, Sezaki, Hara, Umezawa and Nagatsu, 1968.
8) Ayukawa, Hamada, Kojiri, Takeuchi, Hara, Nagatsu and Umezawa, 1969.
9) Taylor, Stubbs and Ellenbogen, 1970.
10) Mizutani, Nagatsu, Asajima and Kinoshita, 1971, 1972.
11) Umezawa, Takeuchi, Iinuma, Suzuki, Ito, Matsuzaki, Nagatsu and Tanabe, 1970.
12) Ohno, Okamoto, Kawabe, Umezawa, Takeuchi, Iinuma and Takahashi, 1971.
13) Nagatsu, T., Nagatsu, I., Umezawa and Takeuchi, 1971.

biosynthesis of norepinephrine is regulated by the feedback inhibition of tyrosine hydroxylase by norepinephrine *in vivo* (Gordon, Spector, Sjoerdsma and Udenfriend, 1968; Alousi and Weiner, 1966; Roth, Stjärne and Euler, 1966, 1967). Norepinephrine inhibited tyrosine hydroxylase in competition with tetrahydrobiopterin *in vitro* (Nagatsu, T., Mizutani, Nagatsu, I., Matsuura and Sugimoto, 1972).

H 22/54   n-Propyl gallate

Various Fe^{++}-chelating agents inhibit the enzyme. α,α'-Dipyridyl (Nagatsu, Levitt and Udenfriend, 1964a, b), o-phenanthroline, 2,4,5-tripyridyl-s-triazine and bathophenanthroline (4,7-diphenyl-1,10-phenanthroline), which have high affinities for Fe^{++}, were the most effective inhibitors. m-Phenanthroline did not inhibit the enzyme at 1 mM (Taylor, Stubbs and Ellenbogen, 1969). 3-Amino-pyrrolo-[3,4c]isoxazole and derivatives inhibited the enzyme. For example, 3-amino-4H-pyrrole[3,4c]isoxazole-5(6H)-carboxylic acid ethyl ester (CL-65263) inhibited the enzyme by 50% at $1 \times 10^{-4}M$ (Taylor, Stubbs and Ellenbogen, 1968). 4-Isopropyltropolone inhibited the enzyme in vitro and in vivo (Goldstein, Gang and Anagnoste, 1968).

CL-65263   4-Isopropyltropolone

Various naphthoquinones are inhibitors. A new antibiotic, Aquayamycin, discovered from a strain of streptomyces (Sezaki, Hara, Ayukawa, Takeuchi, Okami, Hamada, Nagatsu and Umezawa, 1968), was reported to be a potent inhibitor of tyrosine hydroxylase in vitro (Ayukawa, Takeuchi, Sezaki, Hara, Umezawa and Nagatsu, 1968), inhibiting the enzyme by 50% at $3.7 \times 10^{-7}M$.

The inhibition was noncompetitive with tyrosine. The inhibition by 4×10^{-7} M of aquayamycin increased when the concentration of 6,7-dimethyl-tetrahydropterin increased from $2 \times 10^{-4}M$ to $1 \times 10^{-3}M$, and was reversed by Fe^{++}. The structure of aquayamycin was established as 9-(tetrahydro-4',5'-dihydroxy-6'-methyl-2'H-pyran-2'-yl)-3,4,4a,12b-tetrahydro-3,4a,8,12b-tetrahydroxy-3-methyl-benz[a]anthracene-1,7,12(2H)-trione (Sezaki,

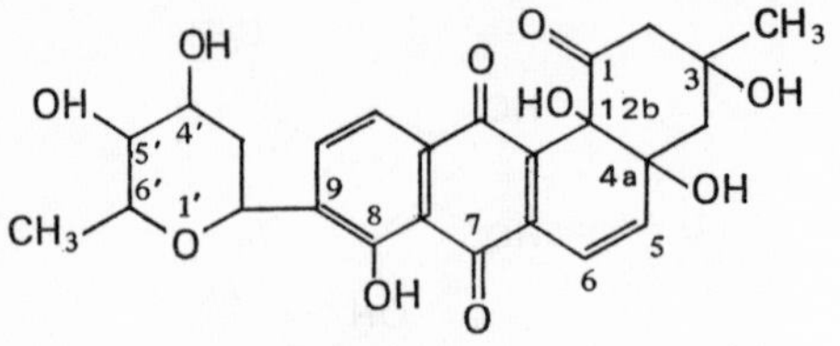

Aquayamycin 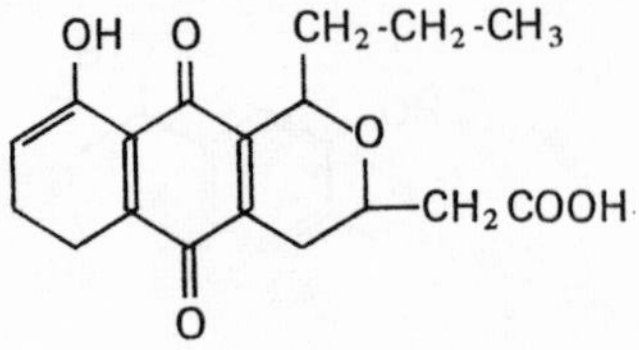   Deoxyfrenolicin

Kondo, Maeda, Umezawa and Ohno, 1970). Deoxyfrenolicin, an analog of frenolicin, which is an antibiotic produced by *Streptomyces fradiae* and has a naphthoquinone structure, was shown to be a potent inhibitor of tyrosine hydroxylase. The inhibition was competitive with tyrosine, increased by high concentrations of the pteridine cofactor, and could not be reversed by Fe^{++}. When administered to rats at 50 mg/kg, deoxyfrenolicin significantly inhibited adrenal tyrosine hydroxylase activity (Taylor, Stubbs and Ellenbogen, 1970). Another quinone-type new antibiotic, chrothiomycin, which had a molecular formula $C_{27}H_{31-33}O_{13}NS$, was also an inhibitor of tyrosine hydroxylase (Ayukawa, Hamada, Kojiri, Takeuchi, Hara, Nagatsu and Umezawa, 1969).

Naphthoquinone pigments in Echinodermata were inhibitors. Echinochrome A and spinochrome A, which are the red pigments of sea urchins, inhibited the enzyme activity (Mizutani, Nagatsu, Asajima and Kinoshita, 1972).

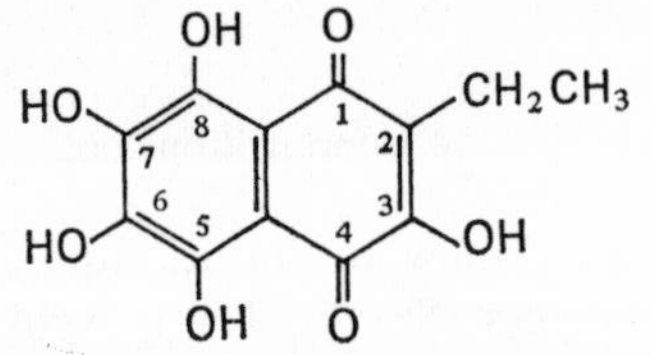

Echinochrome A 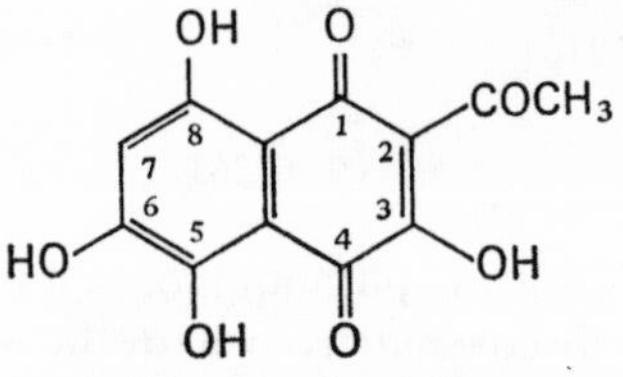   Spinochrome A

Echinochrome A and spinochrome A inhibited by 50% at $2 \times 10^{-4}M$ and $4 \times 10^{-6}M$, respectively. Echinochrome A inhibited noncompetitively with tyrosine or 6,7-dimethyltetrahydropterin, while spinochrome A competitively with tyrosine and uncompetitively with 6,7-dimethyltetrahydropterin. The inhibition by either echinochrome A or spinochrome A was reversed by adding Fe^{++}.

The structure shown below in naphthoquinone derivative appears to be essential for the inhibition of tyrosine hydroxylase.

Oudenone
[(S)-2-(4,5-dihydro-5-propyl-2(3H)-
furylidene]-1,3-cyclopentanedione]

Oudenone, a new tyrosine hydroxylase inhibitor of microbial origin, was discovered (Umezawa, Takeuchi, Iinuma, Suzuki, Ito, Matsuzaki, Nagatsu and Tanabe, 1970), and the structure was determined (Ohno, Okamoto, Kawabe, Umezawa, Takeuchi, Iinuma and Takahashi, 1971). The effect of oudenone on tyrosine hydroxylase was not affected by addition of Fe^{++}. The kinetic study showed the uncompetitive relation between oudenone and tyrosine and the competitive relation between 2-amino-4-hydroxy-6,7-dimethyl-5,6,7,8-tetrahydropteridine and oudenone. Oudenone had a hypotensive effect (Umezawa, Takeuchi, Iinuma, Suzuki, Ito, Matsuzaki, Nagatsu and Tanabe, 1970) and inhibited adrenal tyrosine hydroxylase *in vivo* and caused the reduction of tissue catecholamine levels (Nagatsu, T., Nagatsu, I., Umezawa and Takeuchi, 1971). Oudenone had a more pronounced hypotensive action on spontaneously hypertensive rats (Okamoto and Aoki, 1963) than on normal Wistar rats (Nagatsu, I., Nagatsu, T., Mizutani, Umezawa, Matsuzaki and Takeuchi, 1971).

Tryptophan derivatives, the most potent of which was α-methyl-5-hydroxytryptophan, were reported to inhibit tyrosine hydroxylase. Tyrosine hydroxylase activity was inhibited *in vivo* by a 50 mg/kg does of α-methyl-5-hydroxytryptophan. The administration of this compound resulted in depletion of tissue stores of catecholamines as well as in sedation (Zhelyaskov, Levitt and Udenfriend, 1968). 5-Halotryptophans such as DL-5-bromotryptophan inhibited tyrosine hydroxylase *in vitro* and *in vivo* (McGeer, E. G., McGeer, P. L. and Peters, 1967). α-Methyl-5-hydroxytryptophan was found to lower the brain content of norepinephrine, but did not markedly lower the brain content of dopamine, while α-methyl-*p*-tyrosine lowered the brain contents of both norepinephrine and dopamine (Dominic and Moore, 1969). The two facts that 5-hydroxytryptophan inhibits tyrosine hydroxylase and that norepinephrine inhibits tryptophan hydroxylase (Jequier, Robinson, Lovenberg and Sjoerdsma, 1969), suggest a new insight into the interrelationships of catecholamine and serotonin biosynthetic mechanisms as shown in Fig. 10 (Zhelyaskov, Levitt and Udenfriend, 1968).

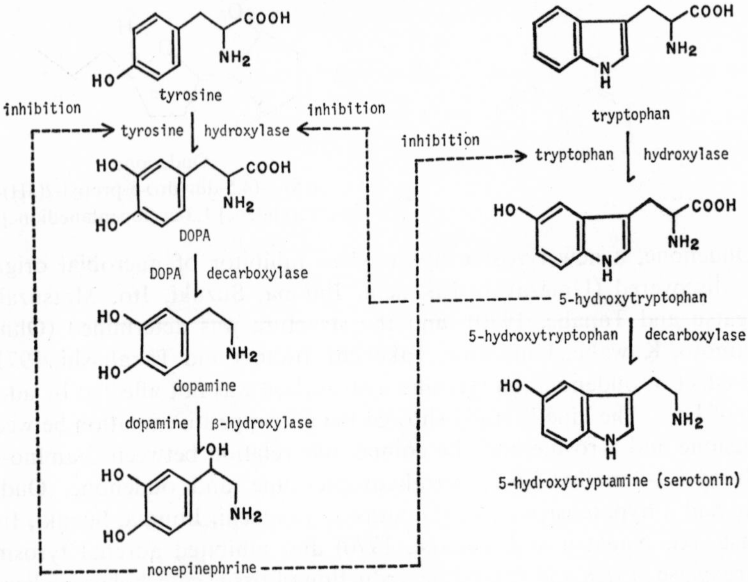

Fig. 10. Biosynthesis of catecholamines and serotonin. The possibility of the mutual regulation of both syntheses (Zhelyaskov, Levitt and Udenfriend, 1968).

E. *Comparison of the properties of tyrosine hydroxylase, tyrosinase and phenylalanine hydroxylase*

It had long been thought before the discovery of tyrosine hydroxylase that tyrosinase is the enzyme responsible for the formation of DOPA in the biosynthesis of catecholamines. It is now obvious that this assumption was wrong, at least in mammals.

Comparison of the properties of three similar enzymes: tyrosine hydroxylase, tyrosinase, and phenylalanine hydroxylase are summarized in Table III. Tyrosine hydroxylase is localized in sympathetic nerve cells and in chromaffin cells as in the adrenal medulla and works only in the formation of catecholamines. The enzyme is specific for L-tyrosine and L-phenylalanine and specifically inhibited by L-α-methyl-*p*-tyrosine.

Phenylalanine hydroxylase is localized exclusively in the liver and is specific for L-phenylalanine. L-α-Methyl-*p*-tyrosine does not inhibit phenylalanine hydroxylase.

Tyrosinase is localized in melanocytes and is responsible for the formation of melanin pigment. It catalyzes two successive reactions: tyrosine → DOPA → dopaquinone. Dopaquinones are polymerized to melanin non-

TABLE III. Comparison of the Properties of Tyrosine Hydroxylase, Phenylalanine Hydroxylase and Tyrosinase.

	Tyrosine hydroxylase[1,2]	Phenylalanine hydroxylase[4]	Tyrosinase[6]
Distribution organs	Adrenal medulla, brain, sympathetically innervated organs (heart, spleen, salivary gland, vas deference, etc.)	Liver, Kidney, Pancreas	Skin, eye, Melanoma
cell type	Sympathetic nerve cell	Liver cell	Melanocyte
Cofactor	Tetrahydropterin (tetrahydrobiopterin?), Fe^{++}?	Tetrahydrobiopterin, Fe^{++}	$DOPA$[7]
Optimum pH	6.0 (5.8–6.3)	7.5	7.0
Substrate	L-Tyrosine ++ L-Phenylalanine ++	L-Phenylalanine +++ L-Tryptophan +	L-Tyrosine + D-Tyrosine + Tyramine + DOPA +++
K_m (M)	L-Tyrosine (DMPH$_4$) 1×10^{-4} L-Phenylalanine (DMPH$_4$) 3×10^{-4} DMPH$_4$ 5×10^{-4} L-Tyrosine[3] (tetrahydrobiopterin) 2×10^{-5} Tetrahydrobiopterin[3] 1×10^{-4}	L-Phenylalanine[5] 1.4×10^{-4} L-Tryptophan 1.7×10^{-3} DMPH$_4$ 1×10^{-4}	L-Tyrosine 6×10^{-4} D-Tyrosine 8×10^{-3} L-DOPA 5×10^{-4} D-DOPA 4×10^{-3}
Inhibitors			
L-α-Methyl-p-tyrosine	+++	0	0
DOPA or other catechols	+	+	0
Fe^{++}-chelating agents, such as α,α'-dipyridyl	++	++	0
Cu-chelating agent, such as diethyldithiocarbamate	0	0	+++
Melanin pigment formation	0	0	+

1) Nagatsu, Levitt and Udenfriend, 1964 b.   2) Ikeda, Levitt and Udenfriend, 1965.   3) Shiman and Kaufman, 1970.
4) Kaufman, 1962 c.   5) Sato, Jequier, Lovenberg and Sjoerdsma, 1967.   6) Pomerantz, 1963.
7) Pomerantz and Warner, 1966.

enzymatically. Tyrosinase is not inhibited by DOPA, but DOPA is the best substrate and an activator, and is thought to be the cofactor of tyrosinase-catalyzed tyrosine hydroxylase reactions (Pomerantz and Warner, 1966). If DOPA is both required and synthesized by tyrosinase it is possible that an independent route to the synthesis of DOPA occurs in melanoma, perhaps via tyrosine hydroxylase (Pomerantz and Warner, 1966). Fe^{++}-chelating agents, such as α,α'-dipyridyl, do not inhibit tyrosinase, but Cu-chelating agents, such as diethyldithiocarbamate, inhibit tyrosinase. Tyrosinase is responsible for the synthesis of catecholamines in insects (Sekeris and Karlson, 1966) and in banana plant (Nagatsu, I., Sudo and Nagatsu, T., 1972).

I. 3. 5. PHYSIOLOGICAL ROLE

Tyrosine hydroxylase was established as the rate-limiting step of catecholamine biosynthesis (Levitt, Spector, Sjoerdsma and Udenfriend, 1965). The end product, norepinephrine, inhibited the initial enzyme, tyrosine hydroxylase (Nagatsu, Levitt and Udenfriend, 1964b). Increase in the norepinephrine synthesis by the release of tissue norepinephrine was confirmed in the intact rat during exercise and exposure to cold (Gordon, Spector, Sjoerdsma and Udenfriend, 1966), in the rat heart on electrical stimulation of the stellate ganglia (Gordon, Reid, Sjoerdsma and Udenfriend, 1966), in the hypogastric nerve vas deference preparation of guinea pig by nerve stimulation (Alousi and Weiner, 1966), in isolated guinea pig vas deference and bovine splenic nerve by nerve stimulation (Roth, Stjärne, and Euler, 1966, 1967), and in the rat submaxillary gland by sympathetic nerve stimulation (Sedvall and Kopin, 1967). All these results suggest that norepinephrine biosynthesis is regulated by the feedback inhibition of tyrosine hydroxylase by norepinephrine.

Tyrosine hydroxylase isolated from the pheochromocytoma, a human tumor which is characterized by a high rate of synthesis and secretion of catecholamines, appears to be less sensitive to the inhibition by norepinephrine (Roth, Stjärne, Levine and Giarman, 1968; Nagatsu, T., Yamamoto and Nagatsu, I., 1970). It remains for further investigation to determine whether the uncontrolled excessive production of norepinephrine in the pheochromocytoma is partly due to altered sensitivity of tyrosine hydroxylase to norepinephrine inhibition or not.

There have been several reports indicating that tyrosine hydroxylase may be an inducible enzyme. Its activity in the adrenal gland and heart of rabbits with neurogenic hypertension increased about 2-fold, probably due to the increase in the amount of enzyme (DeQuattro, Nagatsu, Maronde and

Alexander, 1969). After the electrical stimulation of the hypogastric nerve of the isolated guinea pig vas deference preparation, synthesis of norepinephrine was increased. Norepinephrine, $6 \times 10^{-6}M$, did not affect the increased rate of synthesis seen during the post-nerve stimulation period, but with puromycin, $1.8 \times 10^{-4}M$, partial inhibition was achieved. However, the *in vivo* tyrosine hydroxylase activity did not increase, and it is possible that the results could be due to altered substrate availability or changes in endogenous inhibitor concentrations (Weiner and Rabadjija, 1968). Destruction of peripheral sympathetic nerve endings with 6-hydroxydopamine caused a disappearance of cardiac tyrosine hydroxylase, accompanied by a 2-fold increase in adrenal tyrosine hydroxylase activity in the adrenal gland which might be the result of synthesis of new enzyme protein or activation of the preexisting enzyme (Mueller, Thoenen and Axelrod, 1969a). Reserpine and phenoxybenzamine increased the activity of adrenal tyrosine hydroxylase, and reserpine also increased the activity of tyrosine hydroxylase in the superior cervical ganglion. This increase in enzyme activity was prevented by interruption of nerve impulses by decentralization (Thoenen, Mueller and Axelrod, 1969). After the administration of reserpine, the *in vitro* tyrosine hydroxylase activity increases in rat, guinea pig, mouse and rabbit adrenal gland, in rat superior cervical ganglia and in rabbit brain stem. The results indicate that prolonged periods of drug-induced sympathoadrenal hyperactivity can increase the amount of tyrosine hydroxylase in adrenergic areas of the central and peripheral nervous system (Mueller, Thoenen and Axelrod, 1969b). Evidence was presented indicating the local synthesis of induced tyrosine hydroxylase in the nerve terminals rather than the peripheral movement of the completed enzyme from the nerve cell body (Thoenen, Mueller and Axelrod, 1970a). A small but significant increase in tyrosine hydroxylase activity of the whole brain was found in the electroshock-treated rats, and in the brainstem (24%) and cortex (20%) of such animals (Musacchio, Julou, Ketty and Glowinski, 1969). The activities of tyrosine hydroxylase, phenylethanolamine *N*-methyltransferase, and monoamine oxidase increased in the adrenal glands of mice subjected to psychosocial stimulation (Axelrod, Mueller, Henry and Stephens, 1970).

When large doses of L-DOPA (1000 mg/kg) were given to rats daily for four or seven days, the levels of tyrosine hydroxylase in the adrenal were lowered in comparison to controls. These findings may be a further indication of the existence of a regulatory mechanism which modifies endogenous levels of tyrosine hydroxylase in response to changes in the biosynthetic demand for norepinephrine (Dairman and Udenfriend, 1971).

Inhibitors of tyrosine hydroxylase were shown to have hypotensive effects. After repeated injections (4×150 mg/kg i.p. every six hours) or oral administration (3×3000 mg/kg every eight hours) of α-methyl-p-tyrosine to groups of genetic hypertensive, normotensive, or chronic renal hypertensive rats, there were significant falls in blood pressure in all cases (Laverty and Robertson, 1967). Inhibition of tyrosine hydroxylase by α-methyl-p-tyrosine is an effective means of controlling hypertension in patients with pheochromocytoma (Sjoerdsma, 1967). Oudenone, a new microbial product that inhibits tyrosine hydroxylase, was found to have a hypotensive effect (Umezawa, Takeuchi, Iinuma, Suzuki, Ito, Matsuzaki, Nagatsu and Tanabe, 1970). Oudenone inhibited tyrosine hydroxylase competitively with the tetrahydropteridine (DMPH$_4$) cofactor.

I. 4.   DOPA Decarboxylase (DDC)
(Aromatic L-Amino Acid Decarboxylase)

3,4-Dihydroxy-L-phenylalanine carboxylyase [EC 4. 1. 1. 26]. Trivial name: DOPA decarboxylase, Dihydroxyphenylalanine decarboxylase.

This enzyme, discovered in 1938 (Holtz, Heise and Lüdtke, 1938; Holtz, 1939), is not specific for L-DOPA, but decarboxylates aromatic L-amino acids such as 5-hydroxytryptophan, phenylalanine, tryptophan, and tyrosine. Therefore, the name "aromatic L-amino acid decarboxylase" was proposed (Udenfriend, 1962a). The enzyme has been extensively studied, and several reports have been published on it (Holtz, 1959; Sourkes, 1966; Udenfriend, 1962a). It was completely purified from hog kidney, and its physicochemical properties elucidated (Christenson, Dairman and Udenfriend, 1970).

L-3,4-Dihydroxyphenylalanine   Dopamine
(DOPA)

I. 4. 1. TISSUE DISTRIBUTION
DOPA decarboxylase is widely distributed in a number of mammalian organs; guinea pig and rat liver, guinea pig stomach, rat and dog brain and the kidneys from many species (Lovenberg, Weissbach and Udenfriend, 1962). Adrenal medulla (Langemann, 1951) and the sympathetic

nerve (Goodall and Kirshner, 1958) also contain the enzyme. It was reported to be present almost entirely in the soluble fraction (Blaschko, Hagen and Welch, 1955). However, on careful homogenization of brain (dog, rat and guinea pig) as much as 60% of DOPA decarboxylase activity could be found in synaptosomes (Udenfriend, 1966a). 5-Hydroxytryptophan decarboxylase activity was also found in brain synaptosomes (Rodriguez de Lores Aenaiz and de Robertis, 1964). Although DOPA decarboxylase [E. C. 4. 1. 1. 26] and 5-hydroxytryptophan decarboxylase [E. C. 4. 1. 1. 28] have been given different EC numbers, both enzyme activities have been reported as associated with a single protein (Christenson, Dairman and Udenfriend, 1970). If DOPA decarboxylase is entirely localized in the cytoplasma, it would be necessary for the enzymatically formed dopamine to be taken up by a particle-bound dopamine-β-hydroxylase (Kirshner, Rorie and Kamin, 1963).

Decarboxylation of DOPA was demonstrated in various human tissues (liver, kidney, lung, heart and brain) obtained at autopsy. Addition of pyridoxal phosphate to the incubation medium markedly increased DOPA decarboxylation in some but not all tissues. In contrast to observations in animal tissues, DOPA decarboxylation was generally higher in fetal tissue than in adult tissue (Vogel, McFarland and Prince, 1970). The enzyme was also found in human pheochromocytoma and human argentaffinoma (Hagen, 1962).

I. 4. 2. ASSAY METHOD
See section III. 3.

I. 4. 3. PURIFICATION
DOPA decarboxylase was partially purified from guinea pig kidney (Clark, Weissbach and Udenfriend, 1954; Lovenberg, Weissbach and Udenfriend 1962) and from rat liver (Awapara, Sandman and Hauly, 1962). Dopa decarboxylase in hog kidney has been purified up to 99% pure preparations (Christenson, Dairman and Udenfriend, 1970). A purification procedure from hog kidney by Christenson, Dairman and Udenfriend (1970) is described below in a form of a flow chart.

All procedures were carried out at 0–5°C.

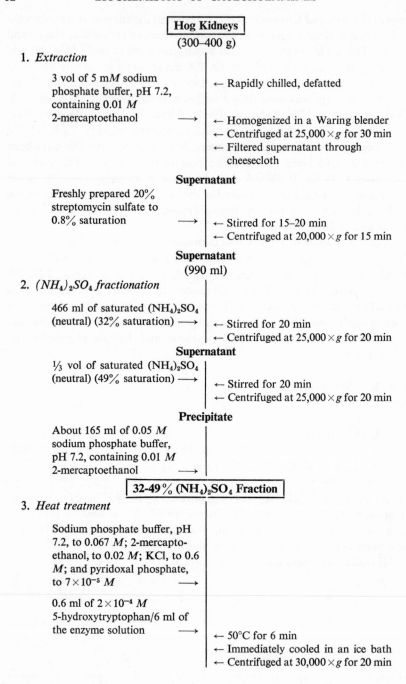

Hog Kidneys
(300–400 g)

1. *Extraction*

3 vol of 5 mM sodium
phosphate buffer, pH 7.2,
containing 0.01 M
2-mercaptoethanol $\longrightarrow$

← Rapidly chilled, defatted

← Homogenized in a Waring blender
← Centrifuged at $25,000 \times g$ for 30 min
← Filtered supernatant through
cheesecloth

Supernatant

Freshly prepared 20%
streptomycin sulfate to
0.8% saturation $\longrightarrow$

← Stirred for 15–20 min
← Centrifuged at $20,000 \times g$ for 15 min

Supernatant
(990 ml)

2. *(NH_4)$_2$SO$_4$ fractionation*

466 ml of saturated (NH$_4$)$_2$SO$_4$
(neutral) (32% saturation) $\longrightarrow$

← Stirred for 20 min
← Centrifuged at $25,000 \times g$ for 20 min

Supernatant

⅓ vol of saturated (NH$_4$)$_2$SO$_4$
(neutral) (49% saturation) $\longrightarrow$

← Stirred for 20 min
← Centrifuged at $25,000 \times g$ for 20 min

Precipitate

About 165 ml of 0.05 M
sodium phosphate buffer,
pH 7.2, containing 0.01 M
2-mercaptoethanol $\longrightarrow$

32-49% (NH$_4$)$_2$SO$_4$ Fraction

3. *Heat treatment*

Sodium phosphate buffer, pH
7.2, to 0.067 M; 2-mercapto-
ethanol, to 0.02 M; KCl, to 0.6
M; and pyridoxal phosphate,
to 7×10^{-5} M $\longrightarrow$

0.6 ml of 2×10^{-4} M
5-hydroxytryptophan/6 ml of
the enzyme solution $\longrightarrow$

← 50°C for 6 min
← Immediately cooled in an ice bath
← Centrifuged at $30,000 \times g$ for 20 min

Supernatant

(about 280 ml)

      ← Dialyzed against two changes of 4 *l*
        each of 5 mM sodium phosphate
        buffer, pH 7.2, containing 0.01 M
        2-mercaptoethanol

| **Dialyzed Heat Supernatant** |

(about 310 ml)

4. *Alumina Cγ treatment*

0.2 N acetic acid to bring
to pH 5.8   ⟶   ← Centrifuged at 20,000 × g for 20 min

Supernatant

A 3% suspension of alumina
Cγ (about 0.4 mg per 280 nm
one optical density unit) ⟶ ← Stirred for 20 min
            ← Centrifuged

Alumina Cγ Precipitate

150 ml of 0.01 M 2-mercapto-
ethanol   ⟶   ← Resuspended
            ← Washed and centrifuged

Washed Alumina Cγ Precipitate

200 ml of 0.1 M sodium
phosphate buffer, pH 7.2,
containing 0.01 M
2-mercaptoethanol ⟶ ← Centrifuged

| **Alumina Cγ Eluate** |

5. *Polyethylene glycol-6000*
precipitation

A 40% solution of polyethylene
glycol-6000 to a final concentration of 12.5% ⟶ ← Stirred for 20 min
            ← Centrifuged at 40,000 × g for 45 min

Supernatant

(290 ml)

140 ml of DEAE-cellulose
suspension (about
27 mg/ml)   ⟶   ← Mixed for 20 min
            ← Filtered with a coarse sintered glass
              funnel

100 ml of 0.01 *M* sodium
phosphate buffer, pH 7.2,
containing 0.01 *M*
2-mercaptoethanol   ⟶ | ← Washed

100 ml of 0.05 *M* sodium
phosphate buffer, pH 7.2,
containing 0.6 *M* NaCl and
0.01 *M* 2-mercaptoethanol ⟶ | ← Suspended
                                ← Centrifuged at 25,000 × *g* for 20 min

Supernatant

| ← Dialyzed against two changes of 2 *l*
  each of 0.05 *M* sodium phosphate
  buffer, pH 7.2, containing 0.01 *M*
  2-mercaptoethanol

Dialyzed Supernatant

6. *DEAE-Sephadex column*
   chromatography

DEAE-Sephadex A-50, 2.5 × 30 cm Column
equilibrated with 0.05 *M* sodium phosphate buffer, pH 7.2, containing 0.01 *M* 2-mercaptoethanol, and rinsed with two small aliquots of the same buffer

A linear gradient of 0–0.5 *M*
NaCl in a total volume of
1,000 ml of the same buffer
solution   ⟶ | ← Flow rate 8–10 ml/hr; fraction size,
                                10 ml

DEAE-Sephadex Eluate
(about 0.25 *M* NaCl eluate)

7. *Hydroxyapatite column*
   chromatography (I) | ← Concentrated by ultrafiltration to
                                 about 10 ml
                               ← Dialyzed overnight against 1 *l* of
                                 0.01 *M* sodium phosphate buffer,
                                 pH 7.2, containing 0.01 *M*
                                 2-mercaptoethanol

Hydroxyapatite, 1.5 × 27 cm Column
(Bio-Gel HTP, 20 g, washed with 400 ml of water at room temperature with very gentle stirring at least five times; the fine particles
decanted off), equilibrated with 0.01 *M* sodium phosphate buffer,
pH 7.2, containing 0.01 *M* 2-mercaptoethanol, and washed with at
least 500 ml of the same buffer over a period of at least 24 hr

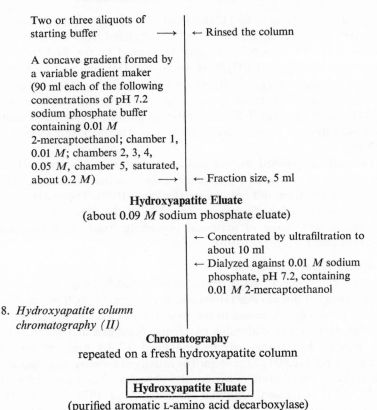

Two or three aliquots of
starting buffer   ⟶   ← Rinsed the column

A concave gradient formed by
a variable gradient maker
(90 ml each of the following
concentrations of pH 7.2
sodium phosphate buffer
containing 0.01 M
2-mercaptoethanol; chamber 1,
0.01 M; chambers 2, 3, 4,
0.05 M, chamber 5, saturated,
about 0.2 M)   ⟶   ← Fraction size, 5 ml

Hydroxyapatite Eluate
(about 0.09 M sodium phosphate eluate)

← Concentrated by ultrafiltration to
   about 10 ml
← Dialyzed against 0.01 M sodium
   phosphate, pH 7.2, containing
   0.01 M 2-mercaptoethanol

8. *Hydroxyapatite column*
   chromatography (II)

Chromatography
repeated on a fresh hydroxyapatite column

Hydroxyapatite Eluate
(purified aromatic L-amino acid decarboxylase)

The purification was about 300-fold with recoveries from 5 to 14%. The
final specific activities ranged from 7,500 to 9,500 nmoles/min/mg (37°C) and
the molecular activity was about 1,000 mole/mole enzyme. The purified
enzyme was relatively stable and was 97–100% pure, as estimated by polyacrylamide gel disc electrophoresis (Christenson, Dairman and Udenfriend, 1970). The enzyme was partially purified from dog brain. The
original specific activity of the enzyme obtained from brain was only about
1/40 of that obtained from guinea pig kidney (Lovenberg, Weissbach and
Udenfriend, 1962).

I. 4. 4. PROPERTIES

A. *Physico-chemical properties*
Purified hog kidney enzyme had a $S_{20,w}$ of 5.82±0.03, and its molecular

weight was calculated to be 112,000 from sedimentation equilibrium using a partial specific volume of 0.742 ml/g, calculated from the amino acid composition. The molecular weights determined by the Archibald technique were 108,000 and 107,000 (Christenson, Dairman and Udenfriend, 1970). Polyacrylamide gel electrophoresis in the presence of sodium dodecyl sulfate produced three bands, corresponding to molecular weights of about 57,000, 40,000 and 21,000. This suggests that purified preparations contain multiple forms of the enzyme (Christenson, Dairman and Udenfriend, 1970).

The partially purified enzyme had an absorption maximum at 415 nm. On addition of pyridoxal-5-phosphate, enzyme activity increased but the absorption spectrum did not change (Fellman, 1959). The excitation and emission spectra of the fluorescent derivative of the enzyme-bound material agreed with those of pyridoxal phosphate standards (Christenson, Dairman and Udenfriend, 1970).

B. *Cofactor and requirement*

A number of observations suggest that pyridoxal-5-phosphate is the prosthetic group of this enzyme (Holtz and Bachmann, 1952). Some pyridoxal phosphate was tightly bound to the apoenzyme as a Schiff's base, whereas another portion was dialyzable (Awapara, Sandman and Hanly, 1962). The purified hog kidney enzyme contained 0.7–1.1 mole of pyridoxal phosphate per 112,000 g of protein. The activity of the enzyme preparations was activated on addition of pyridoxal-5-phosphate 2 to 5-fold at 5×10^{-6}–$1 \times 10^{-4}M$ (Christenson, Dairman and Udenfriend, 1970). The enzyme is inhibited by aldehyde reagents such as hydroxylamine ($5 \times 10^{-5}M$).

The substrate, DOPA, inhibits its own decarboxylation by combining irreversibly with the coenzyme, pyridoxal-5-phosphate. DOPA, dopamine

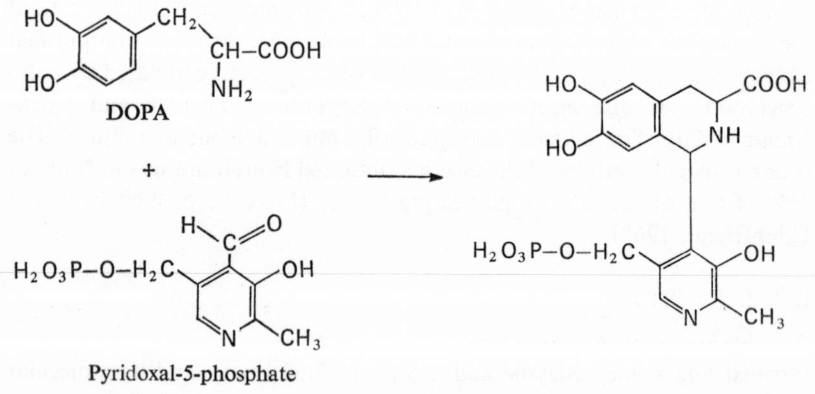

DOPA

+

Pyridoxal-5-phosphate

and norepinephrine form Schiff's bases with pyridoxal-5-phosphate which are easily transformed into tetrahydroisoquinoline derivatives (Schott and Clark, 1952). Pyridoxal phosphate at concentrations above $1 \times 10^{-4}M$ inhibited the purified hog kidney enzyme. This inhibition may be due to the formation of the tetrahydroisoquinoline derivative, since $1 \times 10^{-3}M$ pyridoxal phosphate did not inhibit the enzyme with phenylalanine as substrate. Phenylalanine does not form the tetrahydroisoquinoline derivative (Christenson, Dairman and Udenfriend, 1970).

No metal requirement was shown for the enzyme (Lovenberg, Weissbach and Udenfriend, 1962). The ions, Fe^{++}, Fe^{+++}, K^+, Mg^{++}, Ca^{++} and Al^{+++} had little effect, whereas Cu^{++}, Zn^{++} and Hg^{++} were strongly inhibitory at 1 mM. The metal-chelating agents such as sodium diethyldithiocarbamate, 2,2'-bipyridine, cupferron, 1,10-phenanthroline, sodium EDTA, and 1,5-diphenylcarbohydrazide had no significant effect at 0.1 mM (Christenson, Dairman and Udenfriend, 1970).

C. *Specificity*
DOPA decarboxylase has a wider specificity. The following L-amino acids are decarboxylated by the enzyme purified from guinea pig kidney in decreasing order: DOPA, *o*-tyrosine, *m*-tyrosine, 5-hydroxytryptophan, tryptophan, phenylalanine, *p*-tyrosine, α-methyl-DOPA, α-methyl-5-hydroxytryptophan, and histidine. Throughout the purification procedure, enzyme activity in all the substrates always appeared in the same fractions and showed a similar degree of purification. This indicates that the decarboxylation of all the natural aromatic L-amino acids is catalyzed by an enzyme (Lovenberg, Weissbach and Udenfriend, 1962). The activity of the purified hog kidney enzyme toward histidine was very low but detectable (Christenson, Dairman and Udenfriend, 1970).

The DOPA-decarboxylase from adrenal medulla showed no action on histidine, tyrosine or tryptophan (Hagen, 1962). The DOPA decarboxylase purified from larvae of *Calliphora erythrocephala* acted on DOPA and 5-hydroxytryptophan, but not on other aromatic amino acids (Sekeris, 1963).

D. *Kinetics*
K_m values and V_{max} of aromatic L-amino acids are shown in Table IV (Christenson, Dairman and Udenfriend, 1970).

The optimum pH for the guinea pig enzyme was about 8.5 for natural amino acids, phenylalanine and tryptophan with the exception of DOPA (pH 6.7–7.0). DOPA and its decarboxylation product dopamine are unstable at alkaline pH. The enzyme was inhibited by *p*-chloromercuribenzoate, iodoacetamide, and N-ethylmaleimide but no stimulation of activity

TABLE IV. K_m of Various Substrates for Aromatic L-Amino Acid Decarboxylase from Hog Kidney (Christenson, Dairman and Udenfriend, 1970).

Substrate	K_m (M)	V_{max}[a]
DOPA	1.9×10^{-4}	8,900
5-Hydroxytryptophan	1×10^{-4}	850
Phenylalanine	4.2×10^{-2}	590
Tryptophan	1.0×10^{-2}	230
Tyrosine	8.4×10^{-3}	30

[a] nmoles/mg of protein/min (37°C).

was observed by the addition of sulfhydryl compounds to the incubation (Lovenberg, Weissbach and Udenfriend, 1962; Christenson, Dairman and Udenfriend, 1970).

E. Inhibitors

In an attempt to produce chemical sympathectomy at the DOPA decarboxylase stage, inhibitors of DOPA decarboxylase were widely screened (Clark, 1959; Sourkes, 1966). The following compounds are examples of DOPA decarboxylase inhibitors: α-methyl-DOPA (Sourkes, 1954; Sourkes and D'Iorio, 1963); α-methyl-5-hydroxytryptophan (Lovenberg, Barchas, Weissbach and Udenfriend, 1963); MK-485, the hydrazino analog of α-methyl-DOPA (Hansson, Fleming and Clark, 1964; Porter, Watson, Titus, Totaro and Byer, 1962); NSD-1034, N-m-hydroxybenzyl-N-methylhydrazine (Drain, Horlington, Lazare and Poulter, 1962; Hansson, Fleming and Clark, 1964); 3,4,4'-trihydroxy-3'-carboxychalcone (5-(3,4-dihydroxycinnamoyl)-salicylic acid) (Clark, 1959); Ro4-4602, N-(DL-seryl)-N'-(2,3,4-trihydroxy-benzyl) hydrazine (Hansson, Fleming and Clark, 1964; Pletscher and Gey, 1963; Pletscher, Burkard and Gey, 1964).

The mechanism of inhibition of α-methyl-DOPA appears to be complicated. It was first reported that inhibition was competitive with respect to the substrate (Sourkes, 1954) and, subsequently, it was reported that the character of the inhibition varies with the addition sequence of the substrate and inhibitor to the enzyme. When both were added simultaneously, the inhibition was competitive. When α-methyl-DOPA was preincubated with the enzyme, the inhibition was non-competitive. With simultaneous addition of the inhibitor and substrate, exogenous pyridoxal phosphate decreased the degree of inhibition which, however, retained competitive character. When inhibitor was preincubated with the enzyme before adding the substrate in the absence of added coenzyme, the degree of inhibition was increased several fold and the character of the inhibition was non-competitive. Upon the addition of pyridoxal phosphate, much of the inhibition produced by preincubation with the inhibitor was reversed (Udenfriend, 1962a). Based on these findings, a mechanism of inhibition involving the stable formation of a ternary complex among the inhibitor, enzyme and enzyme-bound pyridoxal phosphate was proposed (Udenfriend, 1962a).

It appears that since DOPA decarboxylase is active in tissues inhibition of the enzyme *in vivo* and the resultant reduction of the tissue catecholamine levels by DOPA decarboxylase inhibitors are difficult to achieve. It was found that α-methyl-DOPA reduced tissue norepinephrine levels in animals, including man, and effectively lowered blood pressure (Sjoerdsma, Oates, Zaltzman and Udenfriend, 1960). However, it was subsequently found that L-α-methyl-DOPA is itself decarboxylated by the enzyme and that it is the corresponding amine which is responsible for the release of tissue catecholamines and the resultant hypotensive effect in man. L-α-Methyl-DOPA is now used as an effective antihypertensive drug.

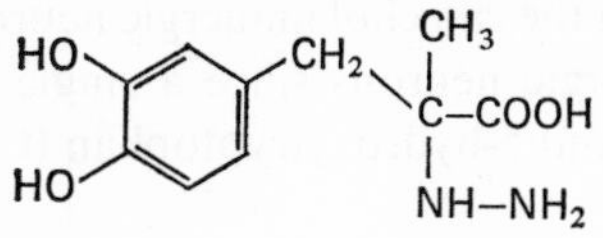

α-Methyl-DOPA hydrazine

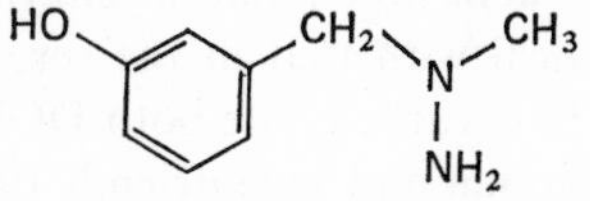

NSD-1034
N-m-Hydroxybenzyl-*N*-methylhydrazine

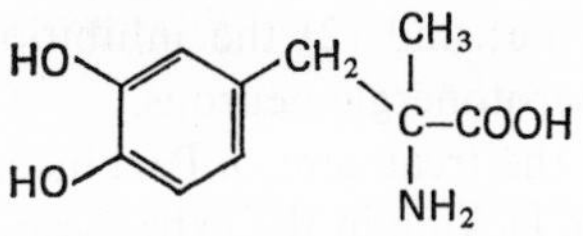

α-Methyl-DOPA

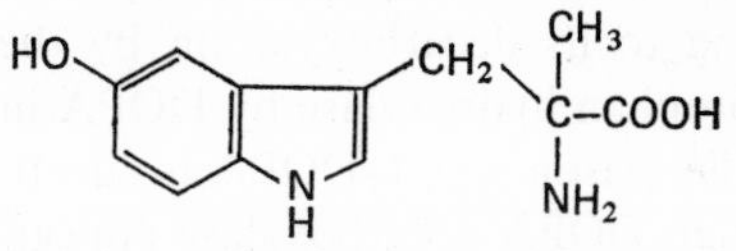

α-Methyl-5-hydroxytryptophan

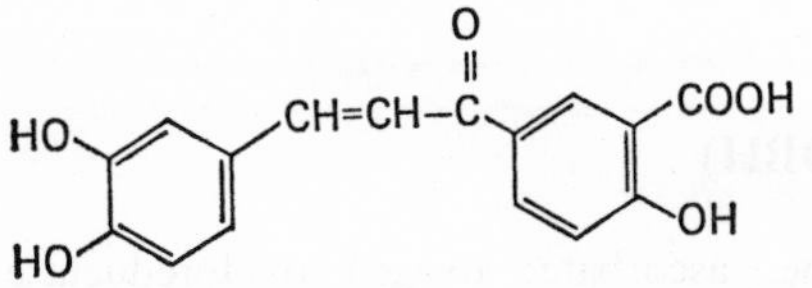

5-(3,4-Dihydroxycinnamoyl)-
salicylic acid

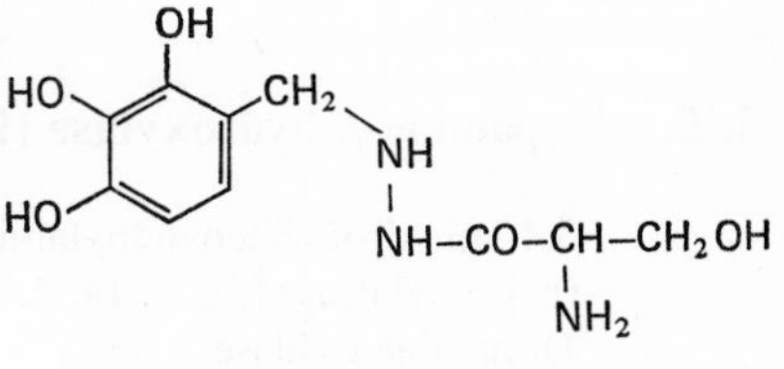

Ro4-4602
N-(DL-Seryl)-*N'*-(2,3,4-tryhydroxy-
benzyl) hydrazine

L-DOPA is an effective drug for use in treating Parkinsonism. DOPA decarboxylase inhibitor, such as Ro4-4602, which inhibits peripheral enzyme *in vivo*, but not in the brain (Pletscher and Gey, 1963), can reduce the necessary dosage of DOPA when the inhibitor and L-DOPA are administered together (Birkmayer and Mentasti, 1967; Tissot, Gaillard, Guggisberg, Ganthier and de Ajuriaguerra, 1969).

F. *Physiological role*

DOPA decarboxylase has a wide substrate specificity as aromatic L-amino acid decarboxylase. The enzyme appears to be distributed intraneuronally in the sympathetic neurons and serotonergic neurons as well as extraneuronally. The intraneuronal enzyme in the sympathetic nerves may work specifically for the biosynthesis of catecholamines in the formation of dopamine from DOPA, while the intraneuronal enzyme in the serotonergic neurons may work for the biosynthesis of serotonin in its formation from 5-hydroxytryptophan. The physiological role of the extraneuronal enzyme is not clear, but may be different from tissue to tissue.

It should be noted that the enzyme in the catecholaminergic neurons may be identical with that in the serotonergic neurons since a single enzyme proved to decarboxylate both DOPA and 5-hydroxytryptophan (Christenson, Dairman and Udenfriend, 1970).

Administration of a large amount of L-DOPA as in the treatment of Parkinsonism caused the decrease of serotonin. The reason may be due to: (1) the replacement of 5-hydroxytryptophan by DOPA and the subsequent replacement of serotonin by dopamine formed in the serotonergic neurons owing to its decarboxylation by the enzyme; and (2) the inhibition of tryptophan hydroxylase by DOPA in the serotonergic neurons.

The reason why L-DOPA is effective for the treatment of Parkinsonism though DOPA decarboxylase appears to be lacking in the extrapyramidal region of the brain of the patients may be explained by the formation of dopamine by the extraneuronal DOPA decarboxylase near the receptor site in the neostriatum of the brain.

I. 5.   Dopamine-β-hydroxylase (DBH)

> 3,4-Dihydroxyphenylethylamine, ascorbate: oxygen oxidoreductase (hydroxylating) [EC 1. 14. 2. 1]. Trivial name: Dopamine hydroxylase, Dopamine oxidase.

Dopamine-β-hydroxylase, which catalyzes the conversion of dopamine to norepinephrine, is an ascorbate-requiring copper-containing oxygenase

(Kaufman, 1966b). Enzyme activity is stimulated by the addition of dicarboxylic acids, such as fumaric acid (Fig. 11.).

Dopamine-β-hydroxylase was first isolated and characterized in 1960 (Levin, Levenberg and Kaufman, 1960) and, subsequently, purified to a single homogeneous protein (Friedman and Kaufman, 1965a).

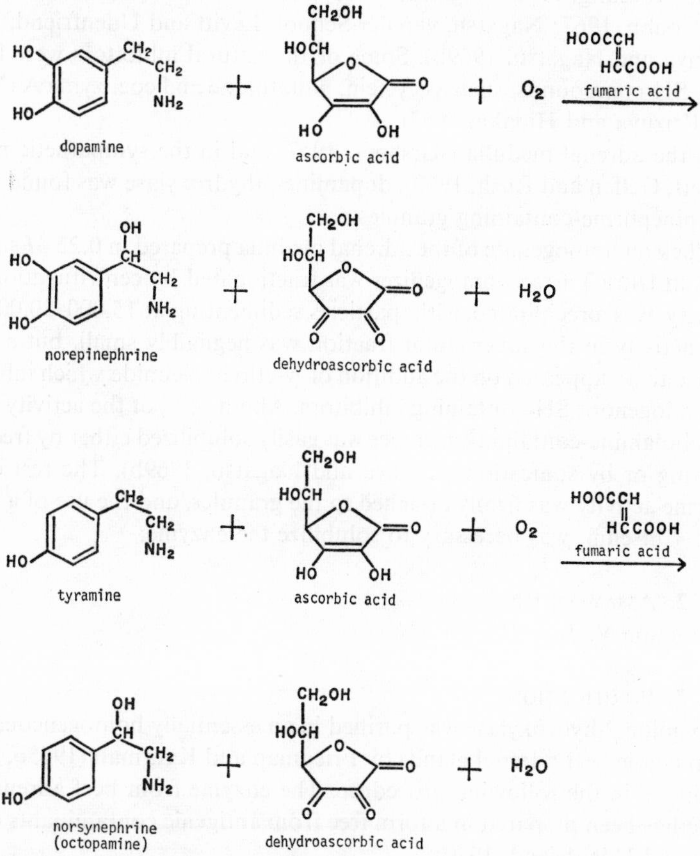

Fig. 11. Reaction of dopamine β-hydroxylase (Kaufman, 1966a).

I. 5. 1. TISSUE DISTRIBUTION

Dopamine-β-hydroxylase is an intraneuronal enzyme in the sympathetic nervous system and enzyme activity was found in the adrenal medulla (Levin, Levenberg and Kaufman, 1960), in the brain (Udenfriend and Creveling, 1959), and various sympathetically innervated organs such as the heart (Potter and Axelrod, 1963b; Nagatsu, van der Schoot, Levitt and Udenfriend, 1968). The enzyme activities of crude preparations from organs were very low because of the presence of endogenous inhibitors. The enzyme activity appeared after endogenous inhibitors were removed through a certain degree of purification (Levin, Levenberg and Kaufman, 1960; Creveling, 1962; Nagatsu, Kuzuya and Hidaka, 1967; Austin, Livett and Chubb, 1967; Nagatsu, van der Schoot, Levitt and Udenfriend, 1968; Kuzuya and Nagatsu, 1969b). Some of the natural inhibitors were found to be SH-compounds, such as cystein, glutathione and coenzyme A (Nagatsu, Kuzuya and Hidaka, 1967).

In the adrenal medulla (Kirshner, 1957) and in the sympathetic nerves (Livett, Geffen and Rush, 1969), dopamine-β-hydroxylase was found in the norepinephrine-containing granules.

When an homogenate of the adrenal medulla prepared in 0.25 M sucrose with an Ultra Turrax homogenizer was fractionated by centrifugation, the activity was precipitated with particles sedimenting at 15,000–20,000 × g. The activity in the supernatant fraction was negligibly small, but a fairly high activity appeared on the addition of N-ethylmaleimide which inhibited the endogenous SH-containing inhibitors. About 50% of the activity in the catecholamine-containing granules was easily solubilized either by freezing-thawing or by sonication (Kuzuya and Nagatsu, 1969b). The rest of the enzyme activity was firmly attached to the granules, and the use of a detergent, Cutscum, was necessary to solubilize the enzyme.

I. 5. 2. ASSAY METHOD
See section V. 3.

I. 5. 3. PURIFICATION
Dopamine-β-hydroxylase was purified in an essentially homogeneous form from whole beef adrenal glands by Friedman and Kaufman (1965b, 1971), as shown in the following procedure. The enzyme from beef adrenal medulla has been prepared in a form free from antigenic contaminants (Hartman and Udenfriend, 1970).

Purification was carried out at a temperature of 2–4°C and glass-distilled water was used throughout. Dialysis was performed for 3 hr against at least a 40-fold excess of the same buffer changed once. All buffers were prepared by diluting 1 M potassium phosphate buffer, pH 6.5, to desired concentrations.

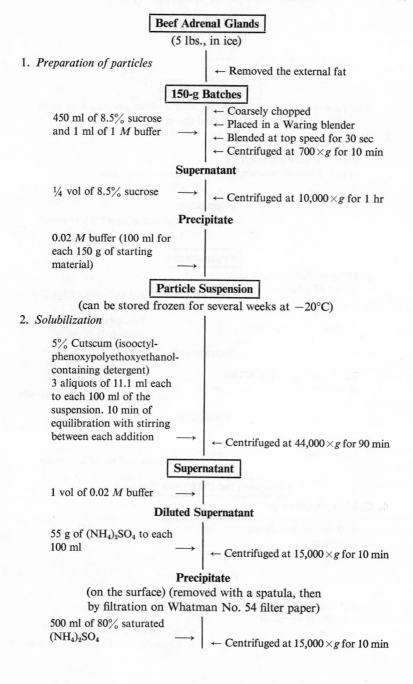

Beef Adrenal Glands
(5 lbs., in ice)

1. *Preparation of particles*

← Removed the external fat

150-g Batches

450 ml of 8.5% sucrose
and 1 ml of 1 M buffer   ⟶

← Coarsely chopped
← Placed in a Waring blender
← Blended at top speed for 30 sec
← Centrifuged at 700 × g for 10 min

Supernatant

¼ vol of 8.5% sucrose   ⟶

← Centrifuged at 10,000 × g for 1 hr

Precipitate

0.02 M buffer (100 ml for
each 150 g of starting
material)   ⟶

Particle Suspension
(can be stored frozen for several weeks at −20°C)

2. *Solubilization*

5% Cutscum (isooctyl-
phenoxypolyethoxyethanol-
containing detergent)
3 aliquots of 11.1 ml each
to each 100 ml of the
suspension. 10 min of
equilibration with stirring
between each addition   ⟶

← Centrifuged at 44,000 × g for 90 min

Supernatant

1 vol of 0.02 M buffer   ⟶

Diluted Supernatant

55 g of $(NH_4)_2SO_4$ to each
100 ml   ⟶

← Centrifuged at 15,000 × g for 10 min

Precipitate
(on the surface) (removed with a spatula, then
by filtration on Whatman No. 54 filter paper)

500 ml of 80% saturated
$(NH_4)_2SO_4$ ⟶

← Centrifuged at 15,000 × g for 10 min

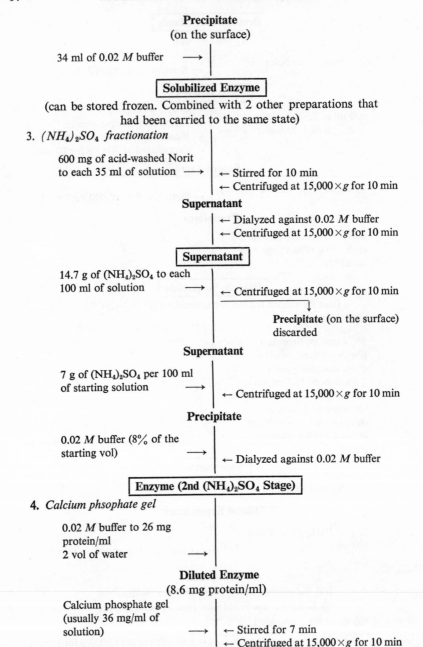

Precipitate
(on the surface)

34 ml of 0.02 M buffer $\longrightarrow$

Solubilized Enzyme

(can be stored frozen. Combined with 2 other preparations that had been carried to the same state)

3. *(NH₄)₂SO₄ fractionation*

600 mg of acid-washed Norit
to each 35 ml of solution $\longrightarrow$ ← Stirred for 10 min
     ← Centrifuged at 15,000 × g for 10 min

Supernatant

   ← Dialyzed against 0.02 M buffer
   ← Centrifuged at 15,000 × g for 10 min

Supernatant

14.7 g of (NH₄)₂SO₄ to each
100 ml of solution $\longrightarrow$ ← Centrifuged at 15,000 × g for 10 min

Precipitate (on the surface)
discarded

Supernatant

7 g of (NH₄)₂SO₄ per 100 ml
of starting solution $\longrightarrow$ ← Centrifuged at 15,000 × g for 10 min

Precipitate

0.02 M buffer (8% of the
starting vol) $\longrightarrow$ ← Dialyzed against 0.02 M buffer

Enzyme (2nd (NH₄)₂SO₄ Stage)

4. *Calcium phsophate gel*

0.02 M buffer to 26 mg
protein/ml
2 vol of water $\longrightarrow$

Diluted Enzyme
(8.6 mg protein/ml)

Calcium phosphate gel
(usually 36 mg/ml of
solution) $\longrightarrow$ ← Stirred for 7 min
     ← Centrifuged at 15,000 × g for 10 min

Gel Precipitate

Elution with 100 ml
of 0.02 M buffer $\longrightarrow$ $\leftarrow$ Centrifuged

Elution with 100 ml
of 0.05 M buffer $\longrightarrow$ $\leftarrow$ Centrifuged

Elution with 100 ml
of 0.10 M buffer $\longrightarrow$ $\leftarrow$ Centrifuged

Elution with 100 ml
of 0.20 M buffer $\longrightarrow$ $\leftarrow$ Centrifuged

The Active Eluate
(usually 0.05 and 0.10 M)

0.02 M buffer to 6–8 mg
protein/ml $\longrightarrow$

Enzyme (Calcium Phosphate Gel Eluate)

5. *Alcohol fractionation*

Ethanol ($-20°C$) to   15 ml $\longrightarrow$ $\leftarrow$ Centrifuged
each 100 ml of solution
Added successively   18 ml $\longrightarrow$ $\leftarrow$ Centrifuged
dropwise at $-5°C$

               84 ml $\longrightarrow$ $\leftarrow$ Centrifuged

               3 ml $\longrightarrow$ $\leftarrow$ Centrifuged

The Second (13-25% Ethanol) and Third
(25-54% Ethanol) Precipite

5 mM buffer 20–30 ml $\longrightarrow$ $\leftarrow$ Dialyzed overnight

6. *DEAE-cellulose*

DEAE-Cellulose Column
(equilibrated with 5 mM buffer, 1.05 ml of packed volume
per mg protein) (361 mg of protein to 3.4×42 cm column)

Three 10-ml portions
of buffer $\longrightarrow$

Gradient elution (three bottles
of equal diameter containing
equal columns of buffer
(0.005, 0.10 and 0.5 M)
connected in series) $\longrightarrow$ $\leftarrow$ Fraction volume, 7.3 ml
                                   Total eluate volume, 900 ml

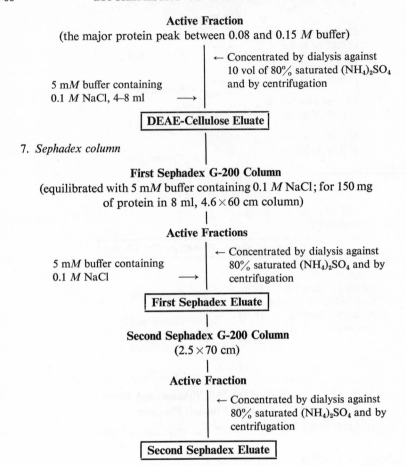

Active Fraction
(the major protein peak between 0.08 and 0.15 M buffer)

← Concentrated by dialysis against
10 vol of 80% saturated $(NH_4)_2SO_4$

5 mM buffer containing   and by centrifugation
0.1 M NaCl, 4–8 ml   ⟶

DEAE-Cellulose Eluate

7. Sephadex column

First Sephadex G-200 Column
(equilibrated with 5 mM buffer containing 0.1 M NaCl; for 150 mg
of protein in 8 ml, 4.6 × 60 cm column)

Active Fractions

← Concentrated by dialysis against
5 mM buffer containing   80% saturated $(NH_4)_2SO_4$ and by
0.1 M NaCl   ⟶   centrifugation

First Sephadex Eluate

Second Sephadex G-200 Column
(2.5 × 70 cm)

Active Fraction

← Concentrated by dialysis against
80% saturated $(NH_4)_2SO_4$ and by
centrifugation

Second Sephadex Eluate

The final enzyme preparation was stored as an ammonium sulfate precipitate. Before using, the precipitate was collected by centrifugation, dissolved in 0.02M buffer, and dialyzed overnight. When stored either as a precipitate or as a concentrated solution, the enzyme lost approximately 20% of its activity per month.

A simpler purification procedure for preparing a partially purified enzyme with a good yield was described by Goldstein, Lauber and Mc-Kereghan (1965) (see procedure A of their methods).

| Calcium Phosphate Gel Eluate |

(Levin, Levenberg and Kaufman, 1965)
Dialyzed and diluted to 0.5 mg protein/ml
20 ml

|

DEAE-Cellulose Column
equilibrated with 0.01 M phosphate buffer, pH 6.8 (2×10 cm)

Wash with 50 ml of
0.01 M buffer $\longrightarrow$

Elution with 0.05 M buffer
containing 0.2 M NaCl
(fraction size, 3 ml) $\longrightarrow$

The Active Fraction

$\leftarrow$ Dialyzed against 0.02 M buffer

DEAE-Cellulose Column
equilibrated with 0.01 M phosphate buffer, pH 6.8 (1×10 cm)

Wash with 10 ml of
0.02 M buffer $\longrightarrow$

Elution with 0.05 M buffer
containing 0.15 M NaCl
(fraction size, 1 ml) $\longrightarrow$

| The Active Fraction |

I. 5. 4. PROPERTIES

The enzyme purified from the bovine adrenal glands by the method of Friedman and Kaufman (1965) was a homogeneous protein as determined by electrophoresis on starch gel (pH 8.9 and 6.5) and by disk electrophoresis (pH 9.5). The enzyme had a $S_{20,w}$ of 8.93 and the molecular weight, determined by equilibrium-ultracentrifugal analysis, was 2.9×10^5. From both these values, it was calculated that the enzyme has a frictional ratio of about 2, which indicates that it is a relatively asymmetrical molecule.

No absorption existed in the visible region and the minimum ratio of absorption at 280 nm: 650 nm was about 200.

Although the amount of copper in the enzyme varied with the preparation and with the length of dialysis against copper-free buffer (16–18 hr), the purest enzyme contained 0.65 to 1 μg of copper per mg of protein (4–7 μmoles per mole). When a concentrated solution of the enzyme was made

1mM with respect to diethyldithiocarbamate, a yellow color developed rapidly. The spectrum of this complex in the visible region was essentially identical to that of the copper-diethyldithiocarbamate complex. Ninety-eight percent of the copper in the enzyme was removed by treatment with cyanide and ammonium sulfate. Only the addition of cupric ions to the cyanide-treated enzyme restored enzyme activity. As additional evidence in support of the idea that dopamine-β-hydroxylase is a copper protein, it was shown that carbon monoxide inhibits the enzyme and that this inhibition is not reversible in light.

The purified enzyme did not have detectable SH groups and it could oxidize ascorbate to dehydroascorbate either anaerobically or aerobically. About 1 μmole of ascorbate was oxidized per μmole of enzyme. The reduced form of the enzyme was formed during the reaction of ascorbate and the enzyme. This reduced enzyme intermediate hydroxylated, aerobically, approximately an equivalent amount of substrate in the absence of a reducing agent. The hydroxylase as isolated by the purification procedure of Friedman and Kaufman (1965b), was in an inactive, oxidized form that requires interaction with ascorbate before it is capable of hydroxylating the substrate. It was found that the protein-bound copper is the site of reduction and its role was studied by means of electron paramagnetic resonance techniques (Friedman and Kaufman, 1966). Most of the protein-bound Cu^{++} is reduced by treatment of the enzyme with ascorbate; a large part of the Cu^{++} in the reduced enzyme was reoxidized during the hydroxylation of the substrate. These results support the concept of a reduction-oxidation role for the protein-bound copper. Fumarate, an activator of dopamine-β-hydroxylase ($+30\%$ activation at $10^{-2}M$), appears to favor the oxidation of Cu^{+} to Cu^{++}. Based on these findings, Friedman and Kaufman (1966) presented the reaction mechanism of dopamine-β-hydroxylase as shown in Fig. 12. A kinetic study supported this hypothesis and the following ping-pong mechanism was proposed (Goldstein, Joh and Garvey III, 1968) (Fig. 13). It was proved that molecular O^{18} is incorporated into a substrate β-phenylethylamine-α-C^{14} to form β-phenylethanolamine containing O^{18}. When the reaction was carried out in a medium of H$_2$O^{18} with air as the gas phase, no O^{18} was found in the β-phenylethanolamine (Kaufman, Bridgers, Eisenberg and Friedman, 1962). Thus dopamine-β-hydroxylase was proved to be a monooxygenase.

In the presence of fumarate, the enzyme catalyzed the hydroxylation of 1,060 moles of dopamine per mole of enzyme per min at 25°C (Friedman and Kaufman, 1965a).

The K_m value based on ascorbate was $6 \times 10^{-4}M$ and maximal activity

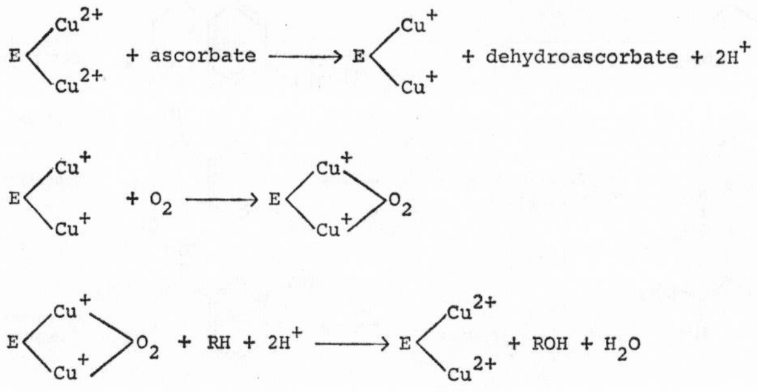

$$E\begin{matrix}Cu^{2+}\\Cu^{2+}\end{matrix} + \text{ascorbate} \longrightarrow E\begin{matrix}Cu^{+}\\Cu^{+}\end{matrix} + \text{dehydroascorbate} + 2H^{+}$$

$$E\begin{matrix}Cu^{+}\\Cu^{+}\end{matrix} + O_2 \longrightarrow E\begin{matrix}Cu^{+}\\Cu^{+}\end{matrix}O_2$$

$$E\begin{matrix}Cu^{+}\\Cu^{+}\end{matrix}O_2 + RH + 2H^{+} \longrightarrow E\begin{matrix}Cu^{2+}\\Cu^{2+}\end{matrix} + ROH + H_2O$$

Fig. 12. The reaction mechanism of dopamine-β-hydroxylase (Friedman and Kaufman, 1966).

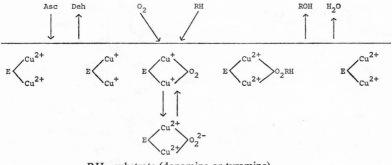

RH=substrate (dopamine or tyramine)
ROH=product (norepinephrine or octopamine)
Asc=ascorbate
Deh=dehydroascorbate

Fig. 13. Schematic presentation of the dopamine β-hydroxylase reaction (Goldstein, Joh and Garvey III, 1968).

was obtained at $9 \times 10^{-3}M$ (Levin, Levenberg and Kaufman, 1960). The K_m value based on dopamine was $6 \times 10^{-3}M$, and based on tyramine, $4 \times 10^{-4}M$ (Creveling, 1962).

The optimum pH for conversion of tyramine to norsynephrine was 5.5, and that for conversion of dopamine to norepinephrine was 6.2 (Creveling, Daly, Witkop and Udenfriend, 1962).

Dopamine-β-hydroxylase not only effects the hydroxylation of dopamine to norepinephrine, but accepts as substrates a wide variety of phenylethylamine derivatives (Creveling, Daly, Witkop and Udenfriend, 1962). The substrates and the products are shown in Fig. 14. Phenylethylamine, tyra-

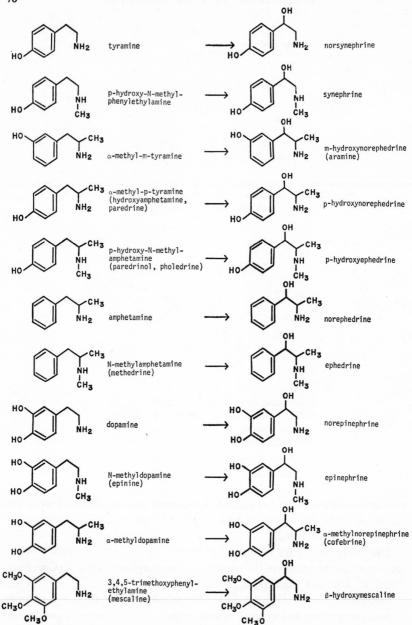

Fig. 14. Substrates and products of dopamine-β-hydroxylase (Creveling, Daly, Witkop and Udenfriend, 1962).

mine, dopamine or epinine was converted to phenylethanolamine, nor-synephrine, norepinephrine, or epinephrine, respectively (Creveling, Daly, Witkop and Udenfriend, 1962; Bridgers and Kaufman, 1962).

In the absence of ascorbic acid, the dopamine-β-hydroxylase catalyzed a dopamine-dependent oxidation of NADH or NADPH, as measured by a decrease in optical density at 340 nm. It was postulated that in the absence of ascorbic acid the catechol grouping of one dopamine molecule is ox-idized to an orthoquinone during hydroxylation of the side chain of an-other dopamine molecule. Thus the catechol grouping of 1 mole of the sub-strate serves as electron donor, forming an orthoquinone. NADH would readily react nonenzymatically with the quinone product, regenerating the substrate dopamine (Levin and Kaufman, 1961).

$$2 \text{ dopamine} + O_2 \xrightarrow{\text{enzymatic}} \text{norepinephrine} + \text{``dopamine-quinone''} + H_2O$$

$$\text{``dopamine-quinone''} + NADH + H^+ \xrightarrow{\text{nonenzymatic}} \text{dopamine} + NAD^+$$

$$\text{Sum:} \quad \text{dopamine} + O_2 + NADH + H^+ \longrightarrow \text{norepinephrine} + NAD^+ + H_2O$$

A similar mechanism was proposed for the hydroxylation of epinine to epinephrine in the absence of ascorbic acid (Bridgers and Kaufman, 1962). However, the enzyme-catalyzed oxidation of ascorbate was so rapid as to preclude any participation of the catechol grouping as a cofactor in side chain hydroxylation.

I. 5. 5. INHIBITORS

Substrate analogues, such as benzylhydrazine and benzyloxyamine were potent inhibitors (Creveling, van der Schoot and Udenfriend, 1962; Niko-dijevic, Creveling and Udenfriend, 1963; van der Schoot, Creveling, Naga-tsu and Udenfriend, 1963).

Copper-chelating agents such as diethyldithiocarbamate and alkylthio-

Phenylethylamine   X=NH: benzylhydrazine   Fusaric acid
                        X=O: benzyloxyamine

urea inhibited the enzyme *in vitro* and *in vivo*. These copper chelating agents reduced the endogenous level of tissue norepinephrine and increased that of tissue dopamine (Green, 1964; Jonsson, Grobecker and Gunne, 1967; Johnson, Boukma and Kim, 1969; 1970). Tropolone and other chelating agents were also inhibitory (Goldstein, Lauber and McKereghan, 1964). Disulfirum via its reduced metabolite diethyldithiocarbamate was an effective inhibitor of dopamine-β-hydroxylase *in vivo* (Goldstein, Anagnoste, Lauber and McKereghan, 1964; Goldstein and Nakajima, 1967).

Reserpine inhibited dopamine-β-hydroxylase by blocking the dopamine-uptake mechanism in the amine-storing granules where the enzyme is localized (Kirshner, 1962; Rutledge and Weiner, 1966; Stjärne, 1966b). However, β-hydroxylation of α-methyl-*m*-tyramine and α-methyldopamine took place despite the blockade of the storage mechanism by reserpine (Meisch, Carlsson and Waldeck, 1967). Dopamine itself was shown to exhibit two properties when administered *in vivo*; the release of norepinephrine from sympathetic tissue and the stimulation of its synthesis (Harrison, Levitt and Udenfriend, 1963).

Various SH compounds, such as cysteine, glutathione, and coenzyme A, inhibited the enzyme. The inhibition was found to be due to chelating action on the protein-bound copper. Cu^{++} partly reversed the inhibition. The inhibition of the enzyme by the endogenous inhibitors in the adrenal medulla and in the brain was completely reversed by the addition of *N*-ethylmaleimide, which is a SH-reacting agent. *N*-Ethylmaleimide itself did not affect the activity of the purified dopamine-β-hydroxylase. By the addition of *N*-ethylmaleimide to a crude enzyme preparation of adrenal medulla marked dopamine-β-hydroxylase activity was observed not only in the catecholamine-granules but also in the soluble fraction (Nagatsu, Kuzuya and Hidaka, 1967; Kuzuya and Nagatsu, 1969b). The addition of Cu^{++} or *p*-chloromercuribenzoate also activated the enzyme in the crude adrenal preparation (Duch, Viveros and Kirshner, 1968).

Fusaric acid (5-butylpicolinic acid) inhibited the enzyme by 50% at 10^{-7} *M in vitro* and showed a potent hypotensive action (Hidaka, Nagatsu, Takeya, Takeuchi, Suda, Kojiri, Matsuzaki and Umezawa, 1969). Picolinic acid and all 5-alkylpicolinic acids inhibited dopamine-β-hydroxylase reaction. The activities were dependent on the number of carbon atoms in the 5-alkyl group, and the 5-butyl and 5-pentyl compounds showed stronger inhibition than the others. By increasing the number of carbons in 5-alkyl group to four or five, the hypotensive effect became stronger, and the 5-butyl- and 5-pentylpicolinic acids showed stronger hypotensive effect than the 5-propionyl-, 5-ethyl- and 5-methylpicolinic acids. The inhibition of dopamine-β-hydroxylase by 5-alkylpicolinic acid was uncompetitive with the substrate tyramine but was competitive with the cofactor ascorbic acid. The chelation of 5-alkylpicolinic acid with copper in dopamine-β-hydroxylase seems to be its inhibitory mechanism (Suda, Takeuchi, Nagatsu, Matsuzaki, Matsumoto and Umezawa, 1969). Fusaric acid inhibited dopamine-β-hydroxylase *in vivo* and lowered endogenous levels of norepinephrine and epinephrine in the adrenal glands, the heart, the brain, and the spleen. Maximum depletion of norepinephrine and epinephrine was observed between 3 and 6 hr after the administration of fusaric acid (Nagatsu, Hidaka, Kuzuya, Takeya, Umezawa, Takeuchi and Suda, 1970),

I. 5. 6. PHYSIOLOGICAL ASPECTS
Although various phenylethylamine substrates can be converted to β-hydroxyderivatives, the main dopamine-β-hydroxylase reaction *in vivo* may be the conversion of dopamine to norepinephrine. It was once suggested that the hydroxylation of dopamine is the rate-limiting step in the formation of both norepinephrine and epinephrine (Blaschko, 1956). However, the activity per gram of tissue was sufficient to lead to the formation of all the epinephrine and norepinephrine known to be present in beef adrenal medulla within 0.25 min, even assuming no loss of enzyme during the purification procedure (Levin, Levenberg and Kaufman 1960). Tyrosine hydroxylase was established as the rate-limiting step of catecholamine biosynthesis (Levitt, Spector, Sjoerdsma and Udenfriend, 1965), however, a potent inhibitor of dopamine-β-hydroxylase *in vivo* would be able to reduce endogenous levels of norepinephrine, though the enzyme itself could not produce the rate-limiting step.

In guinea pig adrenals dopamine-β-hydroxylase activity was very low at birth but reached adult values within five days after birth. The enzyme activity was unaffected by even severe ascorbic acid deficiency (Nagatsu, van der Schoot, Levitt and Udenfriend, 1968). This eliminates the possibility of a specific role of ascorbic acid as a cofactor of dopamine-β-hydroxylase *in vivo*. Alternatively it may indicate that even a marked degree of ascorbic acid deficiency is not enough to make dopamine-β-hydroxylase rate-limiting in the overall conversion of tyrosine to norepinephrine. Rats that were fed a diet deficient in copper for 7–13 weeks showed a greatly decreased rate of conversion of parenterally administered C^{14}-dopamine to cardiac C^{14}-norepinephrine as compared with control animals (Missala, Lloyd, Gregoriads and Sourkes, 1967). During the acetylcholine-stimulated secretion of catecholamines in perfused isolated bovine adrenal glands, dopamine-β-hydroxylase was released into the perfusion fluid together with the catecholamines and a protein specifically found in the catecholamine storage vesicles (chromogranin) (Viveros, Arqueros and Kirshner, 1968). These results support the hypothesis that during secretion from the adrenal gland, the entire soluble content of the storage vesicle is discharged directly to the exterior of the cell (exocytosis, Douglas, 1968).

A specific and potent antibody to the dopamine-β-hydroxylase prepared from bovine adrenal medulla was produced in rabbits. The antibody markedly inhibited dopamine-β-hydroxylase from bovine, dog, guinea pig adrenals and human pheochromocytoma. The specificity of the antibody was demonstrated by the lack of inhibition of tyrosine hydroxylase and DOPA decarboxylase, the other two enzymes in the pathway of catecholamine biosynthesis (Gibb, Spector and Udenfriend, 1967; Hartman and Udenfriend, 1970). The dopamine-β-hydroxylase in the adrenal medulla was immunologically cross-reactive with that in sympathetic nerves. Various sympathetic nerves in the sheep, including fibers from the superior cervical and coeliac ganglia, were ligated and fluorescence antibody techniques were used to locate the enzyme. Immuno-sera of antigens of dopamine-β-hydroxylase from sheep adrenal medulla and of catecholamine-binding protein reacted strongly with the cytoplasm of cell bodies in the superior cervical and stellate ganglia and less strongly with sympathetic nerve fibres emanating from these ganglia. In constricted sympathetic nerves, there was a large increase in dopamine-β-hydroxylase and the catecholamine-binding protein fluorescence which was localized proximal to the constriction in the region where specific catecholamine fluorescence was also observed (Livett, Geffen and Rush, 1969). These results support the hypothesis that the site of synthesis of dopamine-β-hydroxylase is in the cell body and that it is transported to the axonal terminals by axoplasmic flow. To prove this hypothesis, the norepinephrine content and dopamine-β-hydroxylase activity were determined on both sides of a ligature in dog splenic nerves, and in the proximal segment of the nerve (above the ligation), there was an increase in the norepinephrine content and dopamine-β-hydroxylase activity (Laduron and Belpaire, 1968a).

I. 6.   Phenylethanolamine-N-methyltransferase (PNMT)

S-Adenosylmethionine: phenylethanolamine N-methyltransferase [EC 2. 1. 1]. Trivial name: Phenylethanolamine-N-methyltransferase.

The formation of epinephrine by N-methylation of norepinephrine was first proved after the incubation of homogenized adrenal tissue with norepinephrine and ATP added (Bülbring, 1949). It was subsequently found

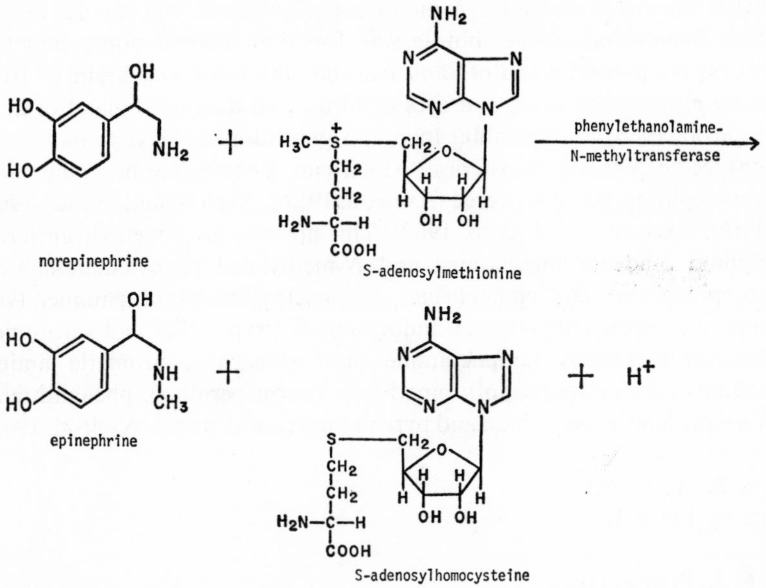

Fig. 15.   Reaction of phenylethanolamine N-methyltransferase (Axelrod, 1962b).

that the methyl group of methionine is incorporated into epinephrine (Keller, Boissonnas and du Vigneaud, 1950) and that the methyl donor for the N-methylation of norepinephrine is S-adenosylmethionine (Kirshner and Goodall, 1957b) (Fig. 15).

The enzyme that converts norepinephrine to epinephrine was partially purified and characterized in adrenal glands of monkeys (Axelrod, 1962b). The enzyme shows an absolute specificity towards phenylethanolamine derivatives including norepinephrine. Because of its substrate specificity, this enzyme was named phenylethanolamine-N-methyltransferase (Axelrod, 1962b). A review concerning this enzyme was published by Axelrod (1966, 1971b).

I. 6. 1. TISSUE DISTRIBUTION

Phenylethanolamine-N-methyltransferase was found in the soluble supernatant fraction of the adrenal medulla of rabbit, rat, monkey, cow, guinea pig and cat. A measurable amount of enzyme activity was found in rabbit heart, and in rabbit and rat brain (Axelrod, 1962b; McGeer, P. L. and McGeer, E. G., 1964; Ciaranello, Barchas, Byers, Stemmle and Barchas,

1969). Phenylethanolamine-*N*-methyltransferase was not found in any other mammalian tissue, but it was found in several nonmammalian tissues; the parotid gland of *Bufo marinus*, the heart and brain of frogs (*Rana pipiens*), the brain and eyes of birds, and the pineal gland of quail (Axelrod, 1966). In the rabbit lung and parotid gland of *Bufo marinus*, a nonspecific *N*-methyltransferase, which can *N*-methylate norepinephrine to epinephrine, was discovered (Axelrod, 1962c; Axelrod and Lerner, 1963; Märki, Axelrod and Witkop, 1962). This nonspecific *N*-methyltransferase required *S*-adenosylmethionine and *N*-methylated phenylethanolamines (norepinephrine and epinephrine), phenylethylamines (dopamine, tyramine, and phenylethylamine), indoleamines (tryptamine and serotonin), phenylpropylamines (amphetamine and ephedrine), aromatic amines (aniline and *p*-aminophenol), piperidines (normeperidine), phenanthrenes (normorphine, norcodeine), and pyrrolidines (nornicotine) (Axelrod, 1966).

I. 6. 2. ASSAY METHOD
See section VII. 4.

I. 6. 3. PURIFICATION
A partial purification from the monkey adrenal medulla was the first procedure described (Axelrod, 1962b) followed by the description of a homogeneous preparation obtained from the bovine adrenal medulla (Connett and Kirshner, 1970). The purification procedure by Connett and Kirshner (1970) is shown below in the form of a flow chart.

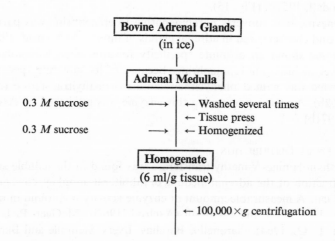

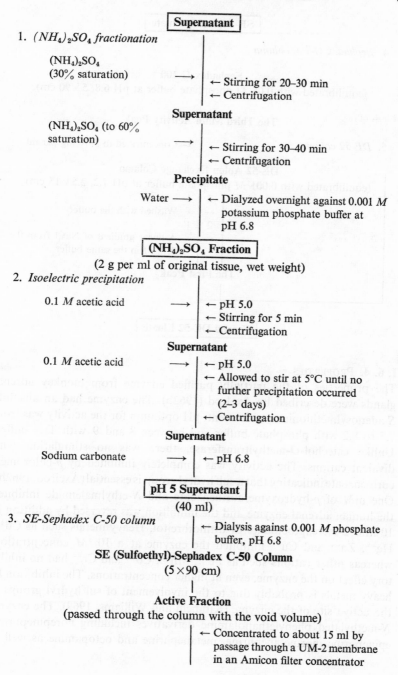

1. *(NH₄)₂SO₄ fractionation*

Supernatant

(NH₄)₂SO₄
(30% saturation) ⟶ ← Stirring for 20–30 min
← Centrifugation

Supernatant

(NH₄)₂SO₄ (to 60%
saturation) ⟶ ← Stirring for 30–40 min
← Centrifugation

Precipitate

Water ⟶ ← Dialyzed overnight against 0.001 M
potassium phosphate buffer at
pH 6.8

(NH₄)₂SO₄ Fraction

(2 g per ml of original tissue, wet weight)

2. *Isoelectric precipitation*

0.1 M acetic acid ⟶ ← pH 5.0
← Stirring for 5 min
← Centrifugation

Supernatant

0.1 M acetic acid ⟶ ← pH 5.0
← Allowed to stir at 5°C until no
further precipitation occurred
(2–3 days)
← Centrifugation

Supernatant

Sodium carbonate ⟶ ← pH 6.8

pH 5 Supernatant

(40 ml)

3. *SE-Sephadex C-50 column*
← Dialysis against 0.001 M phosphate
buffer, pH 6.8

SE (Sulfoethyl)-Sephadex C-50 Column
(5 × 90 cm)

Active Fraction

(passed through the column with the void volume)

← Concentrated to about 15 ml by
passage through a UM-2 membrane
in an Amicon filter concentrator

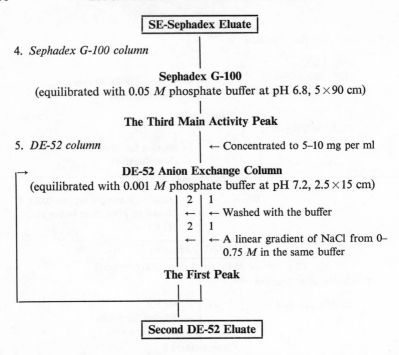

4. *Sephadex G-100 column*

Sephadex G-100
(equilibrated with 0.05 *M* phosphate buffer at pH 6.8, 5×90 cm)

The Third Main Activity Peak

5. *DE-52 column*   ← Concentrated to 5–10 mg per ml

DE-52 Anion Exchange Column
(equilibrated with 0.001 *M* phosphate buffer at pH 7.2, 2.5×15 cm)

2 | 1
← | ← Washed with the buffer
2 | 1
← | ← A linear gradient of NaCl from 0–
0.75 *M* in the same buffer

The First Peak

Second DE-52 Eluate

I. 6. 4. PROPERTIES

The properties of the partially purified enzyme from monkey adrenal glands were described by Axelrod (1962b). The enzyme had an absolute *S*-adenosylmethionine requirement. pH optimum for the activity was from 7.5 to 8.2 with phosphate buffer and between 8 and 9 with Tris buffer. Unlike catechol-*O*-methyltransferase, there was no stimulation with divalent cations. The activity was completely inhibited by *p*-chloromercuribenzoate indicating that a sulfhydryl group is essential (Axelrod, 1962b). One m*M* of *p*-hydroxymercuribenzoate and *N*-ethylmaleimide inhibited the human adrenal enzyme and the inhibition was reversed by addition of 10 m*M* 2-mercaptoethanol or dithiothreitol. Heavy metals such as Cd^{++}, Hg^{++}, Zn^{++} and Cu^{++} inhibited the enzyme at a $10^{-5}M$ concentration, whereas other cations such as Fe^{++}, Mn^{++}, Co^{++} and Cr^{++} had no inhibitory effect on the enzyme, even at higher concentrations. The inhibition by heavy metals is probably due to the involvement of sulfhydryl groups at the active site of the enzyme (Kitabchi and Williams, 1969). The enzyme *N*-methylated phenylethanolamine derivatives including norepinephrine, epinephrine, normetanephrine, metanephrine and octopamine as well as neo-synephrine and norephedrine. None of the phenylethylamine derivatives were N-methylated. Both dextro- and levo-phenylethanolamines were N-methylated but the levo-isomers were better substrates. The enzyme added an additional methyl group to secondary amines, such as epinephrine, metanephrine, and neo-synephrine. N-Methylepinephrine was found in the adrenal glands of cattle, rats, rabbits, and monkeys (Axelrod, 1960a). N-Methylmetanephrine which was found in urine was elevated in urine with pheochromocytoma (Itoh, Yoshinaga, Sato, Ishida and Wada, 1962). Substrate specificity was in the decreasing order: ($-$)-normetanephrine, ($\pm$)-phenylethanolamine, ($\pm$)-m-hydroxyphenylethanolamine, ($-$)-norepinephrine, ($\pm$)-octopamine, ($+$)-norepinephrine, ($-$)-norephedrine and ($-$)-epinephrine (Axelrod, 1966).

Details of the properties of the homogeneous enzyme preparation from beef adrenal medulla were reported by Connett and Kirshner (1970). The purified preparation was homogeneous as shown by chromatography on DE-52, disc electrophoresis and sucrose density gradient centrifugation. When the enzyme solution was concentrated, a precipitate which had no enzyme activity was formed. The maximum concentration which was stable in solution was about 2 mg per ml. The patterns observed in the ultracentrifuge showed an initial, fairly symmetrical peak which rapidly widened as it moved down the cell; the sedimentation coefficient was 3.0 S. The calculated S value of the sucrose density gradient was 2.98. An approximate molecular weight value of 38,000 was obtained by the sucrose density gradient method using hemoglobin as the reference protein.

Using Whittaker's data to plot a standard curve, a column (1.25 × 98 cm) of Sephadex G-100 equilibrated with 0.05 M phosphate buffer, pH 6.8, at 5°C, gave a molecular weight of 38,100. Using a column (1.25 × 98 cm) of Sephadex G-200 equilibrated with 0.05 M phosphate buffer, pH 6.8, at 5°C, a value of 28.05 A for the Stokes radius of the purified enzyme was obtained. From the Stokes radius of 28.05 A and the assumption $\bar{v} = 0.725$ ml/g, a molecular weight of 38,200 and a value of f/f_{min} of 1.21 were obtained. There was no indication of a cofactor requirement for the enzyme. A optimum pH of 7.9 was observed in either the phosphate or the borate buffer. The enzyme was shown to have two essential sulfhydryl groups and was stable at 39°, but unstable at 45°. Normetanephrine ($2.5 \times 10^{-3}M$) had no stabilizing effect, but S-adenosylmethionine ($1 \times 10^{-3}M$) established protection against heat denaturation. The enzyme was inhibited by norepinephrine at concentrations higher than approximately 25–50 μM. The degree of inhibition by excess norepinephrine was affected by the concentration of S-adenosylmethionine in the reaction mixture. In the presence of about 25–50 μM of norepinephrine, about 50 μM of S-adenosylmethionine gave nearly maximum velocity. With partially purified rabbit or bovine enzyme, excess ($\pm$)-normetanephrine also inhibited the activity, but at concentrations higher than 1 mM in the presence of 13.3 μM S-adenosylmethionine. In contrast, ($-$)-norepinephrine gave a maximum activity at about 30 μM, and ($+$)norepinephrine at about 300 μM. ($-$)-Norepinephrine was the most active substrate at low concentrations and had the lowest K_m value, indicating that ($-$)-norepinephrine is a natural substrate in the adrenal gland (Fuller and Hunt, 1965). The K_m for human adrenal phenylethanolamine-N-methyltransferase was also found to be lower for norepinephrine ($8 \times 10^{-5}M$) than normetanephrine ($2.5 \times 10^{-4}M$) or phenylethanolamine ($2.0 \times 10^{-3}M$) (Kitabchi and Williams, 1969). It is suggested that the enzyme operates by a random binding mechanism with a kinetically preferred order of binding in which S-adenosylmethionine is the first preferred substrate. It is also suggested that the enzyme would operate most efficiently under conditions of high S-adenosylmethionine concentration and low norepinephrine concentration (Connett and Kirshner, 1970). Various phenethylamine and phenethanolamine derivatives were inhibitors of the enzyme. Various amines related to transcypromine inhibited the enzyme competitively with normetanephrine (Krakoff and Axelrod, 1967).

Transcypromine

I. 6. 5. PHYSIOLOGICAL ASPECTS

Phenylethanolamine-N-methyltransferase activity was markedly depressed following hypophysectomy. Enzyme activity was restored to normal after administration of ACTH or a dexamethasone, potent glucocorticoid. Enzyme activity stimulation by glucocorticoids was blocked by the concurrent administration of puromycin or actinomycin D. Glucocorticoids did not stimulate the activity of other adrenal enzymes in catecholamine biosynthesis or metabolism, such as tyrosine hydroxylase, catechol-O-methyltransferase, or monoamine oxidase. It appears that glucocorticoids induced phenylethanolamine-N-methyltransferase by influencing effects at level of RNA transcription from DNA (Wurtman and Axelrod, 1965, 1966).

Phenylethanolamine-N-methyltransferase activity in the adrenals increased rapidly during the late fetal life in rats preceding epinephrine accumulation (Margolis, Roffi and Jost, 1966; Fuller and Hunt, 1967). The developmental increase in enzyme activity and the accumulation of epinephrine were prevented by fetal hypophysectomy (decapitation). Administration of adrenocorticotrophic hormone or cortisol acetate largely reversed the effect of fetal decapitation (Margolis, Roffi and Jost, 1966). The enzyme level showed a steady increase with age when expressed as activity per pair of adrenals. However when the enzyme levels were expressed as a concentration, i.e., per mg adrenal weight or mm^3 of adrenal medullary volume, a steady decline was noted over the 2-to-21-day age period. Since both adrenal weights and medullary volume increased in an almost identical manner, comparable values obtained from either expression (Philpott, Zarrow, Denenberg, Lu, Fuller and Hunt, 1969).

The repeated administration of low doses of glucocorticoids depressed the activity of phenylethanolamine-N-methyltransferase in the rat adrenal medulla and also decreased its epinephrine content. This inhibition could be blocked by the concurrent administration of small amounts of ACTH. Larger doses, on the other hand, did not depress enzyme activity and the epinephrine content in the adrenal medulla, even though they caused even greater atrophy of the adrenal (Wurtman, Noble and Axelrod, 1967). Destruction of sympathetic nerve terminals with 6-hydroxydopamine produced a small (19%) but statistically significant increase in adrenal phenylethanolamine-N-methyltransferase activity in normal and hypophysectomized rats. This increase was abolished by transection of the splenic nerves supplying the adrenal glands. The restitution of the enzyme activity by dexamethasone in hypophysectomized animals was not affected by adrenal denervation. Based on these results, Thoenen, Mueller and Axelrod (1970 b) concluded that the normal levels of the enzyme in the adrenal medulla are maintained by adrenocortical glucocorticoids whereas an increase above the normal level can be produced by a (reflex) increase in splanchnic nerve activity.

I. 7. Side Biosynthetic Pathway of Catecholamines

It is well established that the main pathway of catecholamine biosynthesis is: tyrosine → DOPA → dopamine → norepinephrine → epinephrine. However, since the substrate specificities of catecholamine-synthesizing enzymes are low, except for the first enzyme, tyrosine hydroxylase, various alternate side pathways of catecholamine biosynthesis are probable, as

shown in Fig. 16. Various intermediates in these side pathways were discovered. Octopamine (norsynephrine) was discovered in urine (Kakimoto
and Armstrong, 1962a).

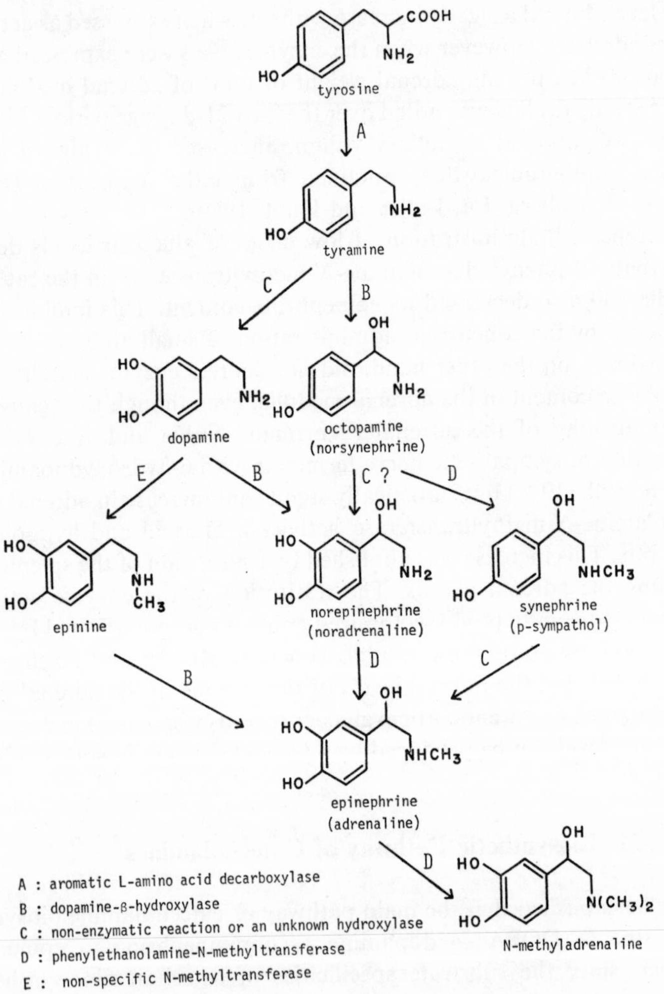

A : aromatic L-amino acid decarboxylase
B : dopamine-β-hydroxylase
C : non-enzymatic reaction or an unknown hydroxylase
D : phenylethanolamine-N-methyltransferase
E : non-specific N-methyltransferase

Fig. 16.   Alternate side pathway for catecholamine biosynthesis (Axelrod,
1963a).

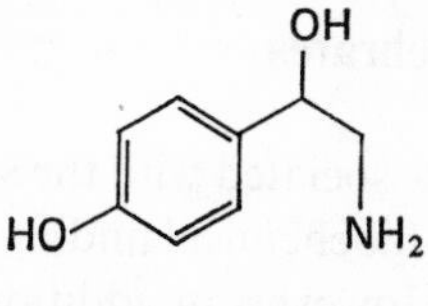

Octopamine (norsynephrine)

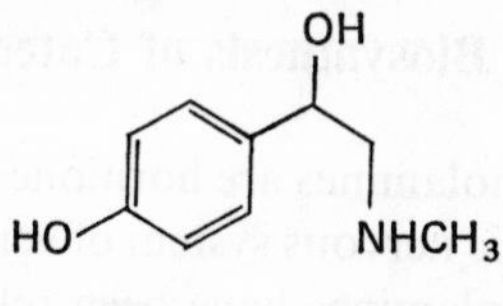

Synephrine (p-sympathol)

Synephrine was also discovered in human urine (Pisano, Oates, Karmen, Sjoerdsma and Udenfriend, 1961). Epinine, together with dopamine, norepinephrine and epinephrine, was discovered either in excised parotid gland of the South American toad (*Bufo marinus*) and in the secretions obtained by pressing the glands of live animals (Märki, Axelrod and Witkop, 1962). N-Methyladrenaline was detected as a normal metabolite of the adrenal gland of monkey, rat, rabbit, guinea pig and beef (Axelrod, 1960a). When tyramine-2-C^{14} or octopamine-7-H^3 was given to rats, radioactive norepinephrine and normetanephrine were highly labeled, but adrenal catecholamines were not labeled (Creveling, Levitt and Udenfriend, 1962). The results suggest that tyramine may be converted to norepinephrine via octopamine, or possibly via dopamine. The physiological significance of this side path-

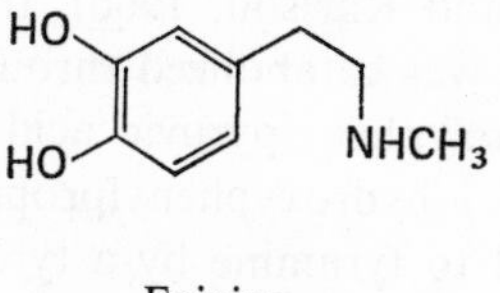

Epinine

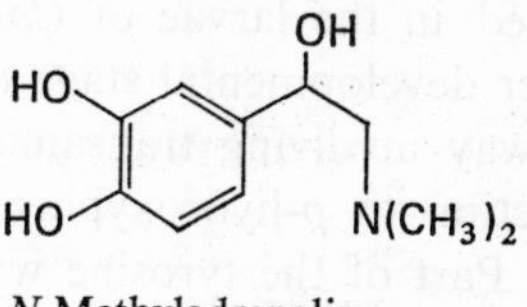

N-Methyladrenaline

way is not clear, but it may be highly significant in evaluating the pharmacological actions of tyramine (Creveling, Levitt and Udenfriend, 1962). An enzyme that forms epinephrine from p- and m-synephrine (sympathol) and dopamine from p- and m-tyramine was found in the microsomes of rabbit liver. The enzyme required the reduced form of NADP and was a nonspecific hydroxylase and formed catechols from the following normally occurring and foreign phenols: p- and m-octopamine, p-hydroxyephedrine, phenol, stilbestrol, N-acetyl-p-aminophenol, estradiol and N-acetylserotonin (Axelrod, 1963a). When p-octopamine was incubated with the catechol-forming enzyme, a small quantity of an unknown catechol compound was formed, but it was different from norepinephrine. From m-octopamine, a small amount of norepinephrine was formed (Axelrod, 1963a).

I. 8.   Biosynthesis of Catecholamines in Invertebrates

Catecholamines are hormones which are normally associated with the sympathetic nervous system of vertebrates. Most of the biochemical findings on catecholamines have been related to vertebrates. However, in addition to all being found in vertebrate groups, catecholamines have also been found in invertebrates, such as insects. Dopamine, norepinephrine and epinephrine were identified in the meal worm, *Tenebrio mollitor*; larvae and adult insects showed higher concentrations than the pupae (Oestlund, 1954). *N*-Acetyldopamine was found in the blowfly, *Calliphora erythrocephala* (Karlson, Sekeris and Sekeri, 1962) and is responsible for the tanning (darkening and hardening) of the cuticle. *N*-Acetyldopaminequinone was formed from *N*-acetyldopamine by the oxidation with a phenoloxidase present in the cuticle (Sekeris and Karlson, 1966).

Catecholamines and catecholamine derivatives were found in different insect species, among them, *Calliphora erythrocephala*, *Tenebrio mollitor*, *Drosophila melanogaster* and *Schistocerca gregaria*. Tyramine, *N*-acetyltyramine and, very probably, the *O*-glucoside of *N*-acetyltyramine were detected (Sekeris and Karlson, 1966).

The biosynthetic pathway of *N*-acetyldopamine from tyrosine was examined in the larvae of *Calliphora* (Sekeris and Karlson, 1966). In the earlier developmental stage of larvae tyrosine was catabolized through a pathway involving transamination to *p*-hydroxyphenylpyruvic acid and reduction to *p*-hydroxyphenyllactic acid and *p*-hydroxyphenylpropionic acid. Part of the tyrosine was decarboxylated to tyramine by a tyrosine decarboxylase and then acetylated to *N*-acetyltyramine (Fig. 17). Tyramine was also hydroxylated to dopamine as the larvae entered their third and last stage. In larvae of the late third instar (an insect in any one of its periods of postembryonic growth between molts), tyrosine was mainly hydroxylated to DOPA, which was further decarboxylated by a DOPA decarboxylase to dopamine. Most of the dopamine was acetylated to *N*-acetyldopamine. *N*-Acetyldopamine was incorporated into the cuticle and used in the sclerotization process or stored as *N*-acetyldopamine-4-*O*-glucoside. A small part of the dopamine was oxidatively deaminated to dihydroxyphenylacetic acid. Part of the dopamine served as precursor to norepinephrine and epinephrine.

Tyrosine hydroxylation reaction in the blowfly (*Calliphora erythrocephala*) was catalyzed by a phenoloxidase showing monophenoloxidase as well as diphenoloxidase activity (Karlson, Mergenhagen and Sekeris,

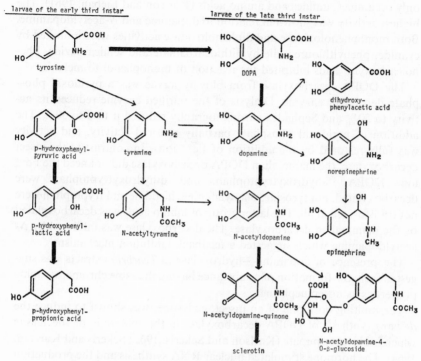

Fig. 17. Biosynthesis and metabolism of catecholamines in *Calliphora*
(Sekeris and Karlson, 1966).

1964; Sekeris and Mergenhagen, 1964). It is thus distinct from the mammalian tyrosine hydroxylase which requires a tetrahydropterin and ferrous ion and catalyzes only the step leading from tyrosine to DOPA (Nagatsu, Levitt and Udenfriend, 1964b). The phenoloxidase existed as an inactive soluble enzyme precursor. It was transformed to the active enzyme by an activator protein (Karlson and Schweiger, 1961). In whole *Calliphora* larvae homogenates, the enzyme was partly soluble but mostly bound to mitochondria and microsomes. It showed high monophenoloxidase and diphenoloxidase activity. A highly purified enzyme was activated with a highly purified activator preparation *in vitro*. The enzyme, so prepared, was soluble and showed only diphenoloxidase activity. If the activation process took place in the presence of fat body mitochondria, a part of the activated enzyme was adsorbed on the mitochondria. Such preparations showed both monophenoloxidase and diphenoloxidase activities. The enzyme acted only on amines, amides and amino acids (Karlson and Liebau, 1961). The highest activity was shown in relation to dopamine and N-acetyldopamine. Both monophenoloxidase and diphenoloxidase activities were inhibited by cyanide, phenylthiourea, diethyldithiocarbamate and semicarbazide. Phenolcarboxylic acids inhibited the reaction of monophenol to melanin.

The DOPA-decarboxylase from blowfly larvae was a pyridoxal phosphate dependent enzyme. Dialysis of the purified enzyme reduced its activity to 50% and Sephadex chromatography reduced it to 0 to 30%. The addition of pyridoxal phosphate partially restored activity, and activity was fully restored by the addition of Fe^{++} ions. In contrast to the insect decarboxylase, the mammalian DOPA decarboxylase did not need the Fe^{++} ion. DOPA, 5-hydroxytryptophan, and dihydroxytryptophan were decarboxylated, but tyrosine, phenylalanine, histidine and tryptophan were not transformed at all. The latter group of amino acids was decarboxylated by the mammalian decarboxylase. The decarboxylase was inhibited by N-acetyldopamine which suggested a feedback inhibition mechanism.

The presence of dopamine-β-hydroxylase in *Tenebrio* extracts was suggested from the formation of a substance having the same chromatographic properties as norepinephrine.

The molting hormone of an insect, ecdysone, was shown to induce the *de novo* synthesis of DOPA decarboxylase in the epidermis of the larvae which is about to pupate (Karlson and Sekeris, 1962; Sekeris and Karlson, 1964). The hormone stimulated nuclear RNA synthesis and the production of a specific messenger RNA controlling the formation of the DOPA decarboxylase.

Phenolcarboxylic acids can regulate the biosynthesis of catecholamines by inhibiting the tyrosine hydroxylation by phenoloxidase. Such acids, products of the catabolic pathway of tyrosine, were found mainly in early stage larvae at a time when the phenoloxidase activity was low. The switching off of tyrosine metabolism from catabolism to decarboxylation by ecdysone led to a decrease in the concentration of carboxylic acids. As a consequence, monophenoloxidase and diphenoloxidase activity of the phenyloxyl oxidase system were enhanced. Catecholamine biosynthesis is also regulated by the feedback inhibition of DOPA decarboxylase by N-acetyldopamine (Sekeris and Karlson, 1966).

Transacetylase, which catalyzes the transfer of acetyl from acetyl-CoA to dopamine as well as tyramine and histamine, was detected in different insect species such as *Calliphora, Tenebrio, Drosophila* and *Schistocerca* (Karlson and Ammon, 1963). The enzyme was detected also in mammalian liver and adrenals (Sekeris and Herrlich, 1964).

I. 9. Biosynthesis of Catecholamines in Plants

The presence of dopamine and norepinephrine in banana tissues was reported by Waalkes, Sjoerdsma, Creveling, Weissbach and Udenfriend (1958), and Udenfriend, Lovenberg and Sjoerdsma (1959). Concerning the enzymes related to the biosynthesis of catecholamines in the banana plant, the presence of a dopamine-β-hydroxylase was reported by Smith and Kirshner (1960, 1962). The properties of the dopamine-β-hydroxylase in banana tissues were different from those of the mammalian enzymes (Levin, Levenberg and Kaufman, 1960; Friedman and Kaufman, 1965a). A partially purified dopamine-β-hydroxylase required only oxygen for activity. No cofactor requirements for the banana enzyme were demonstrated. Biological and fluorometric assays of the norepinephrine produced indicated that the product is a racemic mixture (Smith and Kirshner, 1960). The enzymatic hydroxylation of tyrosine to DOPA in the mammalian sympathetic tissue and in the adrenal medulla is catalyzed by tyrosine hydroxylase which requires a tetrahydropterin as a cofactor (Nagatsu, Levitt and Udenfriend, 1964b). In contrast, the enzymatic tyrosine hydroxylation in banana tissues was catalyzed by a phenoloxidase showing monophenoloxidase as well as diphenoloxidase activity (Nagatsu, I., Sudo and Nagatsu, T., 1972). The banana phenoloxidase was predominantly distributed in the pulp, in contrast to the predominant localization of catecholamines in the peel. The tyrosine hydroxylase activity was found in the soluble fraction and in the particulate fraction. Either L- or D-tyrosine was hydroxylated to DOPA. Formation of DOPA from tyrosine by the banana enzyme was inhibited by diethyldithiocarbamate but not by α,α'-dipyridyl, and it was markedly stimulated by the addition of ascorbate. The banana tyrosine hydroxylase is thus distinct from the mammalian tyrosine hydroxylase which catalyzes only the step leading from L-tyrosine to DOPA and requires a tetrahydropterin and Fe^{++}.

I. 10. Biosynthesis of Catecholamines in Microorganisms

Norepinephrine was isolated from the flagellated protozoan, *Crithidia fasciculate* (0.1–0.2 μg/g wet weight). Epinephrine was not detected. The ciliated protozoan, *Tetrahymena pyriformis*, synthesized norepinephrine (0.25–0.35 μg/g) as well as epinephrine (0.13–0.15 μg/g). DOPA and dopamine were not detected in *Crithidia* and *Tetrahymena* even when DOPA was used as substrate. L-Phenylalanine-C^{14}, L-tyrosine-C^{14} and DL-DOPA-

2-C^{14} were significantly incorporated into the catecholamines in *Tetrahymena*, while only tyrosine and DOPA were incorporated in *Crithidia*, owing to its lack of a phenylalanine hydroxylating system (Janakidevi, Dewey and Kidder, 1966). From the incubation mixture containing a cell-free extract of *Crithidia* with 20 μg of norepinephrine and 20 μg of epinephrine, normetanephrine and 3-methoxy-4-hydroxymandelic acid were identified by paper chromatography (Janakidevi, Dewey and Kidder, 1966).

Chapter II

Metabolism of Catecholamines

Catecholamines are inactivated mainly by catechol-O-methyltransferase (Axelrod, 1957) and monoamine oxidase (Blaschko, Richter and Schlossmann, 1937a). The complete elucidation of the metabolic pathway of catecholamines became possible (Axelrod, 1959) after the discovery of metabolites with a 3-methoxy-4-hydroxyphenyl (vanil) group, such as 3-methoxy-4-hydroxymandelic acid (vanillylmandelic acid) (Armstrong, McMillan and Shaw, 1957), metanephrine, and normetanephrine, and subsequently catechol-O-methyltransferase (Axelrod, 1957).

The main metabolic pathway of catecholamines is shown in Fig. 18. General tyrosine metabolism in relation to catecholamine metabolism is shown in Fig. 19.

II. 1. Metabolic Pathway of Catecholamines

II. 1. 1. METABOLIC PATHWAY OF DOPAMINE

When dopamine-C^{14} was administered to rats (Goldstein, Friedhoff and Simmonds, 1959; Williams, Babuscio and Watson, 1960), 80 % of the dopamine was oxidatively deaminated to 3,4-dihydroxyphenylacetic acid (homoprotocatechuic acid) by monoamine oxidase and 20 % was O-methylated to 3-methoxytyramine (Axelrod, Senoh and Witkop, 1958) by catechol-O-methyltransferase. After the administration of dopamine, 3,4-dihydroxyphenylacetic acid was also O-methylated to 3-methoxy-4-hydroxyphenylacetic acid (homovanillic acid) (De Eds, Booth, Jones, 1957; Goldstein, Friedhoff, Pomerantz and Simmons, 1960) and 3-methoxy-4-hydroxyphenylethanol was also found (Goldstein, Friedhoff, Pomerantz and Simmons, 1960).

6-Hydroxydopamine(3,4,6-trihydroxyphenylethylamine) was formed from dopamine nonenzymatically by air and light (Senoh, Witkop, Creveling and Udenfriend, 1959; Senoh and Witkop, 1959) but it could not be separated from norepinephrine by paper chromatography. The separation was achieved after norepinephrine was converted to β-O-methylnorepinephrine by treatment with methanol-HCl. 6-Hydroxydopamine was prepared by Udenfriend's ascorbate-iron-EDTA system (Udenfriend, Clark, Axelrod and Brodie, 1954). In contrast, enzymatic hydroxylation of dopamine by dopamine-β-hydroxylase was shown to give only norepine-

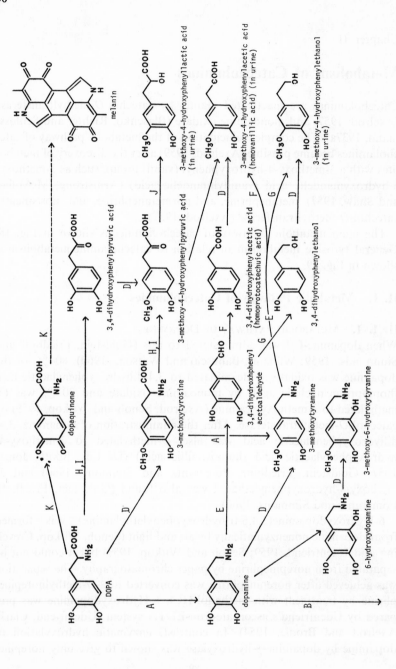

91

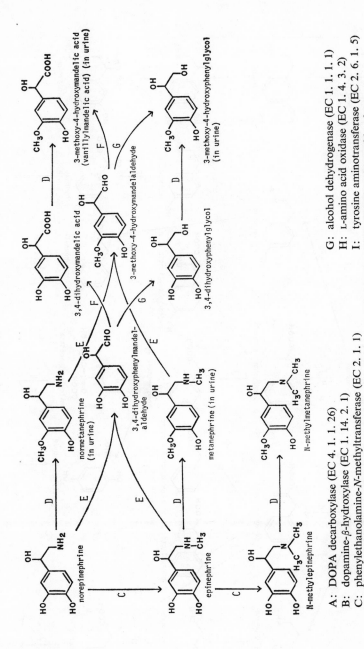

Fig. 18. Metabolism of catecholamines in higher animals.

A: DOPA decarboxylase (EC 4. 1. 1. 26)
B: dopamine-β-hydroxylase (EC 1. 14. 2. 1)
C: phenylethanolamine-*N*-methyltransferase (EC 2. 1. 1)
D: catechol-*O*-methyltransferase (EC 2. 1. 1. 6)
E: monoamine oxidase (EC 1. 4. 3. 4)
F: aldehyde oxidase (EC 1. 2. 3. 1)

G: alcohol dehydrogenase (EC 1. 1. 1. 1)
H: L-amino acid oxidase (EC 1. 4. 3. 2)
I: tyrosine aminotransferase (EC 2. 6. 1. 5)
J: aromatic α-ketoacid reductase
K: *o*-diphenol oxidase (EC 1. 10. 3. 1)

92

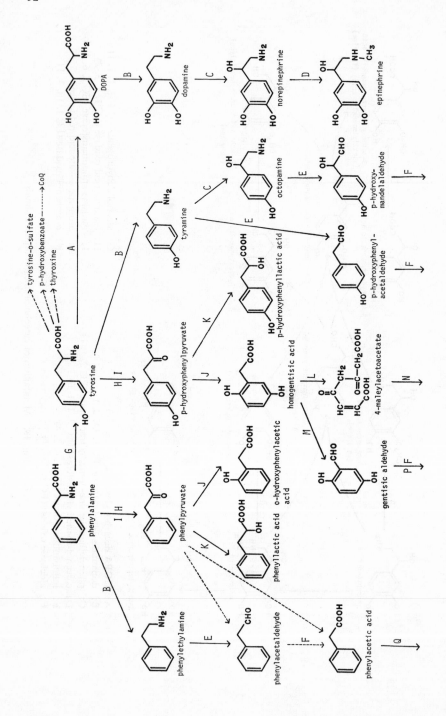

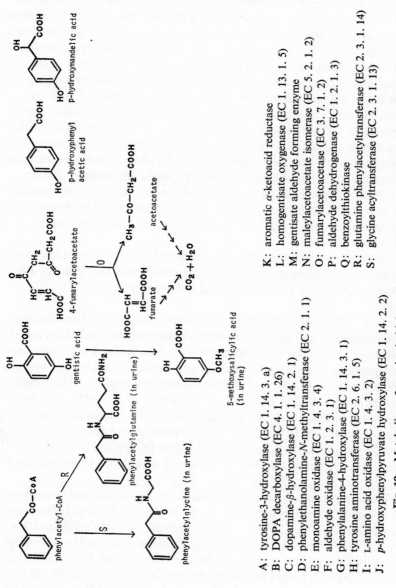

A: tyrosine-3-hydroxylase (EC 1. 14. 3. a)
B: DOPA decarboxylase (EC 4. 1. 1. 26)
C: dopamine-β-hydroxylase (EC 1. 14. 2. 1)
D: phenylethanolamine-N-methyltransferase (EC 2. 1. 1)
E: monoamine oxidase (EC 1. 4. 3. 4)
F: aldehyde oxidase (EC 1. 2. 3. 1)
G: phenylalanine-4-hydroxylase (EC 1. 14. 3. 1)
H: tyrosine aminotransferase (EC 2. 6. 1. 5)
I: L-amino acid oxidase (EC 1. 4. 3. 2)
J: p-hydroxyphenylpyruvate hydroxylase (EC 1. 14. 2. 2)

K: aromatic α-ketoacid reductase
L: homogentisate oxygenase (EC 1. 13. 1. 5)
M: gentisate aldehyde forming enzyme
N: maleylacetoacetate isomerase (EC 5. 2. 1. 2)
O: fumarylacetoacetase (EC 3. 7. 1. 2)
P: aldehyde dehydrogenase (EC 1. 2. 1. 3)
Q: benzoylthiokinase
R: glutamine phenylacetyltransferase (EC 2. 3. 1. 14)
S: glycine acyltransferase (EC 2. 3. 1. 13)

Fig. 19. Metabolism of tyrosine in higher animals in relation to catecholamine metabolism.

phrine by using dopamine-β,β-H^3 and dopamine-α-C^{14} as substrate (Senoh, Creveling, Udenfriend and Witkop, 1959). When dopamine-α-C^{14} was administered to rats, an appreciable fraction was found to be excreted as 6-hydroxydopamine in the urine (Senoh, Creveling, Udenfriend and Witkop, 1959). It remains to be seen whether 6-hydroxydopamine is formed endogenously, but acetylation, paper chromatography, and a differential fluorometric assay of ethylenediamine condensation products did not detect 6-hydroxydopamine in mice hearts at a level of 0.04 μg/g of tissue (Laverty, Sharman and Vogt, 1965). 6-Hydroxydopamine was O-methylated to 3-O-methyl-6-hydroxydopamine with catechol-O-methyltransferase and used for metabolic studies in the rat. The corresponding phenylacetic and mandelic acids as well as the phenylglycol were identified as metabolites (Daly, Benigni, Minnis, Kanaoka and Witkop, 1965).

6-Hydroxydopamine was shown to cause "chemical sympathectomy" by being taken up by the sympathetic nerve terminal and by degenerating the intraneuronal storage site of norepinephrine (Haeusler, Haefely and Thoenen, 1969).

3,4-Dimethoxyphenylethylamine was reported to be excreted into urine, especially in schizophrenic patients (Friedhoff and van Winkle, 1962), however, this could not be confirmed in later experiments.

II. 1. 2. METABOLIC PATHWAY OF NOREPINEPHRINE AND EPINEPHRINE
Norepinephrine and epinephrine have similar metabolic pathways and the following substances were discovered as metabolites from both: normetanephrine (3-methoxynorepinephrine), metanephrine (3-methoxyepinephrine) (Axelrod, 1957), 3-methoxy-4-hydroxymandelic acid (vanilylmandelic acid, VMA) (Armstrong, Shaw and Wall, 1956; Armstrong, McMillan and Shaw, 1957), 3-methoxy-4-hydroxyphenylglycol (Axelrod, Kopin and Mann, 1959), 3,4-dihydroxymandelic acid (Kirshner, Goodall and Rosen, 1958), 3,4-dihydroxyphenylglycol (Kopin and Axelrod, 1960b), N-methylepinephrine (Axelrod, 1960a), and N-methylmetanephrine (Itoh, Yoshinaga, Sato, Ishida and Wada, 1962).

Tracer experiments were carried out in rats using radioactive norepinephrine and epinephrine (Axelrod, Inscoe, Senoh and Witkop, 1958; Kopin, Axelrod and Gordon, 1961), in cats (Axelrod, Weil-Malherbe and Tomchick, 1959; Whitby, Axelrod and Weil-Malherbe, 1961), and in man (Kirshner, Goodall and Rosen, 1958; LaBrosse, Axelrod and Kety, 1958; LarBrosse, Axelrod, Kopin and Kety, 1961) to establish details of the main metabolic pathway of catecholamines (Axelrod, 1959, 1963b, 1965; Daly and Witkop, 1963). However, two points should be noted in the interpretation of the results on the metabolism of radioactive catecholamines. First, the metabolism of exogenously administered catecholamines is different from that of endogenously released catecholamines. Secondly, the metabolism of catecholamines differs according to the animal species.

($\pm$)-Epinephrine-7-H³ (0.3 μg/kg/min and 0.18 μg/kg/min) was administered to a young man by means of intravenous infusion for 30 min, and a 54-hr urine sample was collected for catecholamine metabolites analysis. Results showed that 92.6 % of the administered radioactivity was excreted into the urine, 97 % of the urinary radioactivity was due to epinephrine metabolites, and only 6.8 % of the radioactivity was unchanged epinephrine. More than 80 % of the radioactivity was due to the O-methylated metabolites of epinephrine with catechol-O-methyltransferase. The metabolites were: free metanephrine, 5.2 %; metanephrine glucuronide, 6.0 %; metanephrine sulfate, 29.5 %; 3-methoxy-4-hydroxymandelic acid, 42.4 %; and 3-methoxy-4-hydroxyphenylglycol, 7.1 %. Catechol metabolites were less than 20 %: free dihydroxymandelic acid, 0.7 %; and the conjugated form of dihydroxymandelic acid, 0.9 %. These results showed that the main type of metabolism of epinephrine in the blood is O-methylation with catechol O-methyltransferase. Since catechol-O-methyltransferase is abundant in the liver, circulating catecholamines may be O-methylated in the liver (LaBrosse, Axelrod, Kopin and Kety, 1961). The results are shown in Fig. 20. A general method of determining the relative magnitudes of different pathways of formation of a urinary metabolite from a single precursor substance was used in studying the alternate metabolic pathway of epinephrine in man (Kopin, 1960). The method requires the administration of the precursor and an intermediate labeled with different isotopes, and the determination of the radioactivity of the isotopes in the metabolites. ($-$)-Epinephrine-7-H³ (38.4 μCi) and ($-$)-metanephrine-methoxy-C¹⁴ (4.58 μCi) were used. As shown in Fig. 20, approximately 70 % of the epinephrine in the blood was O-methylated to metanephrine with catechol-O-methyltransferase, and approximately 20 % was deaminated to either 3,4-dihydroxymandelic acid or 3,4-dihydroxyphenylglycol via 3,4-dihydroxymandelaldehyde with monoamine oxidase. Approximately half of the metanephrine was excreted into urine either in a free form or as conjugates of sulfate or glucuronide. The other half was deaminated with monoamine oxidase either to 3-methoxy-4-hydroxyphenylglycol or to 3-methoxy-4-hydroxymandelic acid via 3-methoxy-4-hydroxymandelaldehyde. Most of dihydroxymandelic acid or dihydroxyphenylglycol was O-methylated to 3-methoxy-4-hydroxymandelic acid or 3-methoxy-4-hydroxyphenylglycol with catechol-O-methyltransferase.

96

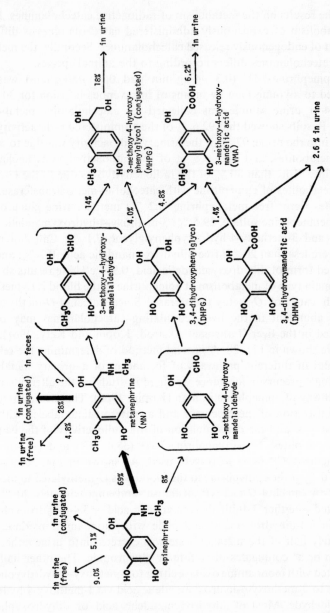

Fig. 20. Metabolism of epinephrine in man (Kopin, 1960; LaBrosse, Axelrod, Kopin and Kety, 1961).

Almost as great a quantity of 3-methoxy-4-hydroxyphenylglycol was excreted in normal human urine as 3-methoxy-4-hydroxymandelic acid (Ruthven and Sandler, 1965; Karoum, Anah, Ruthven and Sandler, 1969). The corresponding alcoholic metabolite of dopamine, 3-methoxy-4-hydroxyphenylethanol, was excreted into urine in a relatively minute concentration (Sandler, 1970). In man, the intermediate aldehyde derived from the oxidative deamination of a phenylethanolamine tends to follow a reductive pathway whereas the aldehyde stemming from a phenylethylamine is predominantly oxidized to its corresponding acid (Sandler, 1970; Breese, Chase and Kopin, 1968).

After intrajugular infusion of $(\pm)$-epinephrine-7-H^3 bitartrate, 10 % of the injected tritium was found in the bile and 72 % in the urine. After intraportal infusion, 31 % was found in the bile and 42 % in the urine. Only metanephrine glucuronide and 3-methoxy-4-hydroxyphenylglycol sulfate were found in the bile. Intestinal reabsorption of epinephrine metabolites was found to be only 13 % and enterohepatic circulation amounted to only 1 % (Hertting and LaBrosse, 1962).

The metabolic pathway of norepinephrine is similar to that of epinephrine. When norepinephrine was administered to man, 3-methoxy-4-hydroxymandelic acid, normetanephrine, and dihydroxymandelic acid were the major metabolites (Goodall, Kirshner and Rosen, 1959). In rat, the main metabolite of norepinephrine was 3-methoxy-4-hydroxyphenylglycol (Axelrod, Kopin and Mann, 1959).

When catechol-O-methyltransferase was inhibited with pyrogallol, the excretion of catecholamine into urine was increased, and the excretion of O-methylated metabolites and the metabolic rate of catecholamines were decreased (Fig. 21) (Kopin, Axelrod and Gordon, 1961). When a monoamine oxidase inhibitor, iproniazid, was administered, the excretion of metanephrine was greatly increased. However, the metabolic rate of catecholamines did not change (Axelrod and Laroche, 1959). These results may have some connection with the pharmacological observation that pyrogallol but not iproniazid increases the physiological response to catecholamines.

Mice weighing approximately 20 g were given 0.5 mg of Regitine intraperitoneally. After 20 min, 1.5 mg of $(-)$-norepinephrine dissolved in 0.5 ml of 0.001 N HCl, was injected intraperitoneally. At selected intervals, each animal, including excreta from the time of injection, was homogenized in a mechanical blender in 100 ml of 10 % trichloroacetic acid, and the residual norepinephrine and 3-methoxynorepinephrine were assayed. By this method, the rate of the formation of normetanephrine and the

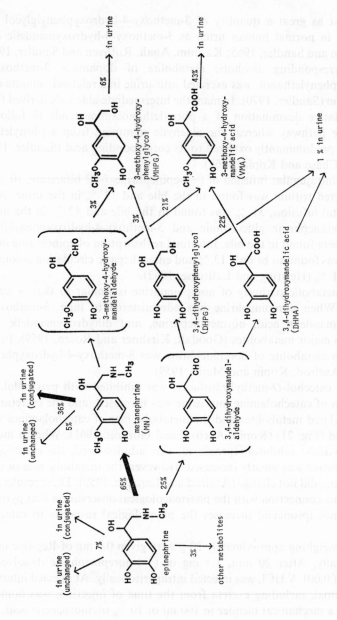

Fig. 21 (a). Metabolism of epinephrine and the effect of metabolic inhibitors in rat (Kopin, Axelrod and Gordon, 1961).

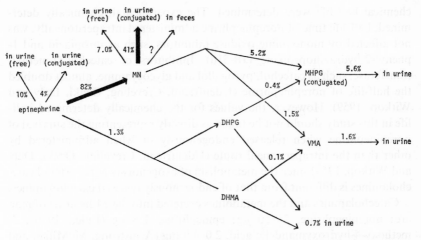

Fig. 21 (b). Iproniazid (a monoamine oxidase inhibitor) treated.

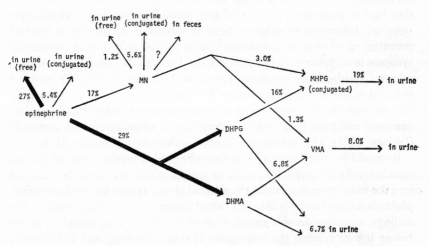

Fig. 21 (c). Pyrogallol (a catechol-*O*-methyltransferase inhibitor) treated.

chemical half-life were determined. The experimental, chemically determined, half-life time of norepinephrine administered intraperitoneally, was
not affected by monoamine oxidase inhibitors, such as iproniazid and 1-
phenyl-2-hydrazinopropane (JB-516). Inhibitors of catechol-O-methyltransferase, such as catechol, pyrogallol and glycocyamine, almost doubled
the half-life of norepinephrine (Udenfriend, Creveling, Ozaki, Daly and
Witkop, 1959). However, the values for the chemically determined half-
life in this study should not be taken as directly representing the survival of
norepinephrine when released endogenously or when administered by
other than the intraperitoneal route (Udenfriend, Creveling, Ozaki, Daly
and Witkop, 1959) since the metabolism of exogenously administered catecholamines is different from that of endogenously released catecholamines.

Catecholamines and the metabolites excreted into the 24-hr urine of man
are: norepinephrine, 25–50 μg; epinephrine, 4–8 μg (Euler, 1956); 3-
methoxy-4-hydroxymandelic acid, 2.0–4.0 mg (Armstrong, McMillan and
Shaw, 1957); normetanephrine, 100–300 μg; and metanephrine, 100–200
μg (Yoshinaga, Itoh, Ishida, Sato and Wada, 1961; Taniguchi, Kakimoto
and Armstrong, 1964).

Although catechol-O-methyltransferase and monoamine oxidase catalyze the catabolism of norepinephrine and epinephrine, neither of these
enzymes appears to play a major role in the type of transmitter inactivation that is analogous to that of acetylcholinesterase during cholinergic
synapses. Inhibition of either or both enzymes fails to produce a marked
potentiation of neurotransmission similar to that seen during cholinergic
synapses in response to anticholinesterase. The action of the norepinephrine
released at adrenergic terminals appear to be terminated by the physical
removal of the released transmitter from its site of action in the synaptic
cleft through the activity of an uptake system which rapidly transfers extraneuronal norepinephrine into the presynaptic adrenergic nerve terminals
(Iversen, 1969). This uptake mechanism is described in section II. 6.

It should be noted that information obtained from the study of infused
catecholamines is applicable only to amines which are normally released
into the bloodstream, as from the adrenal gland. However, most norepinephrine is released directly into individual tissues from the sympathetic nerve
endings, and considerable metabolism of this amine may therefore occur
before it ever reaches the circulation (Crout, Creveling and Udenfriend,
1961). It was suggested that monoamine oxidase plays the greater role in
the initial metabolism of norepinephrine in the brain and heart of the rat
while catechol-O-methyltransferase is of greater significance in the liver
(Crout, Creveling and Udenfriend, 1961). Although O-methylation with

catechol-O-methyltransferase preceding deamination with monoamine oxidase may be the predominant metabolic pathway towards the exogenously administered catecholamines, oxidative deamination with monoamine oxidase may precede O-methylation during the metabolism of endogenously released catecholamines (Andén, Ross and Werdinius, 1964).

II. 2.   Conjugation of Catecholamines

Catecholamines are excreted into urine as sulfate or glucuronide. Sulfate conjugates were predominant in man (Richter, 1940; Richter and MacIntosh, 1941; Kirshner, Goodall and Rosen, 1959). Catecholamine sulfate was formed from 3′-phosphoadenosine 5′-phosphosulfate (PAPS) through the catalysis of a sulfotransferase system (Goldberg and Delbrück, 1959), Glucuronide conjugation was predominant in rat and rabbit (Dodgson, Garton and Williams, 1947; Clark, Akawie, Pogrund and Geissman, 1951; Elmadjian, Lamson and Neri, 1956). Catecholamine glucuronide was formed from uridine diphosphate glucuronide by a glucuronyltransferase (Dutton and Storey, 1954; Isselbacher and Axelrod, 1955). This type of conjugation reaction of catecholamines was predominant after the oral administration of large amounts of catecholamines, suggesting that it might be a detoxication mechanism. The conjugation reaction by intestinal bacteria should also be considered.

II. 3.   Catechol-O-methyltransferase (COMT)

(EC 2.1.1.6. S-Adenosylmethionine: catechol-O-methyltransferase)

The enzymatic O-methylation of catecholamines was discovered by Axelrod (1957) and the enzyme was named catechol-O-methyltransferase (abbreviated COMT) and partially purified and characterized (Axelrod and Tomchick, 1958; Axelrod, 1962a, 1966). The enzyme subsequently purified from rat liver to a homogeneous stage (Assicot and Bohuon, 1970).

II. 3. 1. REACTION
See the figure on next page.

II. 3. 2. ASSAY METHOD
See section V. 6.

II. 3. 3. TISSUE DISTRIBUTION
The enzyme was present in various tissues, glands, blood vessels, sym-

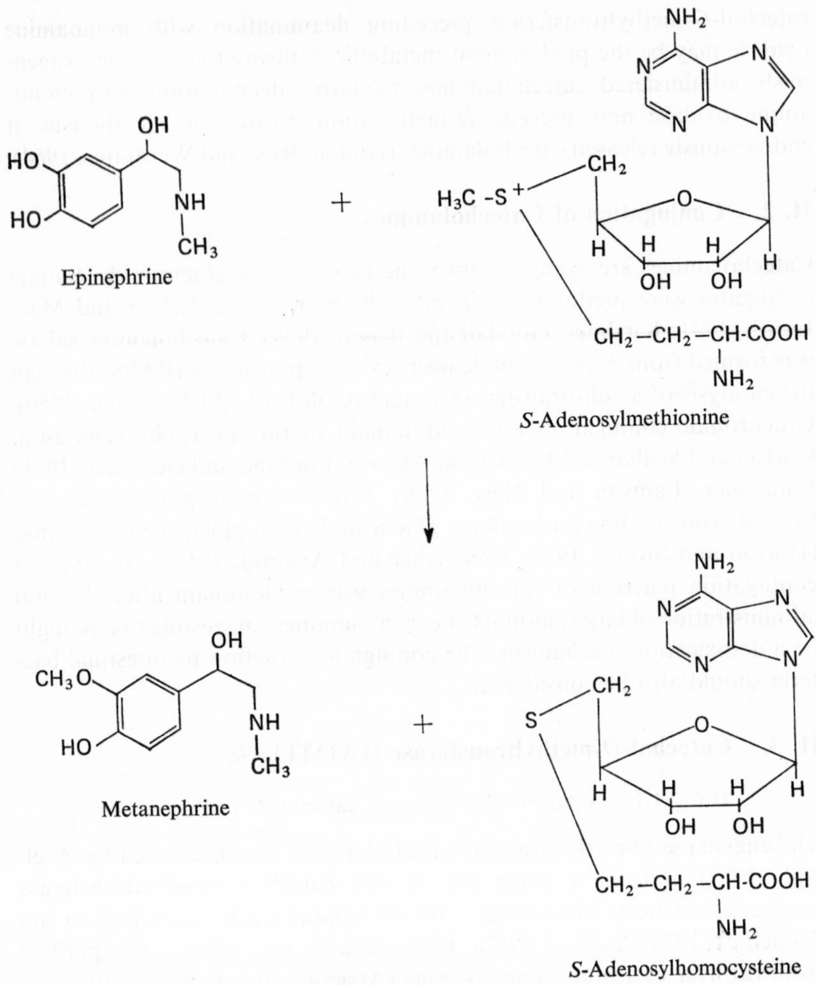

Epinephrine

+

S-Adenosylmethionine

Metanephrine

+

S-Adenosylhomocysteine

pathetic and parasympathetic nerves and ganglia, and all areas of the brain (Axelrod, 1965; Axelrod, Albers and Clemente, 1959). In the brain, the activity was highest in the area postrema and lowest in the cerebellar cortex (Axelrod, Albers and Clemente, 1959). The enzyme activity was also found in amphibian and avian tissues (Axelrod, 1965). The toad venom (the secretion of the parotid glands) of the South American toad (*Bufo marinus*) *O*-methylated enzymatically epinephrine, norepinephrine and dopamine (Märki, Axelrod and Witkop, 1962).

The enzyme was mainly localized in the soluble supernatant fraction (Axelrod and Tomchick, 1958). However, a small amount of this enzyme was also present in the microsomal fraction of the liver (Inscoe, Daly and Axelrod, 1965). The microsomal O-methylating enzyme appeared to be different from the soluble enzyme with respect to pH optima and species distribution. Enzyme activities in rat and rabbit microsomes were approximately equal while the soluble catechol-O-methyltransferase was 50 times greater in the rat than in the rabbit (Inscoe, Daly and Axelrod, 1965).

Another O-methylating enzyme, which can O-methylate diiodophenols, was found in rats (Tomita, Macha and Lardy, 1964).

A catechol-O-methyltransferase in plants O-methylated catechols mainly on the meta position (Finkle and Nelson, 1963). Another plant O-methyltransferase, which is nonspecific and can O-methylate the catechol norbelladine on the para position as well as a variety of catecholamines was also reported (Mann, Fales and Mudd, 1963).

II. 3. 4. PURIFICATION

Catechol-O-methyltransferase was partially purified and characterized from rat liver (Axelrod and Tomchick, 1958), and then further purified approximately 450-fold by salt fractionation, gel filtration, hydroxyapatite treatment, and ion-exchange chromatography. The final enzyme preparation was homogeneous when subjected to disc electrophoresis and sedimentation analysis in the ultracentrifuge (Assicot and Bohuon, 1970).

Purification procedure by Axelrod (1962)

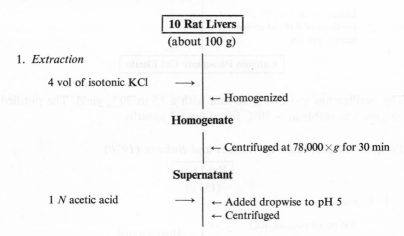

10 Rat Livers
(about 100 g)

1. *Extraction*

4 vol of isotonic KCl   ⟶   ← Homogenized

Homogenate

← Centrifuged at 78,000 × g for 30 min

Supernatant

1 N acetic acid   ⟶   ← Added dropwise to pH 5
    ← Centrifuged

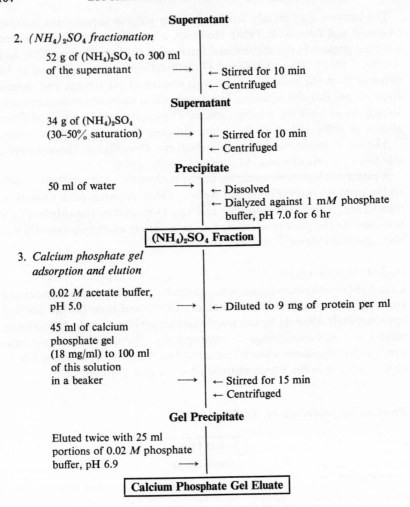

Supernatant

2. *(NH₄)₂SO₄ fractionation*

  52 g of (NH₄)₂SO₄ to 300 ml
  of the supernatant   ⟶   ← Stirred for 10 min
                                 ← Centrifuged

Supernatant

  34 g of (NH₄)₂SO₄
  (30–50% saturation)   ⟶   ← Stirred for 10 min
                                   ← Centrifuged

Precipitate

  50 ml of water   ⟶   ← Dissolved
                                   ← Dialyzed against 1 mM phosphate
                                        buffer, pH 7.0 for 6 hr

(NH₄)₂SO₄ Fraction

3. *Calcium phosphate gel
    adsorption and elution*

  0.02 M acetate buffer,
  pH 5.0   ⟶   ← Diluted to 9 mg of protein per ml

  45 ml of calcium
  phosphate gel
  (18 mg/ml) to 100 ml
  of this solution
  in a beaker   ⟶   ← Stirred for 15 min
                                   ← Centrifuged

Gel Precipitate

  Eluted twice with 25 ml
  portions of 0.02 M phosphate
  buffer, pH 6.9   ⟶

Calcium Phosphate Gel Eluate

The purification was about 30-fold with a 15 to 30% yield. The purified enzyme was stable at −10°C for at least 3 months.

Purification procedure by Assicot and Bohuon (1970)

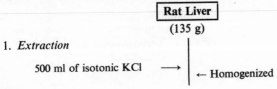

Rat Liver
(135 g)

1. *Extraction*

  500 ml of isotonic KCl   ⟶   ← Homogenized

Homogenate

| ← Centrifuged at 48,000×g for 60 min

Supernatant
(480 ml)

2. *$(NH_4)_2SO_4$ fractionation*

1 *M* acetic acid   ⟶ | ← Added dropwise to pH 5
| ← Allowed to stand for 5 min
| ← Centrifuged at 12,000×g for 10 min

Supernatant

Solid $(NH_4)_2SO_4$ ⎫
10% NH_4OH ⎬   ⟶ | ← 0.3–0.5% saturation at pH 8
            ⎭ | ← Centrifuged

Precipitate

0.01 *M* potassium phosphate
buffer, pH 7.5, the minimal
volume   ⟶ |

|‾$(NH_4)_2SO_4$ Fraction‾|
(stable over a period of at least 4 months at −20°C)

3. *Sephadex G-200 gel filtration*

Sephadex G-200 Column (4×100 cm)
with 3 cm of Sephadex G-15 on the top of the gel

0.01 *M* potassium phosphate
1 m*M* glutathione buffer,
pH 7.5, 1*l* for wash,
then for elution
            ⟶ | ← 4.5 ml fractions, flow rate 30 ml/hr

|‾Sephadex Eluate‾|
(180 ml, fraction 200–240)

4. *Hydroxyapatite treatment*

Hydroxyapatite prepared
from 2 *l* of 0.5 *M* $CaCl_2$
and 2 *l* of 0.5 *M* Na_2HPO_4,
stored at 4°C in 1 *l* of
0.01 *M* phosphate buffer,
pH 6.8. Slurry, 65 ml   ⟶ | ← Stirred for 15 min
| ← Centrifuged at 12,000×g for 15 min

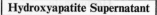

(215 ml, immediately frozen by using a freezing mixture ($-50°C$)
and lyophilized)

5. *DEAE-cellulose chromatography*

Water, the minimal
volume   ⟶

⟵ Dialyzed overnight against 2 *l* of
distilled water

10 ml of Enzyme

DEAE-Cellulose Column
(suspended in 1 mM phosphate buffer, pH 7.5 and equilibrated
with the same buffer, 1.5×4 cm)

Elution with phosphate
buffer 1, 10, 20, 30, 40,
100 mM ⟶

⟵ 2.5 ml fractions, flow rate 1 ml/min

DEAE-Cellulose Eluate
(Main peak: 0.02 M eluate, 3rd protein peak)
(Second peak: 0.03 M eluate, 4th protein peak)

II. 3. 5. PROPERTIES

The physicochemical properties of the enzyme purified by the method of
Assicot and Bohuon (1970) were reported. The enzyme was homogeneous
when subjected to disc gel electrophoresis and sedimentation analysis in the
ultracentrifuge. The sedimentation coefficient was calculated to be $S_{20,w} =$
3.78. The molecular weight, determined by gel filtration, was 240,000. The
purified enzyme dissolved in 0.01 M NaCl had an absorption maximum at
276 nm and the absorbance ratio 280:260 nm was 1.25. No absorption
peak was observed in the visible range from 350 to 800 nm.

The purified enzyme was very unstable, probably due to the oxidation of
SH groups. Variations of pH and ionic strength, addition of substrates, and
addition of the usual protective reagents for sulfhydryl groups were in-
effective. Only dithiothreitol showed a fair stabilization effect on the
enzyme and reactivated the partially inactivated enzyme.

The basic enzymological properties of catechol-O-methyltransferase
have been described in previous reports (Axelrod and Tomchick, 1958;
Axelrod, 1962a). The pH optimum was between 7.3 and 8.2 in phosphate
buffer. S-Adenosylmethionine was the methyl donor. The following cate-

chols were reported to be substrates: $(-)$-epinephrine, $(+)$-epinephrine, $(-)$-norepinephrine, dopamine, DOPA, epinine, $(\pm)$-3,4-dihydroxy-ephedrine, $(\pm)$-3,4-dihydroxyamphetamine, $(\pm)$-3,4-dihydroxybenzoate, 3,4-dihydroxyphenylacetate, 3,4-dihydroxymandelate and catechol. The K_m for epinephrine was $1.2 \times 10^{-4}M$. Monophenolic compounds are not O-methylated by the enzyme. The enzyme had absolute requirements for divalent cations such as Mg^{++}, Mn^{++}, Co^{++}, Zn^{++}, Cd^{++}, Fe^{++} and Ni^{++}. Catechols were generally O-methylated on the hydroxyl group meta to the side chain. m-O-Methylation of epinephrine was to the extent of 90%. Depending on the nature of the side chain, p-O-methylation was observed to occur to the extent of 10–56% (Senoh, Daly, Axelrod and Witkop, 1959). Catechols with the stronger nucleophilic character at the metahydroxy group methylated at this position, whereas compounds predominantly nucleophilic on the parahydroxy group (3,4-dihydroxyacetophenone) methylated to 55% at the para positon to form acetoisovanillone besides acetovanillone.

3-4-Dihydroxy-acetophenone   Acetovanillone   Acetoisovanillone

II. 3. 6. INHIBITORS

The enzyme was inhibited by SH-binding compounds such as p-chloro-mercuribenzoate ($3 \times 10^{-5}M$, 50% inhibition) (Axelrod and Tomchick, 1958). Toropolone derivatives were inhibitors and those with isosteric structures with catecholamines inhibited the enzyme by competing with the catechol substrate and by chelating with the divalent cation (Belleau and Burba, 1961, 1963). Catechol and pyrogallol inhibited the enzyme competitively with the substrates such as norepinephrine and epinephrine (Bacq, Gosselin, Dresse and Renson, 1959; Axelrod and Laroche, 1959). The administration of pyrogallol and quercitin blocked the O-methylation of epinephrine and norepinephrine (Axelrod and Laroche, 1959), and also prolonged the physiological actions of these amines (Bacq, Gosselin, Dresse and Renson, 1959).

II. 3. 7. PHYSIOLOGICAL ROLE

O-Methylation of catecholamines is considered to be the principal pathway for the metabolism of catecholamines, especially when administered exogeneously (Axelrod, Inscoe, Senoh and Witkop, 1958). Approximately 70% of either epinephrine or norepinephrine, which was intraperitoneally administered to rats, was O-methylated. Catechol-O-methyltransferase can O-methylate 3,4-dihydroxyacetophenone, arterenol and adrenalone at the para as well as meta positions *in vivo*. However, no formation of paranephrine from epinephrine could be detected *in vivo*.

Enzymatic demethylation studies *in vitro* showed that in most cases the para O-methyl ethers are demethylated more rapidly than the meta isomers. No interconversion of paranephrine to metanephrine could be observed *in vivo* (Daly, Axelrod and Witkop, 1960). Catechol-O-methyltransferase catalyzed methylation of 5,6-dihydroxyindole and 5,6-dihydroxy-dihydroindole primarily at position 6. Hydroxyindole-O-methyltransferase catalyzed methylation of 5,6-dihydroxyindole mainly at position 5. 5,6-Dihydroxydihydroindole was not a substrate for this enzyme. O-Methylation probably plays a role in melanin formation *in vivo* (Axelrod and Lerner, 1963) (Fig. 22).

II. 4.   Monoamine oxidase (MAO)

(EC 1.4.3.4. Monoamine: oxygen oxidoreductase (deaminating))

The term monoamine oxidase (MAO) is generally used for two groups of enzymes: 1) the mitochondrial monoamine oxidase which catalyzes the oxidative deamination of tyramine, tryptamine, serotonin, dopamine, norepinephrine, epinephrine and other monoamines; 2) the plasma amine oxidase which catalyzes the oxidative deamination of benzylamine, spermine or spermidine.

$$\text{Benzylamine} \qquad \qquad \text{Spermine} \qquad \qquad \text{Spermidine}$$

Benzylamine	Spermine	Spermidine

NH—(CH$_2$)$_3$—NH$_2$ H$_2$N—(CH$_2$)$_3$—NH—(CH$_2$)$_4$—NH$_2$

(CH$_2$)$_4$

NH—(CH$_2$)$_3$—NH$_2$

The latter enzyme, benzylamine oxidase in plasma (Tabor, C. W., Tabor, H. and Rosenthal, 1954; Yamada and Yasunobu, 1962; Blaschko and Bonney, 1962) is a soluble enzyme which has been crystallized from beef

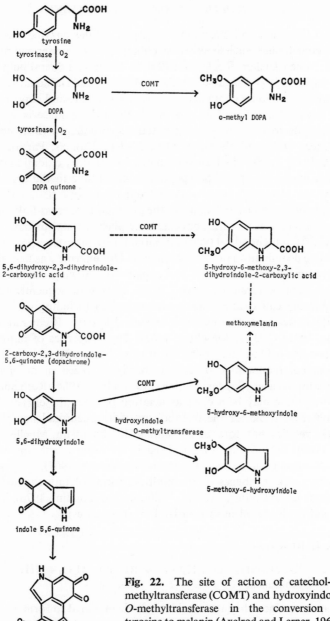

Fig. 22. The site of action of catechol-*O*-methyltransferase (COMT) and hydroxyindole-*O*-methyltransferase in the conversion of tyrosine to melanin (Axelrod and Lerner, 1963).

plasma (Yamada and Yasunobu, 1962). A similar enzyme was found in connective tissues, such as skin (Lovenberg, Dixon, Keiser and Sjoerdsma, 1968), bone (Rucker, Rogler and Parker, 1969), and dental pulp (Nakano and Nagatsu, 1971; Nagatsu, Nakano, Mizutani and Harada, 1972). Plasma benzylamine oxidase contained pyridoxal phosphate and copper (Yamada and Yasunobu, 1963). This type of monoamine oxidase is supposed to participipate in the cross-linking reactions of collagen (Bornstein, Kang and Piez, 1966) and elastin (O'Dell, Elsden, Thomas, Partiridge, Smith and Palmer, 1966), which is presumably initiated by oxidation of specific epsilon amino groups of polypeptide-bound lysine to the corresponding aldehydes. However, lysyl oxidase from connective tissues (Siegel and Martin, 1970) which participates in the production of cross-links in collagen and elastin may be a distinct enzyme from plasma amine oxidase.

The first mitochondrial type of monoamine oxidase is responsible for the oxidative deamination of catecholamines. This enzyme was first discovered as tyramine oxidase, since it was capable of carrying out the oxidative deamination of tyramine (Hare, 1928). It was subsequently found that this enzyme can oxidize various monoamines including catecholamines and it was designated monoamine oxidase (Blaschko, Richter and Schlossmann, 1937a, 1937b; Blaschko, 1963). The properties of mitochondrial monoamine oxidase are described in this chapter. It was suggested that microsomal monoamine oxidase is partly localized in norepinephrine-containing vesicles (Snyder, Fischer and Axelrod, 1965; Roth and Stjärne, 1966) as there may be a close association between the enzyme, which is mainly responsible for the metabolism of intraneuronal norepinephrine, and the vesicles that store catecholamine (de Champlain, Mueller and Axelrod, 1969). The enzyme was localized in the outer membrane of rat liver mitochondria (Schnaitman, Erwin and Greenwalt, 1967).

Recent reports suggested the multiple forms of mitochondrial monoamine oxidase (Collins, Sandler, Williams and Youdim, 1970). This problem will be discussed in section II. 4. 5. (Properties).

II. 4. 1. REACTION

$$R\text{-}CH_2\text{-}NH_2 + O_2 + H_2O \longrightarrow RCHO + H_2O_2 + NH_3$$

Monoamine   Aldehyde

A monoamine substrate is oxidatively deaminated to form an aldehyde, ammonia, and hydrogen peroxide. The formed aldehyde is converted either to acid with aldehyde oxidase or to alcohol with alcohol dehydrogenase (Fig. 23).

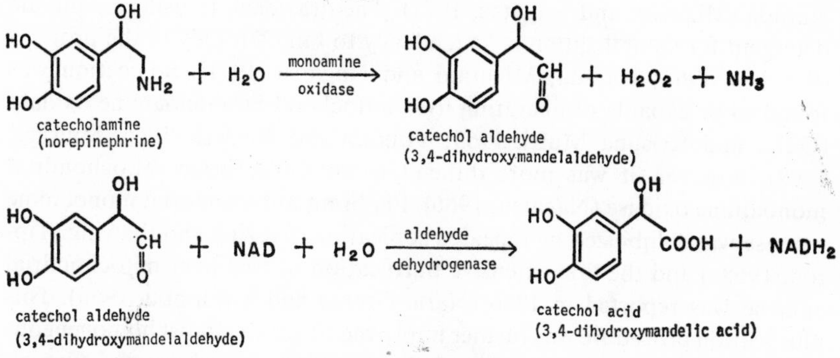

Fig. 23. Oxidation of catecholamine by monoamine oxidase (Leeper, Weissbach and Udenfriend, 1958).

II. 4. 2. Assay Method
See section V. 7.

II. 4. 3. Tissue Distribution

The enzyme was widely distributed in animal tissues and the liver had generally the highest activity towards various monoamine substrates. In man, the parotid and the submaxillary glands had the highest specific activity (Strömblad, 1959; Harada, Oya, Nakano, Kuzuya and Nagatsu, 1971) while enzyme activity in the skeletal muscle and blood seems to be absent. The enzyme was localized in the mitochondria (Cotzias and Dole, 1951; Hawkins, 1952), however, the microsomal fraction of rat liver also contained enzyme activity (Hawkins, 1952a).

II. 4. 4. Purification

Nonionic detergent or prolonged sonication have been used to solubilize mitochondrial monoamine oxidase which is tightly bound to the outer membrane of mitochondria. Among nonionic detergents used were, Cutscum (isooctylphenoxypolyethoxyethanol-containing detergent, Fisher Scientific Co.) (Cotzias, Serlin and Greenough, 1954; Nagatsu, 1966), desoxycholate (Zeller, Barsky and Berman, 1955), cholate (Sakamoto, Ogawa and Hayashi, 1963), OP-10 (Gorkin, 1963), Triton X-100 (Barbato and Abood, 1963; Nara, Gomes and Yasunobu, 1966a), digitonin (Erwin and Hellerman, 1967) and Nonion NS-210 (polyoxyethylenenonyl phenol ether-containing detergent, Nippon Oils and Fats Co., Tokyo) (Harada and Nagatsu, 1969; Nagatsu, Yamamoto and Harada, 1969;

Harada, Mizutani and Nagatsu, 1971). The drawback to using a nonionic detergent for solubilization is its tendency to bind strongly to the proteins (Sourkes, 1968; Harada, Mizutani and Nagatsu, 1971). Sonication was found to be capable of liberating liver mitochondrial monoamine oxidase (Guha and Krishna Murti, 1965; Youdim and Sourkes, 1966; Sourkes, 1968), however, it was more difficult to solubilize brain mitochondrial monoamine oxidase (Nagatsu, 1966). Pig brain mitochondrial monoamine oxidase was solubilized by repeated sonication, freezing and thawing (Tipton, 1968a) and the first extensive purification of beef liver mitochondrial enzyme was reported in 1966 (Nara, Gomes and Yasunobu, 1966). This purification procedure was further improved to get an almost homogeneous preparation (Yasunobu, Igaue and Gomes, 1968; Yasunobu and Gomes, 1971).

Two methods of purification of the enzyme are described in this chapter.

A. *Purification of beef liver mitochondrial monoamine oxidase* (Yasunobu, Igaue and Gomes, 1968; Gomes, Igaue, Kloepfer and Yasunobu, 1969). The specific activity is expressed as 0.001 absorbance unit/min at 25°C with the spectrophotometric method using benzylamine as substrate (Tabor, C. W., Tabor, H. and Rosenthal, 1954).

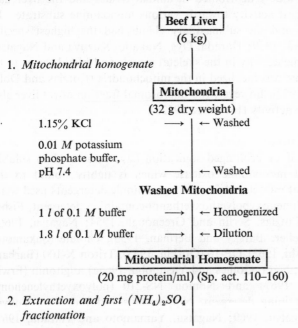

| Beef Liver |
| (6 kg) |

1. *Mitochondrial homogenate*

| Mitochondria |
| (32 g dry weight) |

1.15% KCl   ⟶ | ← Washed

0.01 *M* potassium
phosphate buffer,
pH 7.4   ⟶ | ← Washed

Washed Mitochondria

1 *l* of 0.1 *M* buffer   ⟶ | ← Homogenized

1.8 *l* of 0.1 *M* buffer   ⟶ | ← Dilution

| Mitochondrial Homogenate |
(20 mg protein/ml) (Sp. act. 110–160)

2. *Extraction and first* $(NH_4)_2SO_4$
   fractionation

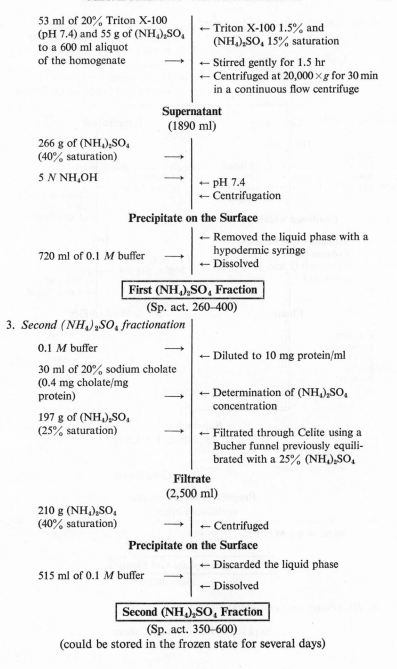

53 ml of 20% Triton X-100
(pH 7.4) and 55 g of $(NH_4)_2SO_4$
to a 600 ml aliquot
of the homogenate   ⟶

← Triton X-100 1.5% and
  $(NH_4)_2SO_4$ 15% saturation

← Stirred gently for 1.5 hr
← Centrifuged at 20,000 × g for 30 min
  in a continuous flow centrifuge

Supernatant
(1890 ml)

266 g of $(NH_4)_2SO_4$
(40% saturation)   ⟶

5 N NH_4OH ⟶

← pH 7.4
← Centrifugation

Precipitate on the Surface

720 ml of 0.1 M buffer   ⟶

← Removed the liquid phase with a
  hypodermic syringe
← Dissolved

First $(NH_4)_2SO_4$ Fraction
(Sp. act. 260–400)

3. *Second $(NH_4)_2SO_4$ fractionation*

0.1 M buffer   ⟶

← Diluted to 10 mg protein/ml

30 ml of 20% sodium cholate
(0.4 mg cholate/mg
protein)   ⟶

← Determination of $(NH_4)_2SO_4$
  concentration

197 g of $(NH_4)_2SO_4$
(25% saturation)   ⟶

← Filtrated through Celite using a
  Bucher funnel previously equilibrated with a 25% $(NH_4)_2SO_4$

Filtrate
(2,500 ml)

210 g $(NH_4)_2SO_4$
(40% saturation)   ⟶

← Centrifuged

Precipitate on the Surface

515 ml of 0.1 M buffer   ⟶

← Discarded the liquid phase

← Dissolved

Second $(NH_4)_2SO_4$ Fraction
(Sp. act. 350–600)
(could be stored in the frozen state for several days)

4. *Calcium phosphate gel treatment*

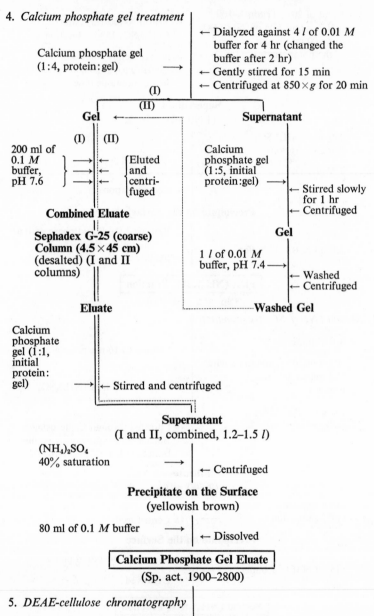

Calcium phosphate gel
(1:4, protein:gel)   ⟶

← Dialyzed against 4 *l* of 0.01 *M*
   buffer for 4 hr (changed the
   buffer after 2 hr)
← Gently stirred for 15 min
← Centrifuged at 850×*g* for 20 min

(I)

(II)

Gel ←   **Supernatant**

(I) (II)

200 ml of
0.1 *M*
buffer,
pH 7.6 ⟶ ← Eluted
   ⟶ ← and
   ⟶ ← centri-
         fuged

Calcium
phosphate gel
(1:5, initial
protein:gel) ⟶
   ← Stirred slowly
      for 1 hr
   ← Centrifuged

Combined Eluate

**Sephadex G-25 (coarse)
Column (4.5×45 cm)**
(desalted) (I and II
columns)

Gel

1 *l* of 0.01 *M*
buffer, pH 7.4 ⟶
   ← Washed
   ← Centrifuged

Eluate

Calcium
phosphate
gel (1:1,
initial
protein:
gel) ⟶ ← Stirred and centrifuged

Washed Gel

Supernatant
(I and II, combined, 1.2–1.5 *l*)

(NH₄)₂SO₄
40% saturation ⟶
   ← Centrifuged

$(NH_4)_2SO_4$

Precipitate on the Surface
(yellowish brown)

80 ml of 0.1 *M* buffer ⟶
   ← Dissolved

Calcium Phosphate Gel Eluate
(Sp. act. 1900–2800)

5. *DEAE-cellulose chromatography*

Sephadex G-25 (coarse) Column
(4.5×45 cm)

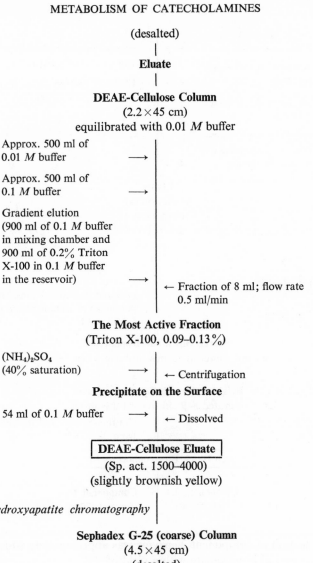

(desalted)

|

Eluate

|

DEAE-Cellulose Column
(2.2 × 45 cm)
equilibrated with 0.01 *M* buffer

Approx. 500 ml of
0.01 *M* buffer   ⟶

Approx. 500 ml of
0.1 *M* buffer   ⟶

Gradient elution
(900 ml of 0.1 *M* buffer
in mixing chamber and
900 ml of 0.2% Triton
X-100 in 0.1 *M* buffer
in the reservoir)   ⟶   ← Fraction of 8 ml; flow rate
0.5 ml/min

The Most Active Fraction
(Triton X-100, 0.09–0.13%)

(NH₄)₂SO₄
(40% saturation)   ⟶   ← Centrifugation

Precipitate on the Surface

54 ml of 0.1 *M* buffer   ⟶   ← Dissolved

| **DEAE-Cellulose Eluate** |
(Sp. act. 1500–4000)
(slightly brownish yellow)

|

6. *Hydroxyapatite chromatography*

Sephadex G-25 (coarse) Column
(4.5 × 45 cm)
(desalted)

|

Eluate
(80–100 ml)

|

Hydroxyapatite Column
(2.9 × 19 cm) which had been equilibrated with 0.01 *M* buffer

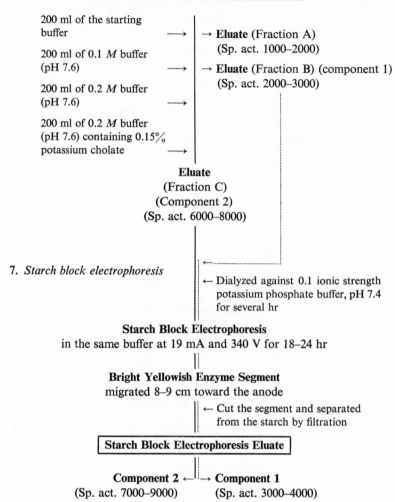

200 ml of the starting
buffer   ⟶   ⟶ **Eluate** (Fraction A)
                                  (Sp. act. 1000–2000)
200 ml of 0.1 *M* buffer
(pH 7.6)   ⟶   ⟶ **Eluate** (Fraction B) (component 1)
                                  (Sp. act. 2000–3000)
200 ml of 0.2 *M* buffer
(pH 7.6)   ⟶

200 ml of 0.2 *M* buffer
(pH 7.6) containing 0.15%
potassium cholate   ⟶

Eluate
(Fraction C)
(Component 2)
(Sp. act. 6000–8000)

7. *Starch block electrophoresis*

← Dialyzed against 0.1 ionic strength
potassium phosphate buffer, pH 7.4
for several hr

Starch Block Electrophoresis
in the same buffer at 19 mA and 340 V for 18–24 hr

Bright Yellowish Enzyme Segment
migrated 8–9 cm toward the anode

← Cut the segment and separated
from the starch by filtration

| **Starch Block Electrophoresis Eluate** |

Component 2 ←⟶ **Component 1**
(Sp. act. 7000–9000)   (Sp. act. 3000–4000)

The purification of component 2 enzyme was approximately 60-fold from
the mitochondrial homogenate with a yield of 5%.

B. *Purification of human and beef brain mitochondrial monoamine oxidase*
   (Harada and Nagatsu, 1969; Nagatsu, Yamamoto and Harada, 1970;
   Harada, Mizutani and Nagatsu, 1971)
Brain mitochondrial monoamine oxidase is more difficult to solubilize than
the liver enzyme and seems to be unstable with ammonium sulfate. The

following partial purification procedure of the brain enzyme was established, and although this method is quite reproducible, the final preparation contains a tightly-bound detergent. Since the detergent is required for solubility, the purified enzyme is not soluble, however, the purified enzyme can retain activity at 0°C.

Enzyme activity was measured by the spectrophotometric method with kynuramine as substrate (Weissbach, Smith, Daly, Witkop and Udenfriend, 1960) (See Section III. 7). When the detergent Nonion NS-210 was used for the solubilization, it interfered with the assay of protein by the Folin phenol reagent (Lowry, Rosebrough, Farr and Randall, 1951), therefore, the protein was estimated based on the nitrogen content determined by the micro-Kjeldahl method and the usual factor of 6.25 was used to convert the nitrogen to protein. However, protein in the fractions separated by chromatography or continuous-flow electrophoresis was determined by the Folin phenol method (Lowry, Rosebrough, Farr and Randall, 1951), using bovine serum albumin as a standard. When turbidity appeared, owing to the presence of detergent, the absorbance was measured after the turbidity was eliminated by centrifugation.

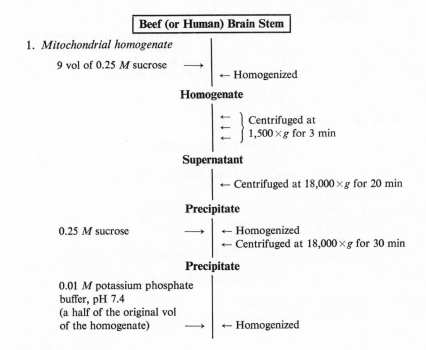

Beef (or Human) Brain Stem

1. *Mitochondrial homogenate*

9 vol of 0.25 M sucrose ⟶ ← Homogenized

Homogenate

← } Centrifuged at
← } 1,500 × g for 3 min
←

Supernatant

← Centrifuged at 18,000 × g for 20 min

Precipitate

0.25 M sucrose ⟶ ← Homogenized
← Centrifuged at 18,000 × g for 30 min

Precipitate

0.01 M potassium phosphate buffer, pH 7.4 (a half of the original vol of the homogenate) ⟶ ← Homogenized

$$\boxed{\textbf{Mitochondrial Homogenate}}$$

(can be stored at $-20°C$)

2. Extraction and $(NH_4)_2SO_4$ fractionation

	← Incubated at 40°C for 10 min with constant stirring
6% (v/v) aqueous solution of Nonion NS-210* to a final conc. of 1% (v/v) ⟶	← Rapidly cooled in an ice bath
	← Dropwise addition with constant gentle stirring
(* polyoxyethylenenonyl phenol ether-containing detergent, Nippon Oils & Fats Co., Tokyo. Cutscum or Triton X-100 can be used, but are less effective)	← Stirring for 1 hr ← Centrifuged at 107,000 × g (max) for 1 hr

Supernatant

Saturated $(NH_4)_2SO_4$ solution (pH 7) to 30% saturation ⟶	← Centrifuged at 9,500 × g for 15 min

Precipitate on the Surface

0.01 M buffer (a minimal volume) ⟶	← Dissolved ← Dialyzed against the same buffer (changed buffer 3 times during 15 hr dialysis) ← Centrifuged

Supernatant

3. DEAE-cellulose chromatography

DEAE-Cellulose Column

$(4 \times 50$ cm$)$

equilibrated with 0.01 M buffer

600 ml of 0.01 M buffer ⟶	← Washed
600 ml of 0.1 M buffer ⟶	← Washed
0.1 M buffer containing 0.4% Nonion NS-210 ⟶	← Elution, fraction size 4 ml

The Most Active Fraction

Saturated $(NH_4)_2SO_4$ solution (pH 7.4) (30% saturation) ⟶	← Centrifuged

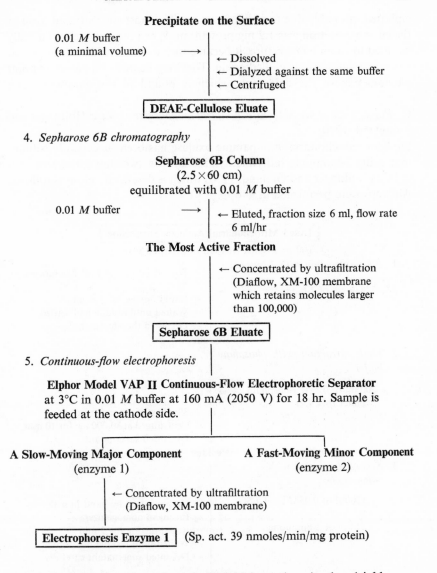

Precipitate on the Surface

0.01 *M* buffer
(a minimal volume)   ⟶   ← Dissolved
                                        ← Dialyzed against the same buffer
                                        ← Centrifuged

| **DEAE-Cellulose Eluate** |

4. *Sepharose 6B chromatography*

Sepharose 6B Column
(2.5 × 60 cm)
equilibrated with 0.01 *M* buffer

0.01 *M* buffer   ⟶   ← Eluted, fraction size 6 ml, flow rate
                                      6 ml/hr

The Most Active Fraction

                                      ← Concentrated by ultrafiltration
                                        (Diaflow, XM-100 membrane
                                        which retains molecules larger
                                        than 100,000)

| **Sepharose 6B Eluate** |

5. *Continuous-flow electrophoresis*

Elphor Model VAP II Continuous-Flow Electrophoretic Separator
at 3°C in 0.01 *M* buffer at 160 mA (2050 V) for 18 hr. Sample is
feeded at the cathode side.

A Slow-Moving Major Component   **A Fast-Moving Minor Component**
(enzyme 1)   (enzyme 2)

          ← Concentrated by ultrafiltration
            (Diaflow, XM-100 membrane)

| **Electrophoresis Enzyme 1** | (Sp. act. 39 nmoles/min/mg protein)

The purification was approximately 40-fold from the mitochondrial homogenate with a yield of 4%.

The enzyme was faintly yellow. The activity was stable at least for 2
weeks at 0°C, but could not be stored in the frozen state. When the enzyme
was extensively concentrated by ultrafiltration, most of the enzyme pre-

cipitated, probably due to polymerization. The most concentrated form of the enzyme solution was 1.2 mg protein/ml. When the enzyme was rapidly warmed to room temperature, it became turbid; the turbidity disappeared when the solution was chilled again. This may be due to a clouding point phenomenon of the detergent, which is bound to the enzyme.

C. *Purification of pig liver mitochondrial monoamine oxidase* (Hollunger and Oreland, 1970).

Pig liver mitochondrial monoamine oxidase has been successfully solubilized using 2-butanone (ethylmethylketone) in a two-step extraction procedure (Hollunger and Oreland, 1970) which is described below as follows. All steps were performed at 4–6°C.

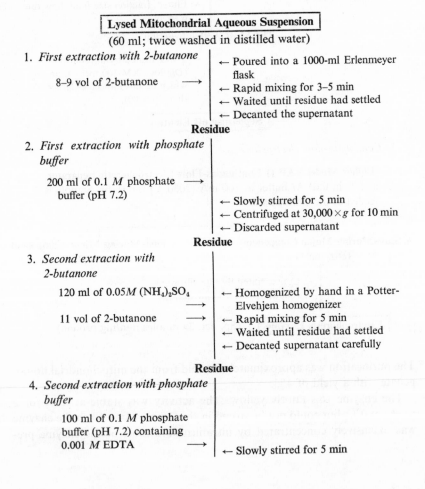

| **Lysed Mitochondrial Aqueous Suspension** |

(60 ml; twice washed in distilled water)

1. *First extraction with 2-butanone*

    8–9 vol of 2-butanone   ⟶

  ← Poured into a 1000-ml Erlenmeyer flask
  ← Rapid mixing for 3–5 min
  ← Waited until residue had settled
  ← Decanted the supernatant

Residue

2. *First extraction with phosphate buffer*

    200 ml of 0.1 M phosphate ⟶ buffer (pH 7.2)

  ← Slowly stirred for 5 min
  ← Centrifuged at 30,000 × g for 10 min
  ← Discarded supernatant

Residue

3. *Second extraction with 2-butanone*

    120 ml of 0.05M $(NH_4)_2SO_4$ ⟶

    11 vol of 2-butanone   ⟶

  ← Homogenized by hand in a Potter-Elvehjem homogenizer
  ← Rapid mixing for 5 min
  ← Waited until residue had settled
  ← Decanted supernatant carefully

Residue

4. *Second extraction with phosphate buffer*

    100 ml of 0.1 M phosphate buffer (pH 7.2) containing 0.001 M EDTA   ⟶

  ← Slowly stirred for 5 min

| ← Centrifuged at 30,000 × g for 10 min

| Supernatant Containing Soluble Monoamine Oxidase |

(yellow, water-clear solution containing 20–35% of the original
mitochondrial monoamine oxidase activity)

This soluble enzyme has been purified and characterized (Oreland, 1971). About 25% of the enzyme was obtained in true solution in the presence of 0.05 M ammonium sulfate using a butanone/water ratio of eleven in the second extraction step (Hollunger and Oreland, 1970). Phosphatidylethanolamine and phosphatidylcholine were largely extracted in the first extraction without the liberation of monoamine oxidase, whereas anionic phospholipids (mainly cardiolipin) was extracted together with monoamine oxidase in the second extraction (Oreland and Olivecrona, 1971). It was further shown that the solubilized enzyme can interact with highly acidic phospholipids either in solution, forming soluble complexes, or with the same phospholipids bound to insoluble membrane residues, and then form insoluble complexes (Olivecrona and Oreland, 1971).

Chicken brain mitochondrial monoamine oxidase was solubilized by using a nonionic detergent, Emulgen 81 (a polyoxyethyleneoctylphenol ether containing detergent), and purified by using ammonium sulfate fractionation and, subsequently, by various column chromatographies such as DEAE-cellulose, DEAE-Sephadex, CM-Sephadex, hydroxyapatite and Sepharose 6B. The purified enzyme had a molecular weight of about 150,000. Disc electrophoresis was used to separate three monoamine oxidases (Hashimoto and Okuyama, 1970).

II. 4. 5. PROPERTIES

Since it was very difficult to solubilize monoamine oxidase from mitochondria, its properties remained uncertain for some time. However recent progress in the solubilization and purification procedures of the enzyme from beef liver mitochondria has made elucidation of the properties possible (Yasunobu, Igaue and Gomes, 1968; Gomes, Igaue, Kloepfer and Yasunobu, 1969). Of two components (components 1 and 2) obtained (Gomes, Igaue, Kloepfer and Yasunobu, 1969), component 2 had the higher enzyme activity. Both components were bright yellow, with absorption maxima at 274, 410 and 450 nm, sedimentation coefficients of 14.4 and 20.6, and molecular weights of about 405,000 and 1,280,000, respectively, for components 1 and 2. Component 1 contained four and component 2 contained 12 FAD or FAD-like substance per mole of enzyme. Many years ago it was thought that there was a possibility that mitochondrial monoamine oxidase might be a flavoprotein (Hawkins, 1952b). The first definite indication that the prosthetic group of the enzyme is a flavin was made in 1966 (Nara, Igaue, Gomes and Yasunobu, 1966). A FAD-like substance was identified in the beef liver enzyme, and evidence indicating that the flavin is involved in the oxidation of substrate was presented (Igaue, Gomes and Yasunobu, 1967). It was also found that the flavin dinucleotide is tightly bound to the enzyme and not freely dissociable, and that the flavin may be covalently attached to the enzyme (Nara, Igaue, Gomes and Yasunobu, 1966).

The flavin peptide derived from monoamine oxidase was isolated by digestion of outer membrane of bovine liver mitochondria with trypsin and chymotrypsin, and the FAD was found to be covalently linked to the peptide chain through the 8α-CH$_3$ group of riboflavin (Kearney, Salach, Walker, Seng and Singer, 1971). The amino acid substituted on the 8α-CH$_3$ group of flavin was cysteine in thioether linkage, and the sequence of the peptide was established as described below (Walker, Kearney, Seng and Singer, 1971).

8α-(S-Cysteinyl)-riboflavin was synthesized and shown to be identical with the flavocoenzyme isolated from liver monoamine oxidase by Walker, Kearney, Seng and Singer (Ghisla and Hemmerich, 1971).

Components 1 and 2 by Gomes, Igaue, Kloepfer and Yasunobu (1969) contained 24 and 106 moles of phospholipid per mole of enzyme, respectively. It was suggested that component 2 may be a trimer of component 1 and that a part of the multiplicity of the enzyme as described below is due to its isolation in different molecular weight forms (Gomes, Igaue, Kloepfer and Yasunobu, 1969). Components 1 and 2 contained, respectively, about 28 and 86 sulfhydryl groups per mole of enzyme or 7 sulfhydryl groups per 100,000 g of protein. It was found that after all the sulfhydryl groups had reacted with p-chloromercuribenzoate, the enzyme was not completely inhibited and that removal of the excess sulfhydryl reagent lead to reactivation of the enzyme. It was suggested, therefore, that sulfhydryl groups are probably required for conformational stability rather than being required for catalysis (Gomes, Naguwa, Kloepfer and Yasunobu, 1969). The optimum pH of components 1 and 2 enzymes was near 9.2, and substrate specificity (%) was also similar: for component 2 enzyme benzylamine, 100; heptylamine, 79; kynuramine, 52; norepinephrine, 46; tryptamine, 32; tyramine, 30; epinephrine, 25; serotonin, 5.

It was first shown that the purified beef liver mitochondrial monoamine oxidase contains about 0.07% of copper and is inhibited by known copper chelating agents, such as cuprizone, neocuproine, 8-hydroxyquinoline, and sodium diethyldithiocarbamate (Nara, Gomes and Yasunobu, 1966). Subsequent higher purifications of the enzyme revealed a decrease in the copper content up to 0.15 μg copper/mg protein, however, the inhibition characteristics of the enzyme inhibited by known metal chelating agents were almost identical. The significance of copper in mitochondrial monoamine oxidase remains to be elucidated, but most likely it is not an essential prosthetic group.

Mitochondrial monoamine oxidase was also highly purified from bovine kidney (Erwin and Hellerman, 1967). The kidney enzyme was solubilized with digitonin, and, subsequently, purified by ammonium sulfate fractionation and calcium phosphate gel-cellulose column chromatography. The purification was 34-fold with a yield of 10%. Absorption and fluorescence spectra indicated strongly that the kidney enzyme is a flavoprotein. Under anaerobic conditions, benzylamine reduced the flavin at 460 nm apparently to 75% of the total reduction observed with sodium dithionite. The enzyme preparation contained approximately 1 mole of flavin per 100,000 g of protein. The flavin prosthetic group could not be characterized precisely due to the tight association of this group with the protein. The kidney enzyme contained 7 to 8 sulfhydryl groups per 100,000 g of protein and the absorption spectrum had a maximum at 410 nm, a plateau at 450 nm and, a shoulder at 485 nm (Erwin and Hellerman, 1967).

The purification procedure of rat and rabbit liver enzyme by Youdim and Sourkes (1966) included solubilization by extensive sonication. Sonication was carried out in a room away from the main laboratory and, during the procedure the operator wore ear-protectors (Sourkes, 1968). About 80 % of the enzyme activity was solubilized and, subsequently, purification by ammonium sulfate fractionation (30–55%), Sephadex G-200, DEAE-Sephadex A-50, and calcium phosphate gel was carried out. A 200-fold purification was achieved with a yield of about 25%. The molecular weight estimated by gel filtration was 290,000 and ultracentrifugation studies showed an estimated molecular weight of about 150,000. It was suggested that a dimer is formed in the course of gel filtration. The rat liver enzyme was pale yellow and the absorption spectrum showed maxima at 410 and 280 nm. The purified rat liver enzyme did not fluoresce appreciably in the visible or ultraviolet ranges, however, if the purified preparation was treated with the proteolytic enzyme, pronase, then a material fluorescing at 520 nm (when activated at 460 nm) was found. When the purified enzyme was precipitated with trichloroacetic acid, some fluorescent material was released. The possibility of two forms of binding of a flavin component in the purified rat liver preparation was suggested.

Tipton (1968a, 1971) reported an extensive purification of pig brain mitochondrial monoamine oxidase. The pig brain enzyme was solubilized by repeating sonication of the frozen (not less than 3 days) mitochondria (45 min), and freeaing (overnight) and thawing six times. 60–80% of the enzyme activity was liberated into the solution. The enzyme was subsequently purified by adjustment to low pH (3.0), treatment with DEAE-cellulose and ethanol precipitation. Purification was about 1,000-fold with a yield of 22% and the molecular weight was estimated to be approximately 102,000 by Sephadex G-200 gel filtration. A smaller amount (less than 10%) of the activity was eluted at the position corresponding to a molecular weight of 435,000. It is suggested that this higher molecular weight form of monoamine oxidase may represent a lipid complex or a tetramer form of the enzyme. The purified enzyme showed a single band in cellulose acetate electrophoresis and a single peak in Sephadex G-200 chromatography. An optimum pH was found near 7.2 and the K_m value toward tyramine was $1.2 \times 10^{-4}M$. Substrate inhibition by tyramine was observed and the K_i value for the substrate acting as an inhibitor was calculated to be $1.7 \times 10^{-2}M$. p-Chloromercuribenzoate at $5 \times 10^{-4}M$ completely inhibited the reaction. The purified enzyme fluoresced at about 520 nm when it was excited at 450 nm. When the enzyme was digested with pronase, the fluorescence intensity increased by about 50%. Based on the fluorescence intensity of the pronase-digested enzyme, a flavin content of 1 mole of FAD per 118,000 g enzyme was calculated. The fluorescent material was liberated from the enzyme either by heating an enzyme solution to 100°C or by treating it with trichloroacetic acid, and identified as FAD by paper chromatography and by titration with D-amino acid apoxidase. By the latter method the molecular weight of the enzyme per FAD molecule was found to be 120,000. The brain enzyme did not contain pyridoxal phosphate. The copper content was 1 g atom per 590,000 g protein. No increase in the activity of the enzyme was observed by preincubating the enzyme with various concentrations of Cu^{++}. The FAD-free apomonoamine oxidase from pig brain mitochondria was prepared by treatment with acid ammonium sulfate (Tipton, 1968b). The apoenzyme was inactive and was partly reactivated by incubation with FAD but not FMN. The dissociation constant for FAD binding to the enzyme was $1.4 \times 10^{-8} M$. Kinetic studies based on initial rate measurements of tyramine oxidation suggested a kinetic mechanism in which a ternary complex between the substrate (tyramine) and oxygen, and the enzyme is not involved (Tipton, 1968b).

The mitochondrial monoamine oxidase in beef or human brain was difficult to solubilize without a detergent (Nagatsu, 1966; Harada and Nagatsu, 1969; Nagatsu, Yamamoto and Harada, 1970; Harada, Mizutani and Nagatsu, 1971). The brain mitochondrial enzyme was extracted with the detergent Cutscum and by sonication (Nagatsu, 1966) or by mild heat treatment and a detergent Nonion NS-210 (Harada and Nagatsu, 1969). The extracted enzyme was subsequently purified by ammonium sulfate fractionation, DEAE-cellulose column chromatography, Sepharose 6B column chromatography, and continuous-flow electrophoresis. A major component (enzyme 1) with a higher specific activity and a minor component (enzyme 2) with a lower specific activity were separated. The properties of both enzymes in relation to kynuramine as substrate including pH-optimum (8.6) and K_m values ($6.7 \times 10^{-5} M$) were similar, but enzyme 1 showed a higher specific activity towards tyramine whereas enzyme 2 showed a higher specific activity towards normetanephrine. Enzyme 1 was faintly yellow and the absorption spectrum exhibited a maximum at 410 nm and a broad shoulder at 480–490 nm. The fluorescence activation spectrum measured at 550 nm showed a maxima at 280, 370 and 460 nm and the fluorescence emission spectrum measured by excitation at 450 nm showed a peak at 520 nm, indicating that enzyme 1 is a flavoprotein. The copper content was less than 0.01 μg/mg protein, and copper chelating agents did not inhibit the enzyme. p-Chloromercuribenzoate and N-ethylmaleimide, however, inhibited the enzyme, indicating the presence of essential SH-group(s). The enzyme preparation contained a tightly-bound detergent which interferes with various analysis of the enzyme. It is hoped that the solubilization of beef or human brain enzyme without a detergent will be accomplished, as with pig brain enzyme (Tipton, 1968b).

Interesting results were reported on the presence of monoamine oxidase isoenzymes. The first direct evidence on the presence of isoenzymes in human and rat liver monoamine oxidase was presented by Collins, Youdim and Sandler (1968). Both human and rat liver mitochondrial monoamine oxidase were solubilized by sonication followed by treatment with cholic acid (1%) (Youdim and Sourkes, 1966) or Triton X-100 (Youdim and Sandler, 1967). Samples (0.1 ml) of enzyme solution mixed with Sephadex G-200 (approx. 40 ml/g) were applied to the top of a 5% (w/v) polyacrylamide gel (Cyanogum 41, British Drug Houses, Ltd.) disc electrophoresis column (0.5 × 7.5 cm). A continuous 0.05 M Tris-HCl buffer system, pH 8.6, was employed. Samples were applied at the cathode to eight tubes at a time and run simultaneously for 2–3 hr at room temperature using a constant current of 6 mA per tube. The protein bands were developed by naphthalene black 12 B-staining. The bands of enzyme activity in the gel columns were separated with a sharp razor. Each band was homogenized in about 1 ml of 0.05 M phosphate buffer, pH 7.4, and after centrifugation at 500 × g for 10 min, the supernatant was retained for protein estimation and enzyme assay with the following substrates: tryptamine-C^{14}, tyramine-C^{14}, kynuramine, and benzylamine. Both human and rat liver solubilized mitochondrial monoamine oxidase consistently separated as four bands of activity migrating towards the anode. The bands showed differing substrate specificity, heat stability, and differing sensitivity to monoamine oxidase inhibitors and pH activity curves.

Further experiments showed at least five bands from human and rat liver monoamine oxidase. The molecular weights of the bands as determined by the gel-filtration method were all within the range of 288,000–320,000. Based on these results, it was suggested that the various bands of activity represent conformational isoenzymes (Collins and Youdim, 1969).

After ultracentrifugation, solubilized and purified rat liver enzyme showed a $S_{20,w}$ of 6.8 and a molecular weight of 155,000, whereas molecular weight determined by gel filtration was about 300,000. Five forms of the enzyme were separated using polyacrylamide gel electrophoresis, and the molecular weight of four of these five forms was about 300,000 by gel filtration, but after exposure to 8 M urea or 1% (w/v) sodium dodecyl sulfate containing 0.1 M 2-mercaptoethanol, a single enzymatically inactive band having a molecular weight of about 75,000 was isolated. When each isoenzyme form was dissociated for 10 min in the presence of 8 M urea and 0.2 M mercaptoethanol followed by dialysis, they reassociated to form all five isoenzymes (Youdim and Collins, 1971).

Four molecular forms of rat brain monoamine oxidase (Youdim, Collins and Sandler, 1969) and of the human brain enzyme (Collins, Sandler, Williams and Youdim, 1970) were separated by polyacrylamide disc electrophoresis. Rat or human brain mitochondria were suspended in Tris-HCl buffer (0.05 M, pH 8.6 or 9.1) containing 1.5% or 1.0% Triton X-100 and benzylamine ($10^{-3}M$). The suspension was subjected to sonication (2–3 hr, 0–5°C, 20 kHz) and the resulting solution fractionated with $(NH_4)_2SO_4$. The precipitate at 30–55% saturation was collected by centrifugation at $12,000 \times g$, dissolved in Tris-HCl and stored at 4°C. The enzyme preparation was further purified by column chromatography on Sephadex G-200. The enzyme activity was eluted as a single sharp peak, and a molecular weight of 230,000 was obtained. Polyacrylamide disc electrophoresis was carried out using Tris-HCl buffer (0.05 M, pH 9.1) as medium. Two hundred microliters of the solubilized enzyme preparation in 0.05 M Tris-HCl buffer, pH 9.1, was introduced onto the gel at the cathode, and a current of 6 mA per tube was applied for 1–2 hr. The gels were developed for monoamine oxidase activity with a solution containing 4 mg of nitro blue tetrazolium, 1 mg of sodium sulfate and 4 mg of tryptamine-HCl in 5 ml of 0.1 M phosphate buffer, pH 7.4 (Glenner, Burtner and Brown, 1957). Two bands, MAO_1 and MAO_2, migrated toward the anode, one, MAO_3, remained at the origin, and the other, MAO_4, migrated towards the cathode. MAO_1 had the highest specific activity towards tryptamine, tyramine and benzylamine. The specific activity of MAO_4 toward dopamine was always greater than that of the other three enzymes.

After a high degree of purification of beef brain monoamine oxidase by solubilization with a detergent, Nonion NS-210, ammonium sulfate fractionation, DEAE-cellulose chromatography and Sepharose 6B chromatography, the enzyme preparation was separated into two components, a slow-moving major component: enzyme 1; and a fast-moving minor component: enzyme 2, which migrated from the cathode to the anode in 0.01 M phosphate buffer, pH 7.4 by continuous-flow electrophoresis. Enzyme 1 had the highest specific activity towards tyramine, whereas enzyme 2 had the highest towards normetanephrine (Harada, Mizutani and Nagatsu, 1971). However, when a detergent is used for the solubilization, it is possible that the different components separated by electrophoresis belong to the same enzyme protein in the mitochondria and are derived through the ability of the detergent to alter the structure of proteins.

In order to eliminate the possibility of detergents altering the tertiary structure of proteins, disintegrated mitochondrial membranes from rat liver by sonication were separated by means of density gradient column electrophoresis. The rates of deamination of monoamines in the fractions after electrophoresis using serotonin, tyramine, p-nitrophenylethylamine, kynuramine, and m-nitro-p-hydroxybenzylamine as substrates, showed that the amine oxidases of rat liver mitochondria may be more or less distinctly separated (Gorkin, 1969).

The two pure enzyme components from beef liver were antigenically indistinguishable (Hartman, Yasunobu and Udenfriend, 1971). About 80% of the beef brain enzyme was also antigenically identical to the liver enzyme. However, the rest of the brain enzyme did not cross-react with antibody to the liver enzyme (Hidaka, Hartman and Udenfriend, 1971).

Another interesting observation is the transformation of mitochondrial monoamine oxidase into a diamine oxidase-like enzyme *in vitro* (Gorkin and Tatyanenko, 1967; Akopyan, Stesina and Gorkin, 1971). After treating rat or bovine liver mitochondrial monoamine oxidase with peroxidized oleic acid in presence of a saturating concentration of serotonin with subsequent dialysis, the maximal specific rate of deamination of tyramine was decreased by about 90% while that of serotonin was decreased only 34%. The enzyme preparation thus obtained also retained, to a considerable degree, the ability to deaminate tryptamine or dopamine. The most striking new property aquired by the modified ("transformed") amine oxidase was its ability to catalyze the deamination of typical substrates of diamine oxidase from animal tissues (histamine), soluble spermine oxidase (spermine), and diamine oxidase from plant tissues (lysine).

Monoamine oxidase is a dehydrogenase. Its reaction mechanism was examined using the enzyme partially purified from the soluble fraction of guinea pig liver and serotonin as substrate. It was separated from aldehyde dehydrogenase, showing that 5-hydroxyindoleacetaldehyde is the intermediate in the oxidation of serotonin to 5-hydroxyindoleacetic acid. The aldehyde was demonstrated by the formation of a colored product with 2,4-dinitrophenylhydrazine and also by its reaction with semicarbazide. The production of 5-hydroxyindoleacetic acid via 5-hydroxyindole-acetaldehyde was dependent on a NAD-linked aldehyde dehydrogenase (guinea pig kidney supernatant from high-speed centrifugation) (Weissbach, Redfield and Udenfriend, 1957). This enzyme system was applied to the metabolism of catecholamines. Catecholamines and their methoxy derivatives, such as (−)-norepinephrine, (+)-norepinephrine, (−)-epinephrine, (+)-epinephrine, 3,4-dihydroxyphenylethylamine, 3-methoxy-4-hydroxyphenylethylamine, 3,4-dimethoxyphenylethylamine, 3-methoxy-(±)-norepinephrine, were oxidized by the monoamine oxidase system. Using norepinephrine or epinephrine as substrate, 3,4-dihydroxyphenyl-glycolic aldehyde was identified as the product, and when sufficient NAD and aldehyde dehydrogenase was present, the formation of 3,4-dihydroxy-mandelic acid was proved (Leeper, Weissbach and Udenfriend, 1958). Based on these results, the reaction sequence in Fig. 23 was established.

In vivo, an intermediate catecholaldehyde, such as 3,4-dihydroxyphenylglycol aldehyde, can be converted either to a catechol acid, such as 3,4-dihydroxymandelic acid, by aldehyde dehydrogenase, or to catechol alcohol, such as 3,4-dihydroxyphenylglycole, by alcohol dehydrogenase (Axelrod, Kopin and Mann, 1959). Oxidation of the dopamine by mono-amine oxidase resulted in the formation of 3,4-dihydroxyphenylacetic acid (Rosengren, 1960).

The general mechanism of action of monoamine oxidase is assumed to be the following equation (Smith, Weissbach and Udenfriend, 1962).

$$
\underset{NH_2}{R-CH-R'} \xrightarrow[MAO]{O_2} \underset{\underset{+}{\overset{\|}{NH}}}{R-C-R'} \xrightarrow{H_2O} \underset{O}{R-C-R'+NH_3}
$$
$$
H_2O_2
$$

N,N-Dimethyltryptamine and N,N-dimethyltryptamine-N-oxide were found to be oxidized by a solubilized and partially purified monoamine oxidase preparation from guinea pig liver mitochondria. The possibility that monoamine oxidase is an oxygenase and the N-oxide an intermediate, was examined by incubating tritium-labeled N,N-dimethyltryptamine and H_2O^{18} with the enzyme preparation from guinea pig liver mitochondria. The results indicated that the N-oxide, although a unique substrate, is not an intermediate in the deamination of N,N-dimethylamines by monoamine oxidase (Smith, Weissbach and Udenfriend, 1962). It appears that the deamination of these N,N-dimethylamines proceeds through an imino compound as in other enzymatically catalyzed deaminations (Smith Weissbach and Udenfriend, 1962).

II. 4. 6. Inhibitors

The clinical application of monoamine oxidase inhibitors started with iproniazid (1-isonicotinyl-2-isopropylhydrazin phosphate), a hydrazine derivative of isonicotinic acid. Iproniazid was the first specific and potent inhibitor of monoamine oxidase discovered (Zeller, Barsky, Fouts, Kirchheimer and Van Orden, 1952; Zeller and Barsky, 1952). Numerous substances belonging to a great variety of chemical classes interfere with monoamine oxidase *in vitro* and in part also *in vivo* (Pletscher, Gey and Zeller, 1960; Pletscher, Gey and Burkard, 1965). Pletscher (1966) has presented a new and extensive review of monoamine oxidase inhibitors.

The structures of typical monoamine oxidase inhibitors are shown in Fig. 24. Hydrazine derivatives, tranylcypromine, pargyline, and modaline in general caused competitive, followed by non-competitive, irreversible inhibition of the enzyme. For this purpose, the drugs, with the exception of tranylcypromine, have to be metabolized to form the actual inhibitors (Pletscher, 1966). Harmaline and related compounds competitively inhibited monoamine oxidase towards serotonin. The inhibition was reversible both *in vitro* and *in vivo* (Udenfriend, Witkop, Redfield and Weissbach, 1958). Procedures based on the measurement of serotonin disappearance in rat liver homogenate *in vitro*, on endogenous brain levels of serotonin, and the conversion of serotonin to 5-hydroxyindoleacetic acid in whole mice were established to detect inhibitors of monoamine oxidase *in vitro* and *in vivo*. By using these procedures in unison, several potent inhibitors of the enzyme were found among many different classes (Ozaki, M., Weissbach, Ozaki, A., Witkop and Udenfriend, 1960). Rats pretreated with harmine (a reversible inhibitor) were effectively protected from the long active inhibitory effects of β-phenylisopropylhydrazine (JB-516), but

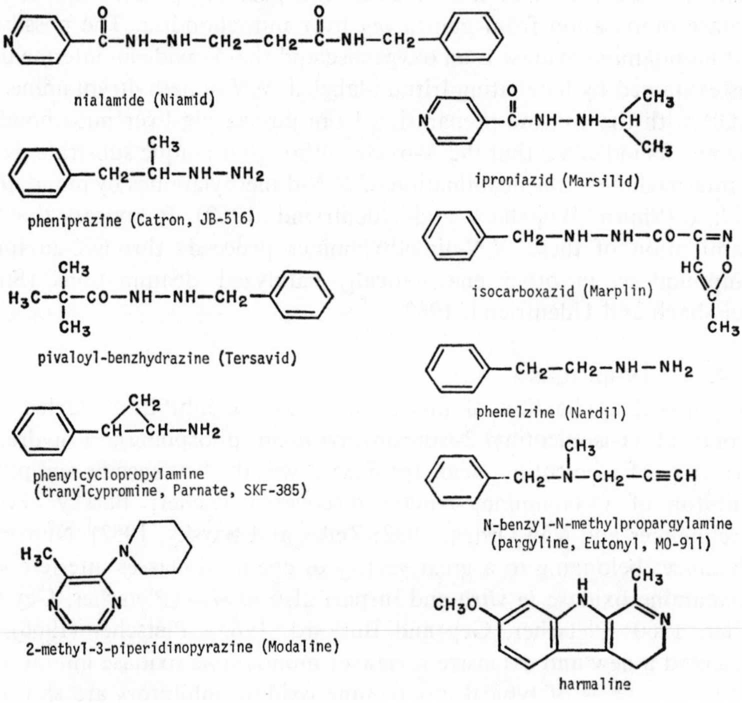

nialamide (Niamid)

pheniprazine (Catron, JB-516)

pivaloyl-benzhydrazine (Tersavid)

phenylcyclopropylamine
(tranylcypromine, Parnate, SKF-385)

2-methyl-3-piperidinopyrazine (Modaline)

iproniazid (Marsilid)

isocarboxazid (Marplin)

phenelzine (Nardil)

N-benzyl-N-methylpropargylamine
(pargyline, Eutonyl, MO-911)

harmaline

Fig. 24. Inhibitors of monoamine oxidase.

not readily from those of phenylcyclopropylamine (Horita and McGrath, 1960). The complete antagonism of β-phenylisopropylhydrazine (JB-516) by harmine resulted because the reversible inhibitors protected the enzyme from β-phenylisopropylhydrazine (Horita and Chinn, 1964).

An irreversible inhibitor, phenelzine-1-C[14], was found to act as a substrate and phenylacetic-1-C[14] acid was identified as the product, suggesting that degradation of the inhibitor was most likely accomplished by oxydative dehydrazination, a reaction mechanism previously not known to have a relationship to monoamine oxidase (Clineschmidt and Horita, 1969a). It was subsequently found that phenylacetic-1-C[14] acid was recovered as a major metabolite in urine from rats receiving phenelzine-1-C[14] intraperitoneally (Clineschmidt and Horita, 1969b).

Monoamine oxidase inhibitors were used clinically for the following disorders: psychiatric disorders, especially depression; angina pectoris and coronary disease; diseases of the gastrointestinal tract; and rheumatoid arthritis. The side effects were: orthostatic or postural hypotension; jaundice and liver toxicity; hypoglycemia and increased appetite; neurological changes ranging from peripheral neuropathy to psychomotor and behavioral syndromes (Giarman, 1959).

II. 4. 7. PHYSIOLOGICAL ROLE

Monoamine oxidase has an important physiological role in the oxidative deamination of biologically active monoamines such as catecholamines and serotonin (Davison, 1958). Both monoamine oxidase and catechol-O-methyltransferase are considered to be important for the metabolism of catecholamines. Upon administration of a monoamine oxidase inhibitor, the tissue levels of catecholamines in the brain were significantly increased (Spector, Prockop, Shore and Brodie, 1958). Rat liver had a high catechol-O-methyltransferase activity, whereas the brain and heart had a high monoamine oxidase activity. The administration of pyrogallol, a catechol-O-methyltransferase inhibitor, did not result in an increase of endogenous catecholamines in the brain and heart, but the administration of a monoamine oxidase inhibitor resulted in an increase. These results suggest that catechol-O-methyltransferase in the liver may be important for the inactivation of catecholamines in the blood, whereas monoamine oxidase may be important in the brain and heart for the metabolism of endogenous catecholamines (Crout, Creveling and Udenfriend, 1961).

The aldehydes formed from norepinephrine and serotonin by monoamine oxidase were found to be totally inactive when assayed on isolated smooth muscle preparations, and this inability was not due to impermeability to the smooth muscle (Renson, Weissbach and Udenfriend, 1964).

Gorkin and Orekhovitch (1967) reported an interesting observation on a new physiological role of monoamine oxidases. The effects of the products of oxidative deamination of tyramine catalyzed by rat liver mitochondrial monoamine oxidase on oxidation of succinate in mitochondrial fragments suggested possible monoamine oxidases participation in the regulation of tissue respiration.

It was suggested that thyroid monoamine oxidase may be a significant source of thyroidal hydrogen peroxide and may play a possible role in iodothyronin biosynthesis (Fischer, Schulz and Oliner, 1966).

It was reported that incubating dopamine with monoamine oxidase *in vitro* produced tetrahydropapaveroline which is a potent hypotensive agent (Holtz, Stock and Westermann, 1964; Kumagai, Matsui, Ogata, Yamada and Fukami, 1968). The formation of 3,4-dihydroxyphenylacetaldehyde from dopamine by monoamine oxidase produced a condensation reaction with dopamine to produce tetrahydropapaveroline. This reaction was demonstrated only *in vitro* (Holtz, Stock and Westermann, 1964) (Fig. 25).

Rat liver monoamine oxidase activity was higher in males than in females. These differences were less than 50% and could be reversed by

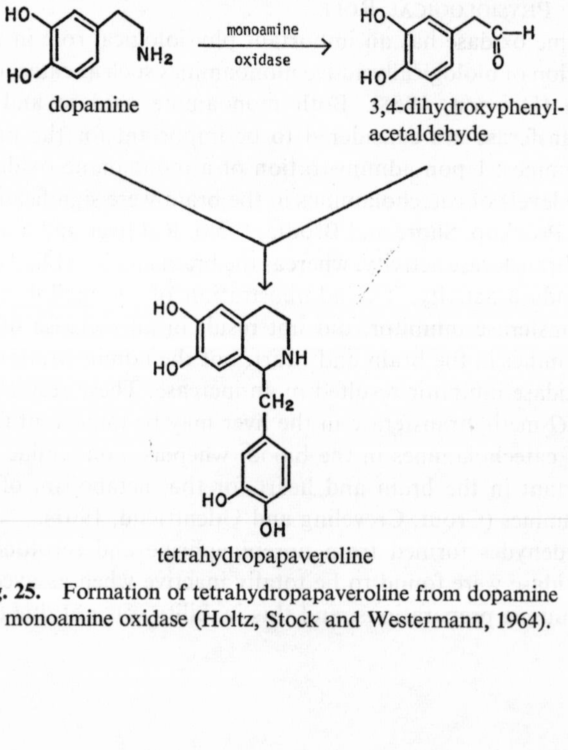

Fig. 25. Formation of tetrahydropapaveroline from dopamine by monoamine oxidase (Holtz, Stock and Westermann, 1964).

regular administration of an opposite sex steroid hormone. When the monoamine oxidase activity of rat heart was inhibited 90%, the rate of disappearance of norepinephrine-H^3 was reduced. However, 50% inhibition had no effect on this rate. It appears that to produce observable changes in cardiac norepinephrine-H^3, more than 50% of the metabolism of the monoamine oxidase activity must be inhibited. Since sex differences in monoamine oxidase activity are less than 50%, these differences are probably of little physiological significance (Wurtman and Axelrod, 1963).

When changes in flavin concentration and monoamine oxidase activity in the brain, liver and kidney during the development of rat was examined, a temporary halt in the development of flavins and monoamine oxidase activity during the first week of postnatal life was found to be characteristic in the brain (Kuzuya and Nagatsu, 1969a).

Reserpine treatment activated mitochondrial monoamine oxidase activity of guinea pig hearts. Reserpine may act on the mitochondrial membrane or structure to increase the penetration of norepinephrine to mitochondrial monoamine oxidase (Izumi, Oka, Yoshida and Imaizumi, 1967, 1969). This observation was confirmed, and reserpine was found to activate rat microsomal monoamine oxidase to a greater extent than the mitochondrial enzyme. It was suggested that oxidative deamination of reserpine-released catecholamine may take place within the microsome-like amine storage granule. Reserpine also inhibited aldehyde dehydrogenase, which may account for the increase of urinary alcohol metabolites of catecholamines after administration (Youdim and Sandler, 1968).

Prolonged isoproterenol administration increased the monoamine oxidase but not the cytochrome oxidase activity of rat salivary glands. It is suggested that the increased monoamine oxidase activity may be related to increased enzyme protein in the stimulated secretory cells (Mueller, de Champlain and Axelrod, 1968).

II. 5. Other Metabolic Pathways of Catecholamines

A catecholamine oxidase which oxidized epinephrine to adrenochrome was found in the salivary gland of cats and other mammals (Axelrod, 1964b). Enzyme activity was measured by trapping the unstable adrenochrome with β-phenylisopropylhydrazine (Fig. 26). The soluble supernatant fraction obtained from 20 mg of tissue was incubated with 0.1 ml of 0.5 M phosphate buffer (pH 7.0), 2 nmoles of epinephrine-H^3, 25 μl of 0.5 M MgCl$_2$ and 0.3 μmole of β-phenylisopropylhydrazine. After 30 min incubation at 37°C, 0.5 ml of 0.5 M borate buffer (pH 10) and 6 ml of

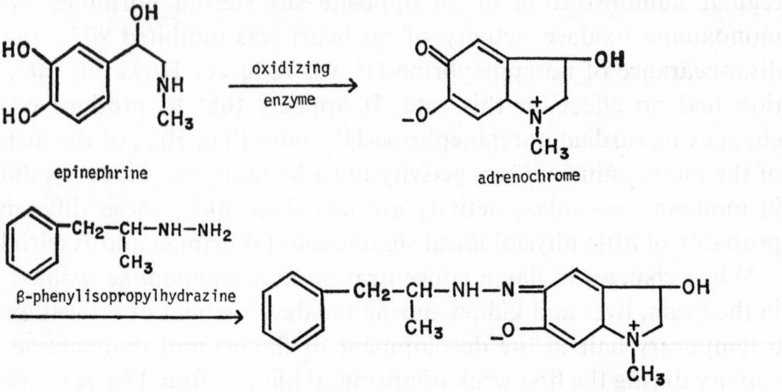

Fig. 26.　The enzymatic formation and trapping of adrenochrome
(Axelrod, 1964b).

toluene isoamyl alcohol (3:2, v/v) were added to the incubation mixture. After shaking for 5 min followed by centrifugation, a 4ml aliquot of the extract was transferred to a vial containing 1 ml ethanol and 10 ml scintillator solution and the radioactivity measured in a scintillation spectrometer. Boiled enzyme (100°C, 3 min) was used for a control incubation. Under the conditions described above, the adrenochrome-H^3 hydrazone was quantitatively extracted. This epinephrine oxidase could oxidize various catechols such as norepinephrine and dopamine. A small amount of serotonin appeared to be metabolized by the enzyme. The K_m value towards epinephrine was $3 \times 10^{-5} M$. The enzyme was highly localized in the parotid and submaxillary glands of cat, and the parotid gland of cat, rat, guinea pig, man and rabbit showed enzyme activity. When epinephrine-H^3 (1.2×10^7 cpm) was injected together with 5 mg/kg of β-phenylisopropyl-hydrazine into the carotid artery of the cat, large amounts of epinephrine and metanephrine were found in the parotid gland 5 min later. However, there was no measurable amount of adrenochrome present in the parotid gland, suggesting that the metabolic role of epinephrine oxidase *in vivo* may not be significant. This enzyme was found in a number of tissues including the skin, lung and various glandular tissues, but no activity was found in the liver and heart.

Enzymatic conversion of metanephrine to normetanephrine was observed by measuring the formaldehyde formed by *N*-demethylation (Axelrod, 1960b). Incubation of metanephrine with rabbit liver microsomes, the soluble supernatant, and NAD resulted in the formation of formaldehyde and normetanephrine. Guinea pig and rat liver also contained the metanephrine N-demethylating enzyme. This N-demethylation reaction could not be found *in vivo*.

N-Acetyldopamine and N-acetylnorepinephrine was found in human urine (Pryor, 1964; Sekeris, 1965). These metabolites are pharmacologically much less active than dopamine and norepinephrine so that the transacetylase (Sekeris and Herrlich, 1964), parallel to the transmethylase, may play an important role in the inactivation of the catecholamines. The presence of the transacetylase in the adrenal glands and the inhibitory action of N-acetyldopamine on DOPA decarboxylase suggest a possible regulatory role of N-acetyldopamine on the biosynthesis of catecholamines in the adrenals (Sekeris and Karlson, 1966).

II. 6. Storage, Release and Uptake of Catecholamines

II. 6. 1. ADRENAL MEDULLA

A. *Catecholamine storage granules in the adrenal medulla*
Epinephrine and norepinephrine in the adrenal medulla were found to be localized in specific intracellular storage granules, chromaffin granules (Blaschko and Welch, 1953; Hillarp, Lagerstedt and Nilson, 1953). The granules contained catecholamines, ATP, a specific protein named chromogranin, lipids and RNA (Hillarp, Högberg and Nilson, 1955; Hillarp, 1958a; Philippu and Schümann, 1963). Since molar ratio of catecholamines to ATP was approximately 4 : 1 (Hagen, 1959; Schümann and Philippu, 1961), one molecule of ATP which has four negative charges can be balanced with one positive charge of four molecules of catecholamines. The molar ratio of pure medullary granules from cattle was 4.5 : 1 (Hillarp, 1958a). If this ratio is valid, then about 10 % of the amines cannot be bound to ATP. This is in accordance with observations that after osmotic lysis of medullary granules of cattle, the entire amount of ATP was released but only 90 % of the catecholamines (Philippu and Schümann, 1964a).

The catecholamine granules were stored at 0°C in isotonic sucrose for several days without losing their catecholamine and ATP content (Schümann, 1966). This fact implies that the storage mechanism is not metabolically dependent. The catecholamine nucleotide complexes were studied by nuclear magnetic resonance spectroscopy (Weiner and Jardetzky, 1964). As a result, the hypothesis that catecholamines together with ATP and perhaps with intragranular protein form a nondiffusible storage-complex within the granules was proposed (Hillarp, 1958a). This hypothesis is summarized in the scheme shown in Fig. 27 (Schümann, 1966; Philippu and Schümann, 1966).

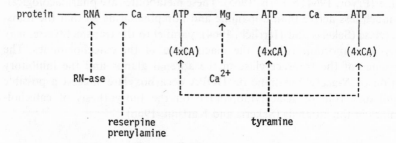

Fig. 27. A hypothesis on the storage complex of catecholamines (CA) with ATP, intragranular protein, RNA, Ca and Mg in the chromaffin granules of the adrenal medulla and on possible reaction mechanism of catecholamine releasers (Schümann, 1966; Philippu and Schümann, 1966).

It was shown that granules isolated from pheochromocytoma were relatively deficient in ATP (Schümann, 1960). Therefore, most catecholamines cannot be stored together with ATP as a complex, and they are probably bound to lipid or lipoprotein material in a granular structure (Euler, 1956; Schümann, 1966).

The interior surface of the chromaffin granules contained dopamine-β-hydroxylase activity (Kirshner, 1962). Dopamine may be taken up into the granules and hydroxylated to norepinephrine. Norepinephrine and epinephrine also were taken up into the granules. This catecholamine uptake process was different from the storage mechanism and was strongly dependent on a metabolic process. The addition of ATP and magnesium greatly accelerated the rate of catecholamine uptake (Carlsson, Hillarp and Waldeck, 1963; Kirshner, 1962) indicating the activation of an active transport mechanism. The catecholamine-containing granules had adenosine triphosphatase activity, the inhibition of which by N-ethylmaleimide suggested a role of the enzyme in the uptake of catecholamines (Kirshner, N., Kirshner, A.G. and Kamin, 1966).

During incubation of the granules at 37°C, a spontaneous release, dependent on temperature, of catecholamines together with ATP took place. The spontaneous release of amines and ATP was accompanied by the same percent loss of RNA. The results suggested that the release is initiated by an enzymatic decomposition of the storage complex. The addition of RNase produced an increased and dose-dependent release of catecholamines, ATP, and RNA to the same degree, but did not change the protein content (Philippu and Schümann, 1963; Schümann, 1966). The granular fraction contained, in addition to catecholamines, ATP, and RNA, sufficient RNase activity to catalyze the spontaneous release of RNA, catecholamines, and ATP at 37°C (Philippu and Schümann, 1964b). Calcium $(2.5 \times 10^{-3} M)$ was capable of releasing proportional amounts of catecholamines and ATP without affecting the RNA content of isolated medullary granules (Philippu and Schümann, 1962; Schümann and Philippu, 1963). Calcium, which was able to liberate catecholamines also from the intact medullary cell (Douglas and Rubin, 1961), was supposed to act directly on the storage complex by displacement of other divalent cations. The granules contained calcium as well as magnesium. One of the divalent cations, calcium plus magnesium, corresponded to 1 mole of ATP (Philippu and Schümann, 1964a). RNase, reserpine, and prenylamine (N-(3,3′-diphenylpropyl)-α-methylphenethylamine, Segontin) released catecholamines, ATP, calcium and magnesium from the granules. In contrast, tyramine released catecholamines exclusively.

Prenylamine

B. *Chromogranins*

Specific proteins, which are called chromogranins, were found in the chromaffin granules of ox, horse and pig adrenal medulla (Blaschko and Helle, 1963; Banks and Helle, 1965; Kirshner, N., Sage, Smith and Kirshner, A.G., 1966). Starch gel electrophoresis showed that the main protein component represented 49 % of the total soluble proteins from ox granules, 59.5 % from horse granules and 73.5 % from pig granules (Winkler, Ziegler and Strieder, 1966).

The identity of the main protein component from chromaffin granules of ox, horse, pig and sheep was proved immunologically (Helle, 1966b). Rabbit antisera was produced against soluble protein from bovine adrenal chromaffin granules, one rapidly reacting antigen was detected by both agar double diffusion and immunoelectrophoresis, while an additional, slowly reacting precipitation line was also observed using the former method. The precipitation line was supposed to be representative of a slow antigen reaction with a slowly diffusing aggregate of the first, strong antigen (Helle, 1966a).

The soluble protein in chromaffin granules may play an important role in the retention of low-molecular-weight components such as catechol-amines, ATP, and Mg^{++}. A nucleotide-free soluble protein preparation was seen to change its sedimentation properties and electrophoretic mobility in the presence of epinephrine, ATP and Mg^{++}. The changes were reversible and indicative of aggregate formation.

During the stimulation periods from isolated bovine adrenal glands dur-ing retrograde perfusion, 6.6 μmoles of catecholamines were secreted to-gether with 1 mg of extra protein in the perfusate. The extra protein re-leased during the stimulation periods was identified as the soluble protein of the chromaffin granules using immunological techniques (Banks and Helle, 1965). The soluble protein fractions of the chromaffin granules of the adrenal medulla were called "chromogranin(s)" (Blaschko, Comline, Schneider, Silver and Smith, 1967). The secretion of chromogranin from the adrenal medulla in the living animal was proved by examining adrenal venous blood from a calf during and between the periods of stimulation of the splanchnic nerve. The ratios of catecholamines (μmoles) to chromo-granin (mg) in the venous plasma during 5 min periods of splanchnic nerve stimulation were 3.3, 11.3 and 4.2. These ratios were of the same order of magnitude as that found for isolated chromaffin granules (10.1 $\pm$ 3.9). It was concluded that the secretion of a soluble protein (chromogranin) from chromaffin granules accompanies that of the catecholamines on stimula-tion of the splanchnic nerve *in vivo* (Blaschko, Comline, Schneider, Silver and Smith, 1967).

The soluble protein chromogranin from chromaffin granules of bovine adrenal medulla was completely purified by chromatography on columns of Sephadex G-75, G-100 or G-200 (Smith and Winkler, 1967b). The purification procedure by Smith and Winkler is shown in the flow chart below (Smith and Winkler, 1967a, b).

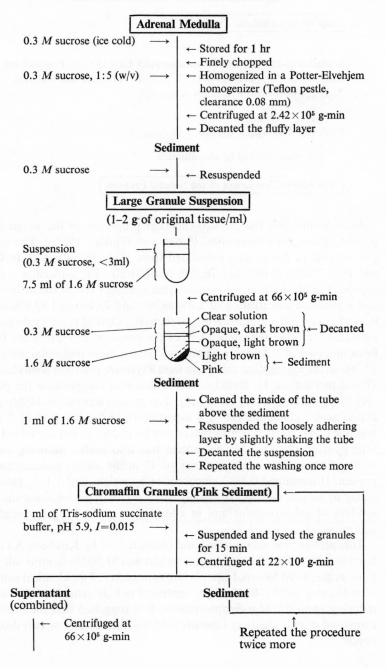

Adrenal Medulla

0.3 *M* sucrose (ice cold) ⟶
- ← Stored for 1 hr
- ← Finely chopped

0.3 *M* sucrose, 1:5 (w/v) ⟶
- ← Homogenized in a Potter-Elvehjem homogenizer (Teflon pestle, clearance 0.08 mm)
- ← Centrifuged at 2.42×10^5 g-min
- ← Decanted the fluffy layer

Sediment

0.3 *M* sucrose ⟶
- ← Resuspended

Large Granule Suspension

(1–2 g of original tissue/ml)

Suspension
(0.3 *M* sucrose, <3ml)

7.5 ml of 1.6 *M* sucrose

← Centrifuged at 66×10^5 g-min

0.3 *M* sucrose
- Clear solution
- Opaque, dark brown ⟩ ← Decanted
- Opaque, light brown

1.6 *M* sucrose
- Light brown ⟩ ← Sediment
- Pink

Sediment

← Cleaned the inside of the tube above the sediment

1 ml of 1.6 *M* sucrose ⟶
- ← Resuspended the loosely adhering layer by slightly shaking the tube
- ← Decanted the suspension
- ← Repeated the washing once more

Chromaffin Granules (Pink Sediment) ←

1 ml of Tris-sodium succinate
buffer, pH 5.9, $I=0.015$ ⟶
- ← Suspended and lysed the granules for 15 min
- ← Centrifuged at 22×10^5 g-min

Supernatant
(combined)

Sediment

← Centrifuged at 66×10^5 g-min

↑
Repeated the procedure twice more

| Supernatant (Soluble Lysate) |

|

Sephadex G-200 Column Chromatography 4.8×150 cm, Tris-sodium succinate buffer, pH 5.9, $I=0.015$, 10 ml/hr, Fraction size$=$6–8 ml, A_{280nm}, Folin-Lowry reaction A_{750nm}

|

Peak No. 2 in A_{280nm} (or No. 1 in A_{750nm})

| ← Concentrated by ultrafiltration

| The Major Component of the Soluble Proteins |

After purification the physico-chemical properties of the major component protein were determined (Smith and Winkler, 1967b). The molecular weights of the protein calculated from $S°_{20,w}$ in buffers of $I=0.015$ and $I=0.3$ were 76,610 and 76,880, respectively. The molecular weights measured by the approach-to-equilibrium method were 70,800 at $I=0.015$ and a protein concentration of 2.05 mg/ml, and 73,400 and 72,600 at $I=$ 0.3 and 2.4 mg/ml and 5.6 mg/ml, respectively. Optical rotatory dispersion indicated that approximately 14 % of the amino acid residues are in the form of an α-helix. Amino acid analysis gave a mean molecular weight of 77,390 on the assumption that there were 8 tyrosine residues, phenylalanine 11 and methionine 13. Based on the amino acid composition the partial specific volume value was 0.717 ml/g. The protein was rich in highly polar amino acids; glutamate (26 %), aspartate (8.35 %), lysine (9.43 %) and arginine (8.49 %). It was also rich in proline (8.56 %), but contained very little cyst(e)ine (0.35 %). The protein was also acidic; allowing for the amide groups, there was an excess of 43 acidic amino residues/mol of protein. It contained 0.5 % glucosamine by weight and 1.1 % galactosamine by weight, i.e., approximately two residues of glucosamine and four residues of galactosamine/mol in addition to about 2 % by weight of neutral sugars.

This protein was also purified and characterized by Kirshner, A.G. and Kirshner, N. (1969). The molecular weight was 81,200 in neutral salt solutions as measured by rapid equilibrium osmometry. Two identical subunits of molecular weight 40,600 were separated in 6 M guanidine-HCl with a reducing agent 0.2 M mercaptoethanol. It is suggested that the protein is composed of two identical subunits held together by one or two disulfide bonds.

C. *Mechanism of secretion of catecholamines from the adrenal medulla*
The mechanism of release of catecholamines from the chromaffin granules
of the adrenal medulla was extensively studied by Douglas (1968). Acetylcholine, which acts on the outside of the plasma membrane, stimulated the
chromaffin cells of the adrenal medulla to liberate the catecholamines,
epinephrine and norepinephrine. The following consequences of exposing
the chromaffin cell to acetylcholine were presented by Douglas (1968).

Interaction between acetylcholine and
the plasma membrane of the chromaffin cell

↓

Altered membrane chemistry (conformation?)

↓

Increased membrane permeability

↓

Entry of sodium and calcium ions

↓

Depolarization (without impulse formation)

↓

Catecholamine secretion

The term "stimulus-secretion coupling" was introduced by Douglas and
Rubin (1961) to embrace all the events occurring in the cell exposed to its
immediate stimulus (acetylcholine) that lead finally to the appearance of
the characteristic secretory product (catecholamines). The ratio of catecholamines to ATP and metabolites recovered in the venous effluent from
the perfused adrenals was similar to that found in the granules. Since
chemical evidences suggest that the membranes of the chromaffin granules
are retained, the chromaffin granules may not be extruded intact during the
secretion. Two possible mechanism of catecholamine secretion from the
adrenal medulla were presented by Douglas (1968). Both mechanisms in-
volve release directly from chromaffin granules to the cell exterior either
through frank rupture of the adherent membranes of chromaffin granule
and cell (exocytosis) or through some greatly increased permeability at the
site of adhesion. In both instances, emptied granule membranes are retained within the cell after evacuation of their soluble contents (Douglas,
1968).

Recent finding of dopamine-β-hydroxylase secretion with norepinephrine after stimulation of the splenic nerve supports the release of norepinephrine from the sympathetic nerve terminals also by exocytosis of synaptic vesicles (Weinshilboum, Thoa, Johnson, Kopin and Axelrod, 1971).

II. 6. 2. SYMPATHETIC NERVES

A. *Catecholamine-storing nerve granules*
Catecholamine-storing granules similar to but smaller than medullary granules were found in bovine splenic nerves and rat spleen (Euler and Hillarp, 1956). The granules contained ATP, and had the same molar ratio of catecholamine to ATP as medullary granules; about 4 : 1 (Schümann, 1958a; Euler, Lishajko and Stjärne, 1963). Just as with the medullary granule membrane, the nerve granule membrane was freely permeable to catecholamines at 0°C (Stjärne, 1964). The catecholamine uptake mechanism in the nerve granule was potentiated by ATP (Euler and Lishajko, 1963a) and inhibited by reserpine (Euler and Lishajko, 1963b; Euler, Stjärne and Lishajko, 1963). Although the properties of the nerve granules are similar to those of adrenal medullary granules, the nerve granules are different in many respects. They were more resistant to osmotic changes and to freezing and thawing (Euler and Lishajko, 1961a; Stjärne, 1964), and the catecholamine turnover rate, as determined by measurement of the rate of exchange of endogenous for exogenous catecholamine on incubation *in vitro* in the presence of $(\pm)$-norepinephrine-H^3, was about 10 times higher in nerve granules (Stjärne, 1964, 1966b). Ca^{++} accelerated the spontaneous rate of amine release in the medullary granules, but had no effect on the nerve or heart granules (Schümann, Schnell and Philippu, 1964).

The dopamine-β-hydroxylase activity was demonstrated in the granules from rat heart (Potter and Axelrod, 1963b), from guinea pig and pig heart (Nagatsu, van der Schoot, Levitt and Udenfriend, 1968), and from rat vas deferens (Austin, Livett and Chubb, 1967).

Incubation of nerve granules with tyrosine did not result in the formation of either dopamine or norepinephrine, either with or without addition of tetrahydropterin (a cofactor for tyrosine hydroxylase). The whole nerve homogenate was capable of synthesizing dopamine or norepinephrine from tyrosine (Stjärne, 1966b). These results suggest that the formation of DOPA from tyrosine *in vivo* may occur on the outside of the granules during the passage of tyrosine through the axonal membrane, while the nerve granules carry out the last two steps in norepinephrine synthesis, the decarboxylation of DOPA and the β-hydroxylation of dopamine (Stjärne, 1966b). On the other hand, there are indications that tyrosine hydroxylase in the caudate nucleus may be localized in the synaptic vesicles of the nerve endings (Fahn, Rodman and Côté, 1969; Nagatsu, T. and Nagatsu, I., 1970). The problem of intracellular localization of enzymes in catecholamine biosynthesis remains to be further elucidated.

B. *Release and uptake of catecholamines in the nerve*

Various agents ("releasers") can cause a net decrease in the norepinephrine content of the nerve granules. On incubation *in vitro* tyramine caused an acceleration of the spontaneous decrease in the catecholamine content of the splenic nerve granules (Euler and Lishajko, 1960; Schümann and Philippu, 1961) and of the bovine medullary granules (Schümann and Philippu, 1961). It is suggested that tyramine acts by competing for uptake into the granules with spontaneously released norepinephrine molecules (Stjärne, 1966a). The spontaneous catecholamine release seems to be a prerequisite for amine uptake (Stjärne, 1966a), as indicated by reserpine experiments which showed that reserpine strongly retards the spontaneous release of norepinephrine from isolated nerve granules (Euler and Lishajko, 1963b). However, reserpine did not affect spontaneous amine release from bovine adrenal medullary granules, but strongly inhibited amine uptake (Kirshner, Rorie and Kamin, 1963).

The norepinephrine uptake mechanism of the nerve granules satisfied Michaelis-Menten kinetics and preferred ($-$)- to ($+$)-norepinephrine and a number of amines competitively inhibited norepinephrine uptake. The preference of ($-$)-norepinephrine to ($+$)-norepinephrine was of the order of 6 to 1 (Stjärne, 1966). After the injection of ($\pm$)-norepinephrine-H^3 to rat, there was more than ten times the amount ($-$)-norepinephrine-H^3 than ($+$)-norepinephrine-H^3 in the rat heart (Maickel, Beaven and Brodie, 1963). Studies in the isolated rat heart perfused with low concentrations of ($-$)- and ($+$)-norepinephrine showed that the rate of uptake of ($-$)-norepinephrine was several times more rapid than that of ($+$)-norepinephrine (Iversen, 1963). The affinity for ($-$)-norepinephrine was almost five times greater than that for ($+$)-norepinephrine (($-$)-norepinephrine : $K_m = 2.7 \times 10^{-7} M$, $V_{max} = 0.20$ $\mu g/min/g$ heart; ($+$)-norepinephrine : $K_m = 1.39 \times 10^{-6} M$, $V_{max} = 0.29$ $\mu g/min/g$ heart) (Iversen, 1967). However, when high concentrations of substrate were used, the rate of uptake was inversely related to the affinity of the substrate for the uptake site in the membrane transport processes (Wilbrandt and Rosenberg, 1961). In the isolated rat heart the rate of uptake of ($+$)-norepinephrine was equal or greater than the rate of uptake of ($-$)-norepinephrine at high concentrations. The demonstration of a stereochemically specific uptake of catecholamines thus depends on the use of small doses of catecholamines (Iversen, 1967).

Compounds more or less closely related to norepinephrine, such as sympathomimetic amines (Musacchio, Kopin and Weise, 1965) and guanethidine (Chang, Costa and Brodie, 1965), were taken up and retained in the granules, either unchanged or after β-hydroxylation.

Guanethidine

The affinity for binding in the nerve granules in the decreasing order was reported as follows: norepinephrine, dopamine, and octopamine. Therefore, it was suggested that the catechol and β-hydroxy groups are important for binding in the nerve granules (Musacchio, Kopin and Weise, 1965; Kopin, 1966). Non-β-hydroxylated derivatives, such as tyramine, were not bound by the storage granules, but were β-hydroxylated to compounds that are stored (octopamine from tyramine) (Kopin, 1966). Such stored compounds, whether formed spontaneously or after the administration of precursors, can be released by nerve stimulation and act as "false neurochemical transmitters" (Kopin, 1966).

In further experiments on the uptake of catecholamines in the isolated perfused rat heart a second type of uptake (Uptake 2) was discovered (Iversen, 1965a, b, 1967). When hearts were perfused with very high concentrations of epinephrine or norepinephrine (1 – 40 μg/ml), a surprisingly rapid uptake of catecholamine occurred. Initial rates of epinephrine uptake in isolated rat heart with increasing epinephrine concentrations showed the emergence of a second type of uptake mechanism (Uptake 2) as the perfusion concentration rose above 0.5 μg/ml. The initial rates of uptake of epinephrine and norepinephrine at various perfusion concentrations were described by Michaelis-Menten kinetics. "Uptake 2" differed in several respects from the uptake mechanism at low catecholamine concentrations (Uptake 1) : (1) Uptake 2 had a higher affinity for epinephrine than norepinephrine, whereas Uptake 1 favoured the accumulation of norepinephrine; (2) In contrast to Uptake 1, the catecholamines accumulated by Uptake 2 disappeared rapidly from the tissue if perfusion was continued with a catecholamine-free medium, although a residue of approximately 2 μg/g tissue remained in the heart even after prolonged periods of wash-out; (3) Uptake 1 had stereo-chemical specificity whereas Uptake 2 proved to have no stereo-chemical specificity; (4) There were striking differences in the drug sensitivities of the two catecholamine uptake processes. In almost every respect the structural requirements for inhibition of Uptake 2 differed from those of Uptake 1 (Iversen, 1967).

The functional significance of two catecholamine uptake mechanisms may be different. Uptake 1 may be an important inactivation process of norepinephrine in the sympathetically innervated tissues in which it is released. Acetylcholinesterase is responsible for inactivation of acetylcholine at the cholinergic nerve endings. In analogy to this, with the inactivation of norepinephrine, monoamine oxidase and catechol-O-methyltransferase were considered to be the enzymes. However, the discovery of a specific and rapid mechanism for the uptake of catecholamines in sympathetic nerve endings led to the view that it is this uptake process which is responsible for the rapid removal of free norepinephrine and epinephrine from the vicinity of adrenergic receptors and from circulation (Iversen, 1965b).

It was once suggested that an uptake of norepinephrine from circulation might serve to replenish the catecholamine stores in tissues. However, it is not likely that this is an important mechanism for maintaining a constant level of norepinephrine in sympathetically innervated tissues. Sympathetic nerve endings contain all the enzymes necessary for the biosynthesis of norepinephrine and can synthesize norepinephrine rapidly enough to maintain it at a constant level. The portions of norepinephrine in rat heart either synthesized locally or taken up from circulation were measured according to the specific activity of norepinephrine after long periods of continuous infusion of norepinephrine-C^{14}. It was concluded that no more than 20% of the norepinephrine in the heart could normally be derived from an uptake from circulation (Kopin and Gordon, 1963; Kopin, Gordon and Horst, 1965). In demedullated animals the norepinephrine content of peripheral tissues was unaffected (Strömblad and Nickerson, 1961; Bhagat and Shideman, 1964). However, under abnormal conditions, the uptake of norepinephrine from the circulation may also be important. It is also possible that the small amounts of epinephrine found in peripheral tissues may originate, at least in part, from an uptake of circulating epinephrine (Strömblad and Nickerson, 1961).

The functional significance of Uptake 2 (Iversen, 1965a) is still unknown. It is possible that Uptake 2 but not Uptake 1 is present over the whole surface of the postganglionic sympathetic neurone (Iversen,

1967). After the administration of large doses of norepinephrine, exogenous norepinephrine accumulated in the cell bodies and preterminal axons; after small dose of norepinephrine, however, an accumulation of norepinephrine was observed only in the terminal regions of the axons (Hamberger, Malmfors, Norberg and Sachs, 1964; Norberg and Hamberger, 1964).

Epinephrine or norepinephrine which is secreted from the adrenal medulla is transported to the target organs by circulation. When norepinephrine-H^3 or epinephrine-H^3 was injected intravenously, a substantial proportion of the injected dose was found to be rapidly transferred from the circulatory system into peripheral tissues (Axelrod, Weil-Malherbe and Tomchick, 1959; Whitby, Axelrod and Weil-Malherbe, 1961, Axelrod, 1963b). The exogenously administered catecholamines were preferentially taken up in various sympathetically innervated organs, such as the heart, spleen, and salivary glands. The smallest uptake was seen in the muscle. The accumulation of norepinephrine in tissues was found to be greater than that of epinephrine.

After the intravenous administration of a relatively smaller dose of nc-epinephrine-H^3 or epinephrine-H^3 (0.1 mg/kg) to mice, the unchanged hormone disappeared in two phases. In the first 5 min after injection, there was a rapid disappearance of the catecholamines and the remaining disappeared slowly thereafter. Detectable amounts of unchanged epinephrine were present in animals killed several hours after the original injection (Axelrod, Weil-Malherbe and Tomchick, 1959; Whitby, Axelrod and Weil-Malherbe, 1961). The specific radioactivity of norepinephrine-H^3 in the organs declined exponentially and biphasically (Axelrod, 1964a). It was found that when a small amount of $(\pm)$-norepinephrine-H^3 (<0.10 μg/kg) was administered, the specific radioactivity of norepinephrine-H^3 in tissues decreased exponentially but in a single phase (Costa, Boullin, Hammer, Vogel and Brodie, 1966).

The catecholamines taken up in the tissues proved to be stored in sympathetic nerves. After surgical sympathectomy by superior cervical ganglionectomy, the uptake of catecholamines in tissues innervated by this ganglion was severely reduced (Hertting, Axelrod, Kopin and Whitby, 1961; Strömblad and Nickerson, 1961; Fischer, Kopin and Axelrod, 1965). The uptake of norepinephrine in sympathectomized heart either by ganglionectomy (Hertting and Schiefthaler, 1964; Hertting, 1965) or by autotransplantation (Potter, Cooper, Willman and Wolfe, 1965) was also severely impaired. The development of the sympathetic nervous system was suppressed by the administration of nerve growth factor antiserum to newborn animals. This procedure is called "immunosympathectomy" (Levi-Montalcini and Angeletti, 1966). The uptake of norepinephrine was markedly reduced in various tissues of immunosympathectomized rats and mice (Sjökvist, Titus, Michelson, Taylor and Richardson, 1965; Zaimis, Berk and Callingham, 1965; Iversen, Glowinski and Axelrod, 1965b). A marked reduction in the endogenous norepinephrine content of various peripheral tissues such as the heart, spleen and lungs in immunosympathectomized mice and rats was reported (Levi-Montalcini and Angeletti, 1962; Zaimis, Berk and Callingham, 1965). However, no changes were detected in the norepinephrine content in the central nervous system of the same animals.

C. *Extragranular pool of norepinephrine*

The presence of an extragranular and intraaxonal pool of norepinephrine *in vivo* is a generally assumed possibility. A small fraction of norepinephrine is always recovered in the soluble supernatant and recovery in a particle-bound form is dependent on the technique of homogenization. Gentle homogenization of bovine splenic nerve tissue with an Ultra Turrax homogenizer was found to yield a recovery of up to 60 % of particle-bound norepinephrine (Stjärne, 1966a). Therefore, a gentler homogenization procedure might lead to a recovery of 100 % of norepinephrine in the particulate fraction. However, some norepinephrine is thought to exist extragranularly in the axons at least temporarily, since otherwise exogenous norepinephrine could never reach the granules (Stjärne, 1966a). "Free" and "extragranular" norepinephrine does not imply a free solution and distribution throughout the axoplasm, but the extragranular norepinephrine may be protected in the axon by a different mechanism, possibly by lipid binding (Euler, 1946a).

II. 6. 3. BRAIN

A. *Catecholamine-storing granules in the brain*

Intracellular distribution of norepinephrine and dopamine in the brain was extensively studied by Whittaker (1966) and de Robertis (1966) and a particular norepinephrine was found in brain homogenate (Weil-Malherbe and Bone, 1957c; Bertler, Hillarp and Rosengren, 1960). Norepinephrine of dog hypothalamus was also found by Whittaker (1966) to be localized in granular fractions containing nerve endings (Chruściel, 1960). A similar finding was obtained with rat brain stem (Levi and Maynert, 1964) and rat whole brain (Potter and Axelrod, 1963b), and was further confirmed by Inouye, Kataoka and Shinagawa (1963). The granular fractions were separated by sucrose density gradient centrifugation, and the norepine-phrine-storing granules were identified as nerve ending particles or "synaptosomes" (Whittaker, Michaelson and Kirkland, 1964) which are derived from pinched-off presynaptic nerve terminals. Nerve ending particles showing the fluorescent histochemical reaction were shown to be concentrated in the synaptosome fraction (Masuoka, 1965).

The subcellular localization of dopamine in caudate nucleus was somewhat equivocal (Laverty, Michaelson, Sharman and Whittaker, 1963) as about 40 % of the dopamine was particle-bound, and only about 25 % of this was recoverable in the synaptosome fraction. The remainder was present in the myelin fraction, the crude nuclear fraction, and the microsomal fraction. This finding, however, is not conclusive evidence against a localization of dopamine in nerve endings (Whittaker, 1966).

Synaptosomes were disrupted by suspension in water (the hypotonic treatment) and separated into a series of fractions containing, respectively, soluble constituents of the synaptosome cytoplasma, synaptic vesicles, external synaptosome membranes and intraterminal mitochondria (Whittaker, 1966; Whittaker, Michaelson and Kirkland, 1964). When a water-treated preparation, prepared in the absence of anticholinesterase was separated on the density gradient, 30–50 % of the stable-bound acetyl-choline was found in the synaptic vesicle fraction (Whittaker, 1966). Significant amounts of stable-bound norepinephrine were also associated with microvesicular storage granules. For dopamine, definite evidence of localization in microvesicular storage granules within nerve terminals is lacking so far (Whittaker, 1966).

Intracellular distribution of catecholamines and the related enzyme was also extensively studied using electron microscopy and subcellular fractionation techniques by de Robertis' group (de Robertis, 1966). In the hypothalamus, two types of vesicles were found by electron microscopy; clear vesicles ranging between 200 and 800 Å with a mean diameter of 510 Å and the granulated vesicles ranging between 700 and 1,700 Å with a mean of about 1,300 Å. These special granulated vesicles of the anterior hypothalamus proved to be catecholamine stores (de Robertis, Pellegrino de Iraldi, Rodríguez de Lores Arnaiz and Zieher, 1965; Matsuoka, Ishii, Shimizu and Imaizumi, 1965). De Robertis' cell fractionation procedure involved a mild homogenization of the brain and the separation of the four primary fractions : nuclear, mitochondrial, microsomal, and soluble. The mitochondrial fraction containing intact nerve endings, free mitochondria and myelin, further separated on a sucrose-density gradient into five sub-fractions. On the other hand, the mitochondrial fraction also subjected to hypotonic treatment, resulting in the swelling and bursting of the nerve endings with release of the synaptic vesicles and other components (de Robertis, 1966) which were further separated by centrifugation. Norepinephrine and dopamine were concentrated in the mitochondrial and microsomal fractions. About 50 % of norepinephrine and 45 % of dopamine were present in the mitochondrial fraction and dopamine was more soluble than norepinephrine. 5-Hydroxytryptophan decarboxylase, which is identical to DOPA decarboxylase, was mainly soluble, but a large portion of the bound enzyme was present in the mitochondrial fraction. Catechol-O-methyltransferase was also mainly soluble, but was also present in the mitochondrial fraction. Monoamine oxidase was mainly found in the mitochondrial fraction. After further subfractionation of the mitochondrial fraction, norepinephrine and dopamine were concentrated in the nerve-endings-rich fraction and there was a higher concentration of norepinephrine. Monoamine oxidase was localized in mitochondria, whereas 5-hydroxytryptophan decarboxylase and catechol-O-methyltransferase were localized in the nerve ending fractions. After hypotonic treatment of the mitochondrial fraction, norepinephrine and dopamine were concentrated in synaptic vesicles released from the nerve endings. 5-Hydroxytryptophan decarboxylase and catechol-O-methyltransferase were found in the soluble fraction while monoamine oxidase remained with the intraterminal mitochondria (de Robertis, 1966). It was concluded that norepinephrine and dopamine (de Robertis, Pellegrino de Iraldi, Rodríguez de Lores Arnaiz and Zieher, 1965) and also 5-hydroxytryptamine (Maynert, Levi and de Lorenzo, 1965) are localized in synaptic vesicles.

The subcellular distribution of tyrosine hydroxylase in the brain remains to be elucidated. Tyrosine hydroxylase in the bovine caudate nucleus was particle-bound and had relatively high specific activities in the nerve ending fractions and in the synaptic vesicle fraction (Fahn, Rodman and Côté, 1969; Nagatsu, T. and Nagatsu, I., 1970).

B. *Synthesis, storage and release of catecholamines in the brain*
Catecholamines cannot get into the brain from the blood because of the presence of the "blood-brain barrier." When norepinephrine-H[3] or epinephrine-H[3] was administered intravenously, the amine did not penetrate into the brain, except into the hypothalamic area where the blood-brain barrier does not exist (Weil-Malherbe, Axelrod and Tomchick, 1959; Weil-Malherbe, Whitby and Axelrod, 1961). Amino acids, such as phenylalanine, tyrosine, or DOPA can pass through the blood-brain barrier. The catecholamines in the brain are synthesized locally from the amino

acid precursor, tyrosine. When catecholamines are administered in the ventricles, they can be taken up by the brain tissues and metabolized. After norepinephrine-C^{14} was injected into the lateral ventricle of a cat, normetanephrine, 3-methoxy-4-hydroxymandelic acid, 3-methoxy-4-hydroxyphenylglycol were identified in the brain (Mannarino, Kirshner and Nashold, 1963). Similar experiments were reported with rat brain by using dopamine-C^{14} and norepinephrine-C^{14} for intraventricular injection (Milhaud and Glowinski, 1962, 1963). Normetanephrine was found in the brain after the administration of a monoamine oxidase inhibitor (Axelrod, 1958).

One hour after the administration of physiological doses (0.13 μg) of norepinephrine-H^3 in the lateral ventricle of the rat brain, the injected norepinephrine disappeared very rapidly from the site of injection; about half of the radioactive norepinephrine was taken up and remained in the brain; the other half disappeared after reaching the systemic circulation as unchanged norepinephrine and metabolites (Glowinski, Kopin and Axelrod, 1965; Glowinski and Axelrod, 1966). The norepinephrine which is taken up by the brain appears to be bound to the tissue and it is possible that the bound norepinephrine is stored in the synaptic vesicles of the nerve endings. The bound norepinephrine disappeared slowly from the brain in a multiple fashion, which suggests that the norepinephrine may be stored in more than one compartment. A large rapidly released store had a half-life of 3 hr, whereas that of a smaller and more firmly bound store was 17 hr.

Endogenous catecholamines in the guinea pig brain were labeled by administering the precursor amino acid L-tyrosine-C^{14} or DL-DOPA-H^3. The half-life of brain dopamine was about 2.5 hr, and that of brain norepinephrine about 4 hr. The rate of synthesis was calculated to be at least 0.03–0.04 μg/g/hr or 2.4 μg/day for the whole guinea pig brain (Udenfriend and Zaltzman-Nirenberg, 1963). Similar results on the disappearance of radioactive norepinephrine formed from radioactive precursors injected peripherally in mouse brain were also reported. DL-DOPA-H^3, L-tyrosine-H^3, and DL-tyrosine-3-C^{14} were administered to male mice intravenously, and the decrease in the specific radioactivities of catecholamines in the brain, heart, liver, spleen and adrenals was measured. The half-lives was 4–8 hr at the initial fast disappearance, and 18 hr at the second slow disappearance. The half-life in the adrenals was about 1 week (Burack and Draskóczy, 1964). The long half-life of epinephrine in the adrenal gland was first discovered by Udenfriend, Cooper, Clark and Baer (1953).

Studies involving the measurement of the radioactive metabolite present in the urine after the administration of norepinephrine-H^3 in the lateral ventricle indicate that there is a blood-brain barrier not only for the entry but also for the excit of the catecholamine (Glowinski, Kopin and Axelrod, 1965; Glowinski and Axelrod, 1966).

Chapter III

Assay Methods for Enzymes Related to Catecholamine Synthesis and Metabolism

III. 1. Assay of Phenylalanine Hydroxylase Activity

Crude phenylalanine hydroxylase enzyme preparations contain both dihydropteridine reductase and the reduced pteridine cofactor. For a purified phenylalanine hydroxylase enzyme preparation, it is necessary to add a preparation of dihydropteridine reductase and a tetrahydropteridine cofactor (also a NADPH-generating system). This tetrahydropteridine-generating system can be replaced by a tetrahydropteridine and certain reductants such as dithiothreitol or mercaptoethanol.

III. 1. 1. ASSAY BASED ON A COLORIMETRIC OR FLUOROMETRIC DETERMINATION OF TYROSINE

A. *Method by Kaufman* (1962 c)
Tyrosine formed from phenylalanine was determined colorimetrically by a nitrosonaphthol procedure of Udenfriend and Cooper (1952b). The incubation mixture (1.0 ml) contained in μmoles: L-phenylalanine, 2; potassium phosphate buffer (pH 6.8), 100; NADP, 0.25; glucose, 250; glusoce dehydrogenase, in excess; sheep liver enzyme (dihydropteridine reductase); a pteridine cofactor (tetrahydrobiopterin); and enzyme solution to be assayed. The mixture was incubated at 25°C for 30 min with shaking in air. The reaction was stopped by the addition of 2.0 ml of 12 % trichloroacetic acid. A zero time control, where the trichloroacetic acid was added prior to any of the enzymes, served as a blank. The precipitated protein was removed by centrifugation, and tyrosine was determined on a 2.0 ml aliquot of the supernatant fluid (see the colorimetric or the fluorometric method for the assay of tyrosine, section IV. 11).

Two potential difficulties in application of the assay method to crude tissue preparations were pointed out. If under the conditions of the assay tyrosine is metabolized much faster than it is formed, hydroxylase activity may not be detected. This can be checked by a control in which tyrosine disappearance is determined under the assay conditions. A second source of error may be encountered if significant amounts of phenolic materials are formed from precursors present in the crude tissue. In this situation, the hydroxylase activity can be checked by the chromatographic procedure described in the next section.

B.   *A direct assay based on the non-enzymatic regeneration of 6,7-dimethyl-tetrahydropterin* (Bublitz, 1969)

This assay is based on the observation that dithiothreitol not only regenerates tetrahydropteridine from dihydropteridine (quinoid form) but also effectively destroys peroxide formed during the aerobic oxidation of the tetrahyropteridine.

phenylalanine + O_2 + 6,7-dimethyltetrahydropterin
$\longrightarrow$ tyrosine + H_2O + 6,7-dimethyldihydropterin (quinoid form)

6,7-dimethyldihydropterin (quinoid form) + dithiothreitol
$\longrightarrow$ 6,7-dimethyltetrahydropterin + oxidized dithiothreitol

The standard system (0.1 ml) contained in μmoles: Tris-HCl (pH 7.2), 100; freshly prepared dithiothreitol, 10; 6,7-dimethyltetrahydropterin (DMPH$_4$), 0.4; L-phenylalanine, 2; and enzyme. The complete system except DMPH$_4$ was incubated for 5 min at 25°C. DMPH$_4$ was then added and the system was incubated for 20 min at 25°C with shaking in air. The reaction was stopped by the addition of 2 ml of 12% trichloroacetic acid. Tyrosine in 2ml aliquots of the deproteinized solution was estimated colorimetrically (Udenfriend and Cooper, 1952b) or fluorometrically (Waalkes and Udenfriend, 1957) (see section IV. 11).

III. 1. 2.   ASSAY BASED ON THE RADIOASSAY OF TYROSINE BY CHROMATOGRAPHIC SEPARATION (1) (Kaufman, 1969)

The incubation mixture (0.2 ml) contained in μmoles: potassium phosphate buffer (pH 6.8), 30; L-phenylalanine-C^{14}, 0.4 (0.2 μCi); NADPH, 0.05; NAD, 0.05; nicotinamide, 1.0; glucose, 10.0; dihydropteridine reductase in excess; glucose dehydrogenase in excess (The glucose dehydrogenase fractions contained catalase. If another reduced pyridine-nucleotide generating system is used, catalase should be added separately.); enzyme solution to be assayed; 6,7-dimethyltetrahydropterin (DMPH$_4$), 0.06; and water made up to a final volume of 0.2 ml. A tube containing the complete reaction mixture but with an extract that had been boiled for 90 sec before the addition of the other components served as the control. The mixture was incubated for 1 hr with shaking at 25°C. The reaction was stopped by the addition of 0.02 ml of 3 M trichloroacetic acid, and the tubes were then placed in an ice bath for 5–10 min. The tubes were then centrifuged and 0.02- to 0.04-ml aliquots of the clear supernatant fluid were applied under a stream of warm air to Whatman 3 MM paper. Tyrosine and phenylalanine standards were spotted on top of a separate aliquot of one of the deproteinized reaction mixtures and after development, the appropriate strip was sprayed with a ninhydrin solution to locate the tyrosine and phenylalanine on the chromatogram. The paper was developed for 15–17 hr at room temperature in 2-propanol/ water/ NH_4OH (8:1:1, v/v/v). After drying in air, the paper was cut into 1.0 × 2.6-cm pieces. The pieces were placed in vials containg 10 ml of Bray's scintillation solution plus 1.0 ml of water, and the radioactivity was determined by a liquid scintillation spectrometer after the paper was suspended in aqueous Bray's solution for 2–3 hr. The amount of enzyme-dependent tyrosine formation was calculated from the radioactivity in the tyrosine area of the chromatogram, corrected for the radioactivity in the same area of the control strip.

This assay procedure was sensitive enough to quantitatively determine hydroxylase activity in the usual 5 to 20 mg liver sample obtained by needle biopsy. Liver samples were placed in a vial with 3 vol of cold 0.12 M KCl and immediately frozen until it was ready to be assayed. For assaying, the tissue-KCl mixture was thawed and transferred to a glass grinder and gently homogenized by hand. Another 15–17 vol of 0.15 M KCl (based on the original weight of liver) were added and the mixture was stirred, transferred to a centrifuge tube, and centrifuged for 20 min at 6,000 × g. The supernatant fluid was used for the assay. For a 60-min incubation period, 0.25 mg of extract protein gave 24.2 nmoles of tyrosine formed. The mean specific activity of phenylalanine hydroxylase in three different control human liver samples obtained by open biopsy was 76 ± 14 μmoles tyrosine formed/g protein/60 min, or 1.27 ± 0.23 nmoles/min/mg protein (Kaufman, 1969).

III. 1. 3. Assay Based on the Radioassay of Tyrosine by Chromato-graphic Separation (2) (Justice, O'Flynn and Hsia, 1967)

Fresh liver was homogenized with three volumes of 0.15 M KCl. The homogenate was centrifuged at 16,000 × g for 15 min, and the supernatant fluid was immediately used for assay. The incubation mixture (0.15 ml) contained in μmoles: L-phenylalanine-U-C^{14} (2 mCi/mmole), 0.01; L-phenylalanine, 0.19; NADH, 0.25; nicotinamide, 0.5; $DMPH_4$, 0.23; enzyme, 0.01 ml; phosphate buffer (0.2 M, pH 7.0). Incubation was carried out at 25°C for 45 min and the reaction was stopped by the addition of 12 % trichloroacetic acid. The reaction mixture was centrifuged at 2,000 × g and 100 μl of supernatant was applied to Whatman paper No. 3. Ascending chromatography was carried out in a solvent system using 2-propanol/

water/ammonium hydroxide (8:1:1, v/v/v) for 18 hr. The paper was cut into strips and scanned for radioactivity using a strip counter. The concentration of L-phenylalanine and L-tyrosine formed during the incubation were calculated from the area subscribed by the curves. The enzyme activity in human liver was reported to be 57.0 $\pm$ 10.0 nmoles/mg protein/60 min, or 0.95 $\pm$ 0.17 nmoles/min/mg protein.

III. 1. 4. A Radioisotope Assay Using *p*-Tritio-L-phenylalanine as a Substrate (Guroff and Abramowitz, 1967; Guroff, 1969b)

This method is based on the use of *p*-tritio-L-phenylalanine as a substrate. After the enzymic reaction the tyrosine which is formed is treated with *N*-iodosuccinimide to produce *m,m*-diiodotyrosine, and the amino acids are removed by adsorption on Dowex 50. The tritium released by the combination of enzymatic hydroxylation and iodination appears as tritiated water and can be used as a measure of the enzyme activity (Fig. 28).

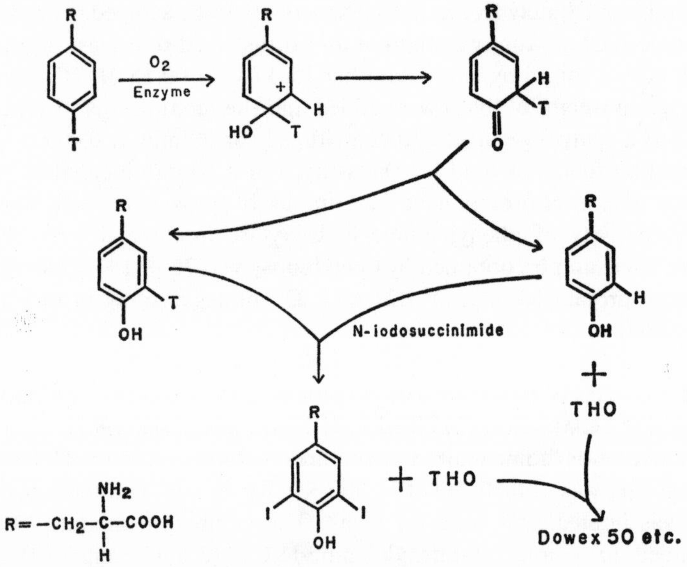

Fig. 28. Phenylalanine hydroxylase assay (Guroff, 1969b).

One μmole of carrier L-phenylalanine was added per mCi of *p*-tritio-L-phenylalanine (5,700 μCi/μmole). The material was then chromatographed on Whatman 3 MM paper in 2-propanol/NH$_3$/H$_2$O (80:10:10, v/v/v). The phenylalanine was eluted from the paper and the eluate was acidified and applied to a 0.5 ml column of Dowex-50-H$^+$. The column was washed with 10 ml of water and the amino acid was eluted with 20 ml of 1 N HCl. The eluate was evaporated to dryness on a rotary evaporator and the residue dissolved in 1 ml of H$_2$O. Finally, 9 ml of alcohol was added and the isotope was stored at $-20°C$.

Commercial N-iodosuccinimide was recrystallized from hot dioxane with the addition of carbon tetrachloride to the end point. The mixture was cooled and the crystals collected. The purified N-iodosuccinimide was washed with carbon tetrachloride and stored at $-20°C$.

The incubation mixture (0.25 ml) contained in μmoles: p-tritiophenyl-alanine (10 μl, between 130,000 and 160,000 cpm); L-phenylalanine, 1; Tris buffer (pH 7.3), 25; NADH, 1; 6,7-dimethyl-tetrahydropterin (DMPH$_4$), 0.15 (in 0.03 ml of 0.1 M mercaptoethanol); enzyme solution to be assayed; and water. Pseudomonas enzyme was activated with Fe^{++} before use (Guroff and Ito, 1965) and incubation was carried out for 10 min at 30°C in air. The incubation mixtures were then heated for 1 min at 100°C, immediately cooled in ice, and kept cold for the remainder of the procedure. Sodium acetate buffer, 0.2 M, pH 5.5, 0.5 ml, was then added. The sample was centrifuged in a refrigerated centrifuge and the supernatant fraction was removed with a transfer pipet; this is unnecessary in assays of the activity of purified enzyme. To the cold supernatant solution, 0.2 ml of a freshly prepared 1 % aqueous solution of N-iodosuccinimide was added. The mixture was allowed to remain at 0°C for 5 min, then 0.05 ml of 30 % trichloroacetic acid was added to each tube.

The colored supernatant portion of each sample was placed on a Dowex 50/charcoal column. To prepare these columns, 1 ml of an 80 % slurry of acid-washed Dowex-50 (H$^+$) was pipetted into a cotton-plugged, disposable Pasteur pipette. After the resin had settled, 0.1 ml of a 10 % slurry of activated charcoal was added. The columns were then washed with 1 or 2 ml of water. The sample was allowed to run into the column. The tubes were each rinsed with 1 ml of water which was then applied to the column. The combined effluent from the sample and the wash were collected in counting vials; 10 ml of Bray's counting solution was added.

It has been found that the hydroxylation of p-tritiophenylalanine proceeds with the direct release of 8 % of tritium from the $para$-position. The remaining 92 % is retained in the product. It has been shown with iodination experiments using m,m-ditritiotyrosine as a model that 81 % of the tritium is released under the conditions of the assay. Therefore, the nmoles of phenylalanine hydroxylated in the isotopic assay was calculated from the cpm using the equation:

$$\text{nmoles} = \frac{\text{cpm of } H_2O \text{ observed}}{\text{sp. act. of phenylalanine added}} \times \left(0.08 + \frac{0.92}{0.81}\right)$$

$$= \frac{\text{cpm of } H_2O \text{ observed}}{\text{sp. act. of phenylalanine added}} \times \frac{1}{0.82}$$

The assay is rapid, sensitive and simple, and is eminently applicable to crude tissue extracts since there is no blank for endogenous tyrosine, no problem from the further metabolism of tyrosine, and no contribution from tyrosine coming from non-hydroxylation routs such as proteolysis during incubation.

III. 2.   Assay of Tyrosine Hydroxylase Activity

Since the activity of tyrosine hydroxylase is very low, the use of sensitive radioassay is necessary. In the case of tissues with a high enzyme activity, fluorescence assay is also applicable.

An serious problem is the selecting of an appropriate blank to eliminate non-enzymic hydroxylation reaction. Boiled enzyme often gives an erroneously high blank, especially when crude tissue preparations such as slices and minces are used (Nagatsu, Levitt and Udenfriend, 1964b). Since the enzyme is stereospecific, the use of D-tyrosine provides the best blank.

As reported by Shiman, Akino and Kaufman (1971), the addition of either catalase or peroxidase can stimulate the reaction. However, the addition of Fe^{++} not only replaces catalase, but produces a more pronounced stimulation, suggesting its cofactor activity (Nagatsu, T., Mizutani and Nagatsu, I., 1972). Another sensitive method based on the enzymatic decarboxylation of C^{14}-carboxyl labeled L-DOPA formed from L-tyrosine-1-C^{14} has been reported (Waymire, Bjur and Weiner, 1971).

III. 2. 1.   TYROSINE-C^{14} METHOD

A. *Principle*
L-Tyrosine-C^{14} is used as a substrate. L-DOPA-C^{14} enzymatically formed is isolated on an alumina column and assayed in a liquid scintillation counter (Nagatsu, Levitt and Udenfriend, 1964a,b).

B. *Materials*
1. *Enzyme sources*. In the case of adrenal homogenate, 15 parts of 0.25 M sucrose was added to 1 part of that tissue. In other organs, such as the brain, heart and spleen, the tissues were minced with scissors, and 3 parts of 0.25 M sucrose was added to 1 part of the tissue. Homogenate was pre-

pared in a Potter homogenizer for 20 sec at 0°C. If the homogenization was not complete, the homogenate was cooled in ice and homogenization repeated using 0.4 ml of the homogenate for the assay. Crude tissue preparations contain natural inhibitors, and, therefore, should be always checked to insure that the velocity is proportional to the enzyme concentration. To avoid the effects caused by natural inhibitors, a partial purification of the enzyme is recommended.

2. L-*Tyrosine* (1 mM). 9.05 mg of L-tyrosine in 50 ml 0.01 N HCl.

3. *Mercaptoethanol* (1 M). 781 mg in 10 ml H_2O.

4. *2-Amino-4-hydroxy-6,7-dimethyl-5,6,7,8-tetrahydropteridine (6,7-dimethyl-5,6,7,8-tetrahydropterin)* (DMPH$_4$) (10 mM). DMPH$_4$·HCl· 1.5 H_2O, 25.85 mg in 10 ml of 1 M mercaptoethanol. This solution was stored in the frozen state at -15°C. When the tetrahydropteridine was added separately from mercaptoethanol, the compound was dissolved in 0.005 M HCl and stored at -15°C. The DMPH$_4$ solutions deteriorated upon repeated freezing and thawing and were therefore prepared and stored only in small amounts (Tietz, Lindberg and Kennedy, 1964). The purity was checked by thin-layer chromatography on silica gel G (Brinkmann) developed by 0.05 M potassium phosphate at pH 6.8 under 100 % nitrogen. The chromatographed product was visualized by fluorescence and by decolorizing 2,6-dichlorophenolindophenol (Bublitz, 1969). The concentration in solution was calculated from the extinction coefficient, 16.0 × 10^3 M^{-1} cm^{-1} at 265 nm (Whiteley and Huennekens, 1967).

5. *Fe^{++}* (10 mM). Freshly prepared. 27.8 mg of FeSO$_4$·7H$_2$O in 10 ml H_2O, or 39.2 mg of FeSO$_4$(NH$_4$)$_2$SO$_4$·6H$_2$O in 10 ml H_2O.

6. L-*Tyrosine-C^{14} (uniformly labeled)*. Specific activity: 500μCi/ μmole. This isotope was purified before use to remove trace contaminants which behaved like DOPA in adsorption by alumina and in chromatographic properties. Impurities were removed by adjustment of tyrosine solutions (3 to 5 ml) to pH 8.5, addition of alumina (0.5 g), and stirring for 10 min. After the solution was decanted, treatment with alumina was repeated two more times. After the final treatment with alumina, the solution was adjusted to pH 6.5 and passed through a column, 0.5 × 3 cm, of Amberlite IRC-50 (Na$^+$) buffered at pH 6.5. Tyrosine is not adsorbed under these conditions and appears in the effluent. The column was washed with 6 ml of H_2O, and the effluent and washings were combined and acidified by adding HCl to a final concentration of 0.1 N. By this procedure, the DOPA impurity in the tyrosine-C^{14}-preparation was reduced to less than 100 cpm per 100,000 cpm of tyrosine (Nagatsu, Levitt and Udenfriend, 1964b). Purification after the alumina treatment can be carried out

also by passing the isotope through a column, 1.5 ml, of Amberlite CG-120 (H^+) or Dowex-50 (H^+). The solution treated with alumina was acidified with acetic acid and poured onto the column. The column was washed with 20 ml of water and 5 ml of 1 N HCl. Elution was made with 10 ml of 1 N HCl. Solutions of purified tyrosine-C^{14} were stable when stored frozen.

7. *Alumina.* Aluminum oxide, acid-washed, for chromatographic use. (See Chapter IV. 1. for the treatment of alumina).

8. *EDTA* (0.2 M). Dissolve 37.2 g disodium ethylenediamine tetra-acetate ($Na_2C_{10}H_{14}O_8 \cdot 2H_2O$) in water (with heating), cool and make to 500 ml.

9. *Sodium acetate* (0.2M). Dissolve 13.6 g sodium acetate ($CH_3CO-ONa \cdot 3H_2O$) in water and diluted to 500 ml.

10. *DOPA carrier* (1000 $\mu g/ml$). 10 mg of DOPA in 10 ml of 0.01 N HCl.

11. *Bray's scintillator* (Bray, 1960). Combine naphthalene 60 g, PPO (2,5-diphenyloxazole) 4 g, POPOP (1,4-di-2-(5-phenyloxazolyl)benzene) 0.2 g, methanol (absolute) 100 ml, ethylene glycol 20 ml, and add *p*-dioxane to 1 *l*.

C. *Procedure*

The incubation mixture (total volume, 1.0 ml) shown in the following table was prepared in a small test tube (9 ml) in an ice bath:

	Volume (μl)	Amount ($\mu moles$)	Final concentration (M)
Sodium acetate buffer (1.0 M, pH 6.0)	200	200	2.0×10^{-1}
Fe^{++}($Fe(NH_4)_2(SO_4)_2$ or $FeSO_4$) (10 mM)	100	1.0	1.0×10^{-3}
Water	to 1000 (total volume)		
Enzyme	An appropriate amount		
$DMPH_4$ (10 mM)		1.0	1.0×10^{-3}
in mercaptoethanol (1.0 M)	100	100	1.0×10^{-1}
Preincubation, 3 min at 30°C in air			
L-Tyrosine and L-Tyrosine-C^{14}(U.L.)	100	0.100	1.0×10^{-4}
(1 mM, 0.5 $\mu Ci/ml$)			
		(0.05 μCi, about 100,000 cpm)	
Total volume	1,000[a]		
Incubation, 15 min at 30°C in air			

[a]The volume of the incubation can be reduced to 0.50, 0.10, or 0.05 ml.

The incubation mixture was preincubated at 30°C in air with shaking for

3 min. The incubation was started by adding L-tyrosine-C^{14} and carried out for 15 min at 30°C with shaking.

The following four kinds of blank were used:

1) D-Tyrosine-C^{14} instead of L-tyrosine-C^{14}.

2) Boiled enzyme blank. Heat the enzyme solution at 80°C for 10 min and add to the incubation mixture. Incubate together with the homogenate samples.

3) Non-incubated zero time blank. Add 200 μg of DOPA and 3 ml of 5 % trichloroacetic acid at zero time.

4) No enzyme blank. Instead of the enzyme solution, add same volume of the solvent such as buffer or sucrose solution. Incubate together with the enzyme samples.

All blanks gave similar values. Blanks 3 or 4 are the most convenient.

The reaction was stopped by adding 200 μg (0.2 ml) of DOPA and 3 ml of 5 % trichloroacetic acid. After 10 min the mixture was centrifuged. The supernatant was decanted into a small 30 ml beaker containing 0.5 ml of 0.2 M EDTA, 10 ml of 0.2 M sodium acetate and 0.4 g of alumina (one rounded spoonful). It was titrated to pH 8.5 using a glass electrode first with 3 N NH$_4$OH, then with 1 N NH$_4$OH under constant stirring. The mixture was stirred for 5 min, and the electrode and the stirring bar were rinsed with a few ml of water. The alumina was allowed to settle for 3–5 min, and the supernatant carefully decanted and discarded (The supernatant was saved for the assay of endogenous tyrosine, when a crude enzyme solution was used.) The alumina was quantitatively transferred with water to a glass column (0.6 cm in diameter). The water was allowed to drain through and the alumina was washed with two 10 ml portions of deionized water. The tip of the column was rinsed with water to remove tyrosine-C^{14} contamination. The column was eluted with 2.0 ml of 0.3 N acetic acid into a small test tube. One ml of the alumina eluate was taken into a counting vial, and 10 ml of Bray's scintillation solution was added and counted with a liquid scintillation spectrometer. A standard made up of one-half the amount of L-tyrosine-C^{14} added into the reaction mixture (0.05 ml) and diluted to 1.0 ml with 0.3 N acetic acid, and 10 ml of Bray's scintillation solution was also counted.

The recovery of DOPA on the alumina column in the above procedure was 65–70 %. Where greater precision was required, a fluorometric assay was carried out to determine the fraction of DOPA carrier isolated. 0.4 ml of alumina eluate was taken and 9.6 ml of H$_2$O was added. As a standard, 200 μg (0.2 ml) of DOPA solution and 1.8 ml of 0.3 N acetic acid were mixed, and then 0.4 ml of the mixture was diluted with 9.6 ml of H$_2$O

(4 μg/ml of solution). As a blank, a mixture of 0.4 ml of 0.3 N acetic acid and 9.6 ml of H_2O was used. The native fluorescence of DOPA at 339 nm with an excitation light at 282 nm was measured by a spectrophotofluorometer. Recovery should be checked when newly prepared alumina is used. Calculation of tyrosine hydroxylase activity:

DOPA formed (nmoles) in 15 min =

$$\frac{(\text{experimental}-\text{blank}) \text{ cpm} \times \dfrac{100}{\text{alumina recovery } \%}}{(\text{L-tyrosine-C}^{14} \text{ standard}) \text{ cpm}} \times [\text{tyrosine}]^* \text{ (nmoles)}$$

III. 2. 2. L-TYROSINE-3,5-H³ METHOD (Nagatsu, Levitt and Udenfriend, 1964c; Levitt, Gibb, Daly, Lipton and Udenfriend, 1967)

A. *Principle*
A simpler procedure for assay of tyrosine hydroxylase is based on displacement of tritium (H³, T) in the following reaction sequence:

$$\text{L-Tyrosine-3,5-T} + \tfrac{1}{2} O_2 \xrightarrow[\text{hydroxylase}]{\text{tyrosine}} \text{L-DOPA-5-T} + T^+$$

$$T^+ + H_2O \longrightarrow H^+ + THO$$

B. *Materials* (see also III. 2. 1.)
Commercially available L-tyrosine-3,5-T (1,000 μCi/μmole), which is prepared by catalytic reduction of 3,5-diiodo-L-tyrosine with tritium gas (2,000 μCi in 2 ml), was acidified with 50 μl of acetic acid and poured on a column of Dowex-50(H+), 0.5 × 3 cm. After the column was washed, with 100 ml of H_2O and 10 ml of 0.5N HCl the tyrosine was eluted with 20 ml of 3 N HCl. The 3 N HCl fraction was evaporated to dryness under a stream of nitrogen or in a flush evaporator at room temperature (Sampls should not be heated since this increases the counts in the blank), taken up in 10 ml of absolute ethanol, and stored at $-20°C$. For routine assay, aliquots of the isotope tyrosine solution (in the case of 0.20 mCi/ml, 20 μl aliquots), were evaporated to dryness under nitrogen gas at room temperature and immediately dissolved in 1.0 ml L-tyrosine (1 mM) solution. This isotope solution can be used for 10 tubes using 100 μl for each tube.

---

* When a crude enzyme preparation containing endogenous tyrosine is used, tyrosine in the enzyme solution should be measured separately. Total tyrosine in the incubation mixture=100 nmoles (including the isotope)+endogenous tyrosine in the enzyme solution.

C. *Procedure*

The incubation mixture shown in the following table was prepared in a small test tube (9 ml tube) in an ice bath:

	Volume (μl)	Amount (μmoles)	Final concentration (M)
Sodium acetate buffer (1.0 M, pH 6.0)	200	200	2.0×10^{-1}
Fe^{++}(Fe(NH$_4$)$_2$(SO$_4$)$_2$ or FeSO$_4$) (10 mM)	100	1.0	1.0×10^{-3}
Water	to 1,000 (total volume)		
Enzyme	An appropriate amount		
DMPH$_4$ (10 mM)		1.0	1.0×10^{-3}
in mercaptoethanol (1.0 M)	100	100	1.0×10^{-1}
Preincubation, 3 min at 30°C in air			
L-Tyrosine-3,5-T	100	0.100	1.0×10^{-4}
		(0.4 μCi)	
Total volume	1,000[a]		
Incubation, 15 min at 30°C in air			

[a] The volume of the incubation can be reduced to 0.50, 0.10, or 0.05 ml.

The incubation mixture was preincubated at 30°C in air with shaking for 3 min. The incubation was started by adding 0.1 ml of L-tyrosine-3,5-T. The reaction mixture was incubated at 30°C for 15 min with shaking, and the reaction was stopped by adding 0.1 ml of 25 % trichloroacetic acid or 0.05 ml of glacial acetic acid. After 10 min, the mixture was centrifuged and the supernatant transferred with a disposable Pasteur pipette to a Dowex-50-H$^+$ column, 0.5 × 2 cm. The test tube containing the protein precipitate was washed with 1 ml water which was added to the column after the initial effluent had passed through. The combined effluents (2 ml) were collected in a counting vial to which 15 ml of a Bray's fluorophor solution for scintillation counting was then added. With whole homogenate or crude enzyme preparations, the addition of the fluorophor solution frequently resulted in slight turbidity which influenced tritium counting. In such cases, internal standards were used to correct for quenching. A reagent blank, in which all additions were made except for the enzyme, was used to correct for small amounts of tritium released non-enzymatically. It was found from double labeling experiments that about 90 % of tritium is in the 3 and 5 positions of tyrosine-3,5-T. The tyrosine standard was prepared by taking 0.1 ml of L-tyrosine-3,5-T solution, 1.8 ml H$_2$O, and 0.1 ml of 25 % trichloroacetic acid. For each 100 equivalents of tyrosine oxidized, 45 will be recovered in water. The recovery of T-labelled water in the 2 ml of effluent used for radioassay was 90 %. Therefore, the amount of tyrosine oxidized was calculated by means of the following equation:

$$\text{tyrosine oxidized} = \frac{\text{cpm water} \times \dfrac{100}{90}}{\text{cpm standard} \times \dfrac{100}{45}} \times [\text{tyrosine}]^* \text{ nmoles}$$

III. 2. 3. FLUORESCENCE ASSAY (Nagatsu and Yamamoto, 1968)
L-Tyrosine was used as a substrate for the assay, and D-tyrosine for the blank. DOPA formed enzymatically only from L-tyrosine was isolated by column chromatography and assayed fluorometrically. This method was less sensitive than the radioassays, but could be applied to adrenal or brain preparations which have high activities. The incubation mixture contained (total volume 1.0 ml): sodium acetate buffer (1 M, pH 6.0), 0.2 ml (200 μmoles); L-tyrosine or D-tyrosine (for the blank) (1 mM), 0.1 ml (0.1 μmole); Fe^{++}(Fe(NH$_4$)$_2$(SO$_4$)$_2$ or FeSO$_4$) (10 mM), 0.1 ml (1.0 μmole); water to a final volume of 1.0 ml; DMPH$_4$ (10 mM) in mercaptoethanol (1 M), 0.1 ml (DMPH$_4$ 1.0 μmole; mercaptoethanol 100 μmoles). The incubation mixture was preincubated at 30°C in air with shaking for 3 min. The incubation was started by adding the enzyme to be assayed. The incubation was carried out at 30°C for 15 min with shaking. For the blank incubation, D-tyrosine was used as substrate instead of L-tyrosine. Ten nmoles of DOPA was added to another blank incubation as internal standard. Reaction was stopped by the addition of 50 μl of glacial acetic acid and the incubation mixture was centrifuged in order to remove protein. The precipitate was washed with 1 ml of 2 % acetic acid and centrifuged. The combined supernatants were passed through two columns fitted together in sequence; the top column contained Florisil (100/200 mesh, 0.6 × 4.0 cm) previously washed with 2 % acetic acid until the effluent was pH 4.0 (Kaufman, 1963a), and the bottom column contained Amberlite CG-120-Na$^+$ (Type I, 0.6 cm × 4.0 cm) previously washed with 5 M NaOH and water. The effluent from the two columns was discarded. Both columns were washed with 5 ml of 2 % acetic acid and the washings were discarded. The Amberlite CG-120 column was then separated and washed with 10 ml of water. DOPA was eluted with 10 ml of 0.1 M

---

* In the case of crude enzymes, measure tyrosine in the enzyme material. [tyrosine]= tyrosine added (100 nmoles)+tyrosine in the enzyme material.

sodium acetate buffer (pH 6.5). The eluate was used directly for the assay of DOPA. However, when greater sensitivity was required, the DOPA was further concentrated on an alumina column. To the Amberlite eluate, 0.5 ml of 0.2 M EDTA and 400 mg of alumina, which had been previously treated with acid were added (Crout, 1961; see IV.I.). The pH was adjusted to 8.5 by the dropwise addition of 3 N NH$_4$OH with constant stirring using a glass electrode. The alumina was allowed to settle and the aqueous phase was decanted and discarded. The alumina was transferred to a column (0.6 cm in diameter) and washed with 10 ml of water. After washing, the DOPA was eluted with 2 ml of 0.3 N acetic acid. To 2.0 ml of the Amberlite column eluate or 1.0 ml of alumina eluate plus 1.0 ml of 1 M sodium acetate, 0.1 ml of 0.25 % K$_3$Fe(CN)$_6$ was added. After 3 min, 1.0 ml of a mixture of 2% ascorbic acid and 20% NaOH (1:9, v/v) was added and the resultant fluorescence was measured with a spectrophotofluorometer at 480 nm, with the excitation light at 356 nm. The DOPA formed enzymatically was calculated from the value of the internal standard by means of the following equation:

$$\frac{F(L) - F(D)}{F(D + IS) - F(D)} \times 10 \text{ nmoles}$$

where $F(L)$=reading of L-tyrosine incubation, $F(D)$=reading of D-tyrosine incubation, and $F(D + IS)$=reading of D-tyrosine plus DOPA (internal standard, 10 nmoles).

Although fluorescence assay is less sensitive than radioassay, it has some advantages. Besides the convenience of the dispensability of a labeled substrate and a liquid scintillation spectrometer, the separate measurement of tyrosine concentration in the homogenate is not necessary for calculation.

III. 2. 4. ASSAY WITH A TETRAHYDROPTERIDINE-GENERATING SYSTEM
Tyrosine hydroxylase activity can be measured by coupling it with dihydropteridine reductase and the NADPH regenerating system (Brenneman and Kaufman, 1964). The incubation mixture (total volume 1.0 ml) contained (in μmoles) potassium phosphate (pH 6.4), 200; NADPH, 0.25; NADH, 0.25; D-glucose, 100; glucose dehydrogenase in excess; dihydropteridine reductase (sheep liver enzyme purified through the first ammonium sulfate step) (Kaufman and Levenberg, 1959), in excess; enzyme to be assayed; DMPH$_4$, 0.05; and L-tyrosine-C^{14} (or L-tyrosine-3,5-T), 1.0 (0.05 μCi). L-DOPA-C^{14} (or tritiated water) formed was isolated and measured as described in sections III. 1. 1 and III. 2. 2.

III. 2. 5. REPORTED ACTIVITIES

The activity of tyrosine hydroxylase is greatly influenced by the addition of cofactors (tetrahydropterin and Fe^{++}), the structure of the tetrahydropterin cofactor, and the purity of the enzyme preparation. Reported values are shown in Table V.

III. 3.   Assay of DOPA Decarboxylase Activity

DOPA decarboxylase activity can be measured by three different procedures: manometric method, sprectrofluorometry, and radioassay. The manometric method is based on the enzymic production of CO_2. (Schales and Schales, 1949; Schales, 1955; Hartman, Akawie and Clark, 1955; Holtz and Westermann, 1956). The formed dopamine can be assayed spectrofluorometrically after separation from DOPA on an Amberlite IRC-50 column (Davis and Awapara, 1960; Lovenberg, Weissbach and Udenfriend, 1962). In radioassays, dopamine-C^{14} formed from DOPA-C^{14} is isolated and the radioactivity measured (Sommerville, 1964; Laduron and Belpaire, 1968b). Another sensitive assay based on $C^{14}O_2$ evolution from (carboxy-C^{14}) DOPA has been reported (Christenson, Pairman and Udenfriend, 1970).

III. 3. 1. FLUOROMETRIC METHOD (Lovenberg, Weissbach and Udenfriend, 1962)

An example of the incubation mixture (total volume, 1 ml) is shown in the following table:

	Volume (μl)	Amount $(\mu moles)$	Final concentration (M)
Phosphate buffer (1.0 M, pH 7.0)	100	100	1×10^{-1}
A monoamine oxidase inhibitor			
(10 mM): Harmaline	30	0.3	3×10^{-4}
(Marsilid or iproniazid)	(100	1.0	1×10^{-3})
Pyridoxal phosphate (1 mM^a)	70	0.07	7×10^{-5}
Water (total volume)	to 1,000		
Enzyme			
DOPA (10 mM^b)	100	1.0	1×10^{-3}

^{a} Mol wt 247.15; 2.47 mg/10 ml water.
^{b} Mol wt 197.19; 19.72 mg/10 ml 0.01 N HCl.

After 3 min at 37°C (20 min incubation can be carried out, when the activity is low), the incubation mixture was heated for 1 min, or 0.5 ml, 25%

TABLE V. Distribution of Tyrosine Hydroxylase.

Enzyme preparation	Cofactor (M)	Tyrosine hydroxylase activity (nmoles/min)	Reference
Bovine adrenal medulla			
Homogenate	THF (5×10^{-3}) Fe^{++} (5×10^{-4})	0.020 (per mg protein)	1)
Supernatant $(NH_4)_2SO_4$ (0–40%)		0.040 2.7	
Homogenate	$DMPH_4$ (1×10^{-3}) Fe^{++} (5×10^{-4})	0.91 (per mg protein)	2)
Particles		2.1	
Supernatant		0.25	
$(NH_4)_2SO_4$ (25–45%)		24	
Homogenate		141 (per g tissue)	
Particles		150	
Supernatant		19	
Bovine caudate nucleus	$DMPH_4$ (1×10^{-3}) Fe^{++} (1×10^{-3})		3)
Homogenate		0.012 (per mg protein)	
Nerve endings		0.017	
Supernatant		0.017	
Synaptic vesicles		0.018	
Rabbit	$DMPH_4$ (1×10^{-3})		4)
Adrenal glands		7.2 ± 0.35 (per g tissue)	
Caudate nucleus		4.7 ± 1.6	
Brain stem		1.1	
Heart (left ventricle)	$DMPH_4$ (1×10^{-3})	0.067 ± 0.008 (per g tissue)	5)
Human pheochromocytoma	$DMPH_4$ (1×10^{-3})		6)
Homogenate		0.10 (per mg protein)	
Supernatant		0.14	
$(NH_4)_2SO_4$ (25–35%) and hydroxyapatite		20.0	

THF = tetrahydrofolate; $DMPH_4$ = 6,7-dimethyltetrahydropterin

1) Nagatsu, Levitt and Udenfriend, 1964 b.
2) Petrack, Sheppy and Fetzer, 1968.
3) Nagatsu, T. and Nagatsu, I., 1970.
4) Nagatsu and Yamamoto, 1968.
5) DeQuattro, Nagatsu, Maronde and Alexander, 1969.
6) Nagatsu, T., Yamamoto and Nagatsu, I., 1970.

TABLE VI. Distribution of DOPA Decarboxylase.

Enzyme preparation	Pyridoxal phosphate (M)	DOPA decarboxylase activity (nmoles/min) (37°C)	Reference
Rat tissue homogenate	2×10^{-5}	2,300 (per g dry weight)	1)
Kidney		2,300	
Liver		1,870	
Small intestine		850	
Brain		170	
Lung		120	
Spleen		20	
Rabbit tissue homogenate	2×10^{-5}		
Kidney		830	
Liver		70	
Small intestine		70	
Brain		20	
Heart		20	
Lung		20	
Spleen		30	
Adrenals		50	
Guinea pig tissue homogenate	2×10^{-5}	2,640	
Kidney		2,640	
Liver		720	
Small intestine		1,230	
Brain		80	
Heart		30	
Lung		20	
Spleen		20	
Adrenals		50	
Rabbit brain stem supernatant	$(-)$	25 ± 1 (per g tissue)	2)
	2×10^{-5}	33 ± 2	

	K_m (×10⁻⁵)			(per mg protein / per g tissue)
Guinea pig kidney				
Supernatant	7×10^{-5}			59 (per mg protein)
Alumina C_γ eluate				630
DEAE-cellulose eluate				3,290
Hog kidney				
Supernatant	8.4×10^{-5}			26.1 (per mg protein)
A homogeneous enzyme				8,670
Dog brain stem				
Supernatant				1.1
Alumina C_γ eluate				6.8
Human tissue homogenate				(per g tissue)
Liver Adult	(−)	0.33	1.1	2.0
	5×10^{-5}	0.53	3.8	6.7
Liver Fetal	(−)	20	24	30
	5×10^{-5}	23	31	33
Heart Adult	(−)	0.07	0.07	0.07
	5×10^{-5}	0.13	0.17	0.47
Heart Fetal	(−)	0.07	0.10	0.27
	5×10^{-5}	0.23	0.27	0.33
Lung Adult	(−)	0.07	0.15	0.33
	5×10^{-5}	0.23	0.60	0.80
Lung Fetal	(−)	0.67	0.92	1.4
	5×10^{-5}	5.8	6.2	6.7
Kidney Adult	(−)	0.20	0.20	0.40
	5×10^{-5}	1.0	1.1	1.3
Kidney Fetal	(−)	8.0	9.5	21
	5×10^{-5}	24	34	34
Brain Adult	(−)	0.07	0.10	0.10
	5×10^{-5}	0.07	0.18	0.33
Brain Fetal	(−)	0.07	0.15	0.20
	5×10^{-5}	0.13	0.42	0.67

3)

4)

5)

1) Davis and Awapara, 1960.   2) Burkard, Pavlin, Pletscher and Gey, 1962.
3) Lovenberg, Weissbach and Udenfriend, 1962.   4) Christenson, Dairman and Udenfriend, 1970.
5) Vogel, McFarland and Prince, 1970.

trichloroacetic acid was added, and diluted to 5 ml with water. The diluted sample was centrifuged and the supernatant passed through an Amberlite IRC-50 column (packed volume, 1 ml) which was buffered at pH 6.5. The resin was washed with 5 ml of 0.1 M phosphate buffer, pH 6.5, and the dopamine eluted with 5 ml of 0.5 N HCl. The acid eluate containing the dopamine was read directly in a spectrophotofluorometer. The uncorrected excitation and fluorescent wave lengths were 280 nm and 330 nm, respectively.

III. 3. 2. RADIOASSAY (Laduron and Belpaire, 1968b)

Dopamine-C^{14} formed from DOPA-C^{14} was extracted with butanol and measured in a liquid scintillation spectrometer. To 0.1 ml of enzyme preparation in a 15 ml glass-stoppered tube, 0.65 ml of 0.5 M phosphate and 0.1 M borate buffer (pH 6.9) containing 0.51 μmole DOPA, 0.5 μCi DOPA-C^{14} (spec. act. 3.93 mCi/mmole), 20 μg pyridoxal phosphate, and 0.75 μmole transcypromine were added. A blank was obtained by adding the enzyme preparation after the incubation period. The samples were incubated at 37°C for 20 min. The reaction mixtures were then immediately chilled at 0°C and 1 g of NaCl and 10 ml of butanol, free of acid (Sommerville, 1964), were added. Before each extraction, butanol was washed with phosphate-borate buffer (pH 6.9). After vigorous shaking, the extraction mixtures were centrifuged at low speed for 5 min. For radioactivity determinations, 1 ml organic phase was mixed with 10 ml Bray's solution and counted in a liquid scintillation spectrometer.

Under these experimental conditions, no difference in the activity of DOPA decarboxylase was observed in an atmosphere of air or nitrogen.

Recoveries of radioactive dopamine (0.1 μCi) added to the incubation mixture ranged from 55 to 60%. An internal standard of labeled dopamine was added to the incubation mixture. The amount of dopamine formed was calculated from the counts of the internal standard.

III. 3. 3. REPORTED ACTIVITIES

DOPA decarboxylase activity in tissue of various mammalian species is shown in Table VI. The activity is expressed in nmoles/min by calculating the reported values.

III. 4. Assay of Dopamine-β-hydroxylase Activity

Either dopamine or norepinephrine is used as substrate. The enzyme activity in the crude tissue preparations is very low owing to the presence of endogenous inhibitors. A certain degree of enzyme purification is necessary to show a maximal enzyme activity. In the case of the adrenal medulla, the endogenous inhibitors were blocked by the addition of N-ethylmaleimide (Nagatsu, Kuzuya and Hidaka, 1967; Kuzuya and Nagatsu, 1969b), or Cu or p-chloromercuribenzoate (Duch, Viveros and Kirshner, 1968). The standard incubation mixture (Creveling, Daly, Witkop and Udenfriend, 1962; Kuzuya and Nagatsu, 1969b) (total volume 1.0 ml) is shown in the following table:

	Volume (μl)	Amount (μmoles)	Final concentration (M)
Phosphate buffer (1.0 M, pH 5.5)	200	200	2×10^{-1}
Fumaric acid (0.2 M)	50	10	1×10^{-2}
(disodium fumarate 324.2 mg/10 ml H$_2$O)			
Ascorbic acid (0.2 M)	50	10	1×10^{-3}
(176 mg/5 ml H$_2$O)			
Catalase (crystalline catalase aqueous solution)	Enough catalase to give maximum stimulation (about 50 μg)		
N-Ethylmaleimide (0.2 M)	200	40	4×10^{-2}
(25 mg/ml H$_2$O)			
Substrate (tyramine or dopamine) (0.1 M)			
Enzyme	100	10	1×10^{-2}
Water (total volume)	to 1,000[a]		

[a] The volume of the incubation can be reduced to 0.50 or 0.10 ml.

Catalase protected the enzyme from inactivation due to H$_2$O$_2$ produced by the presence of ascorbate (Levin, Levenberg and Kaufman, 1960; Creveling, Daly, Witkop and Udenfriend, 1962). Excess catalase inhibited the reaction. Therefore, the amount of catalase to give maximum stimulation must be determined in a pilot experiment with each batch of catalase. In the case of a crude preparation from the adrenal medulla, 40 μmoles of N-ethylmaleimide (0.2 M, 25 mg/ml H$_2$O, 0.2 ml) were included in the incubation mixture (Kuzuya and Nagatsu, 1969b). Incubation was usually carried out at 37° or 25°C in air with shaking for 10–60 min.

III. 4. 1. Assay Using Dopamine as a Substrate

When dopamine is used as substrate, the norepinephrine formed can be measured: 1) by direct spectrofluorometry based on the trihydroxyindole reaction; 2) by paper chromatography; or 3) by periodate oxidation (Levin, Levenberg and Kaufman, 1960).

A. *Chromatographic methods* (Levin, Levenberg and Kaufman, 1960) Dopamine-C^{14} was used as substrate. The reaction was stopped by the addition of a deproteinizing reagent such as trichloroacetic acid, perchloric acid or acid alcohol. The mixture was centrifuged to remove protein. The supernatant was evaporated to dryness under a jet of nitrogen or by lyophilization. When a crude enzyme preparation was used, the purification of norepinephrine formed together with dopamine on an alumina column and the evaporation of the alumina eluate is recommended. The residue was extracted with an acid-alcohol mixture and the extract clarified by centrifugation. The extract was analyzed by paper chromatography, thinlayer chromatography or high-voltage electrophoresis. Radioactive norepinephrine formed from dopamine-C^{14} was determined by counting the chromatograms in a windowless chromatogram scanner or with a liquid scintillation counter. The areas corresponding to norepinephrine were located by spraying the chromatogram with a spray reagent.

The following procedure was described by Levin, Levenberg and Kaufman (1960). The reaction was stopped by the addition of 2 ml of 3 % acetic acid in ethanol (v/v) and the solution heated at 55°C for 5 min to denature protein. The precipitate was removed by centrifugation. The volume of the supernatant liquid was reduced to 0.1 ml under a jet of nitrogen and then lyophilized to dryness. The residue was extracted with 0.1 to 0.3 ml of a solution containing 2 % acetic acid in 60 % ethanol (v/v) and the extract clarified by centrifugation. This extract was used for chromatography, with the addition of carrier norepinephrine if necessary. Descending paper chromatography was carried out in *n*-butanol-HCl (Euler and Hamberg, 1949a) or in phenol-HCl (James, 1948). Radioactive norepinephrine formed enzymatically from dopamine-α-C^{14} was detected by counting paper strips in a windowless paper chromatogram scanner.

B. *Assay of norepinephrine-C^{14} by periodate oxidation* (Levin, Levenberg and Kaufman, 1960)
This method is based on oxidation of the side chain of norepinephrine with sodium periodate. Because of the presence of adjacent amino and hydroxyl groups, the carbon chain of norepinephrine is more susceptible to attack by periodate than is the corresponding chain of dopamine. Dopamine labeled with C^{14} in the terminal position of the side chain was used as substrate for enzymatic reaction, and the norepinephrine formed was treated with periodate to liberate radioactive formaldehyde, which was then trapped and counted. The enzymatic reaction was stopped, the mix-

ture deproteinized and concentrated, and an extract prepared, all in the same manner as for chromatography. This extract was diluted with 8 volumes of water and centrifuged. To 0.35 ml of the supernatant fluid, 0.15 ml of 2 M acetate buffer, pH 4.0, was added. An aliquot was removed and the radioactivity measured. The remainder of the solution was equilibrated at 39°C, and 0.2 ml of saturated sodium periodate was added, followed by 0.1 ml of 1 M formaldehyde as carrier. Exactly 45 sec after the periodate addition, 2.0 ml of an aqueous suspension of acid-washed Norit A (100 mg/ml) was added to stop oxidation. The Norit was removed by centrifugation and by filtration through a sintered glass filter. To the filtrate 1.5 ml of 1 M sodium acetate in 0.5 M HCl, pH 4.5, followed by 6 ml of 0.8 % dimedon were added. The mixture was allowed to stand in the cold for several hours. The precipitate was collected by centrifugation in the cold, washed 4 times with water, suspended in about 1.2 ml of acetone, plated, dried, weighed, and counted. Since all the norepinephrine present does not react in this time, the method measured only relative, and not absolute, amounts of norepinephrine. A correction was made for the small amount of radioactive formaldehyde formed from dopamine by assaying a blank composed of an incubation mixture in which norepinephrine formation has been prevented, either by deproteinizing before incubation, using boiled enzyme or inhibiting the reaction by KCN. The periodate oxidation technique was most useful for measuring relative activity in crude enzyme preparations containing considerable amounts of catecholamines.

C. *Norepinephrine assay by fluorometry* (Levin, Levenberg and Kaufman, 1960)
The reaction was stopped by the addition of 0.2 ml of 0.6 M trichloroacetic acid. After centrifugation, 10 μl aliquot of the supernatant was added to 2.0 ml of 1 M acetate buffer (pH 6.5). Norepinephrine formed from dopamine was assayed according to the fluorometric procedure of Euler and Floding (1955a). This method was used to measure norepinephrine formation with purified enzyme preparations.

III. 4. 2. ASSAY USING TYRAMINE AS A SUBSTRATE
When tyramine or tyramine-H[3] is used as substrate, the norsynephrine (octopamine) formed can be assayed by measuring the p-hydroxybenzaldehyde formed from norsynephrine after oxidation of the side chain with sodium periodate either by spectrophotometry or by radioassay.

A. *Spectrophotometric assay* (Creveling, Daly, Witkop and Udenfriend, 1962)
The reaction was stopped by the addition of 0.2 ml of 3 M trichloro-acetic acid. As a control, the reaction mixture without tyramine was incubated at the same time and the substrate was added after stopping the reaction. When a crude enzyme preparation was used, the acidified reaction mixture was centrifuged and the supernatant was used. A 1.0-ml aliquot of the acidified reaction mixture was transferred to an Amberlite IR-CG-120-H^+ column or a Dowex-50-8X-H^+ column (0.5 × 3 cm). The column was washed with 10 ml of water and the amines (tyramine and norsynephrine) eluted with 3.0 ml of 3 N NH_4OH. An assay of the norsynephrine formed from tyramine was made on an aliquot of the column eluate by periodate oxidation, and the absorbance of the p-hydroxybenzaldehyde formed was measured. Norsynephrine was converted to p-hydroxybenzaldehyde by the addition of 0.3 ml of 2% sodium periodate ($NaIO_4$), and then, excess periodate was reduced with 0.3 ml of 10 % sodium metabisulfite ($Na_2S_2O_5$). A_{330} nm was measured and compared with a norsynephrine standard carried through the entire procedure (recovery 95–100 %). About 0.7 absorbance was achieved with 0.1 μmole of norsynephrine. When higher sensitivity is required the p-hydroxybenzaldehyde is further isolated by solvent extraction. The benzaldehyde was extracted from the solution with 30 ml toluene, and an aliquot of the solvent was re-extracted with 1 ml of 3 N NH_4OH. A_{330} nm was measured.

Assay of dopamine-β-hydroxylase in human blood (Nagatsu and Udenfriend, 1972). This assay method has been found to be applicable for the assay of dopamine-β-hydroxylase in human blood (serum or plasma) by increasing its sensitivity using a microassay system (Nagatsu and Udenfriend, 1972). Human serum or plasma were obtained either by venopuncture or by capillary tubes from finger tip blood. Samples obtained by venopuncture were placed on ice and the serum removed. Finger tip blood samples were obtained in heparinized capillary tubes (Scientific Products Inc.). One end was sealed using a plastic putty (Critoseal, Fisher Scientific) and the capillary tube was centrifuged for 3 min at 11,000 rpm using a microhematocrit centrifuge. Plasma aliquots were removed by using a micropipette.

The standard incubation mixture (total volume 1.0 ml) contained: 2–50 μl of human serum or plasma, as enzyme and water to dilute to 400 μl; 1 M sodium acetate buffer, pH 5.0, 200 μl; 0.2 M sodium fumarate, 50μl; 0.2 M ascorbic acid, 50μl; catalase (1 mg/ml), 50 μl (1,500 units, Sigma); 0.4 M tyramine, 50 μl; 0.02 M pargyline, 50 μl; and 0.2 M N-ethylmaleimide, 150 μl. A sample of boiled enzyme preparation (95°C for 5 min) was used as blank. The reaction mixture was incubated at 37°C for 60 min, in air, in a metabolic shaker. The incubation was stopped by adding 0.2 ml of 3 M trichloroacetic acid, and the mixture was centrifuged at 2,000 rpm for 10 min. The supernatant fluid was transferred to a small column of Dowex-50 (H$^+$) (200–400 mesh) (packed volume, 0.2 ml) which had been prepared in a disposable Pasteur pipette (0.5 cm × 10 cm). The tube and precipitate were washed with 1 ml of water, and the washings were also transferred to the column. The column was washed two more times with 2 ml of water and then the adsorbed amines were eluted with 1.0 ml of 4 N NH$_4$OH. Octopamine in the eluate was converted to p-hydroxybenzaldehyde by the addition of 0.10 ml of 2 % NaIO$_4$.

Excess periodate was then reduced by adding 0.10 ml of 10% Na$_2$S$_2$O$_5$. Absorbancy was measured against water at 330 nm in a microcuvette with a 1 cm light path. When 20 nmoles of octopamine in 1.0 ml of 4 N NH$_4$OH was carried through the oxidation procedure as standard, an absorbancy of 0.43 was observed. The blank value (boiled enzyme) was about 0.05. Enzyme activity was linear with time of incubation up to 60 min at 37°C and with the amount of enzyme up to 50 μl of human serum or plasma. The small Dowex-50 columns after the assay could be regenerated by washing with 2 ml of water twice, and then with 2 ml of 5 N HCl and 2 ml of water twice again.

In the radioassay using phenylethanolamine-N-methyltransferase and S-adenosylmethionine-methyl-C^{14} in the second incubation (Weinshilboum and Axelrod, 1971; Goldstein, Freedman and Bonnay, 1971), saturating amounts of tyramine could not be used, because tyramine was found to inhibit the second enzymatic step in the procedure, N-methyltransferase (Weinshilboum and Axelrod, 1971). In contrast, the present method operates under optimal conditions and gives maximal values. The enzyme activities obtained on 58 normal human sera ranged from 1 to 100 nmoles/min/ml serum but the activity appears to be fairly constant on successive days for an individual. The mean value was 42 nmoles/min/ml.

B. *Radioassay* (Friedman and Kaufman, 1965b)

The following procedure was described by Friedman and Kaufman (1965b). Tyramine-H^3 (uniformly labeled) with a specific activity of 1.5 μCi per μmole was used as substrate. The reaction was stopped with 1 ml of 6% metaphosphoric acid. The precipitated protein was removed by centrifugation. To 1.0-ml aliquots of the supernatant fluid 0.25 ml of 15 N NaOH and 0.30 ml of 2 % NaIO$_4$ were added. The mixture was allowed to stand for 4 min at room temperature. Exactly 0.30 ml of 10 % $NaHSO_4$ was then added, followed by 1 ml of 5 N HCl. One ml of the reaction mixture was removed and shaken vigorously for 5 min with 5 ml of toluene to extract the p-hydroxybenzaldehyde formed. Four ml of the toluene extract was mixed with 5 ml of the toluene-phosphor solution, and radioactivity was determined in a scintillation counter. Internal standards were used to correct for any quenching.

III. 4. 3. RADIOASSAY USING PHENYLETHANOLAMINE-N-METHYLTRANSFERASE (PNMT) (Molinoff, Weinshilboum and Axelrod, 1971)

A highly sensitive radioassay for the determination of dopamine-β-hydroxylase activity in homogenates of adrenal gland, heart, salivary glands, stellate ganglion, and in human and rat serum has been described (Molinoff, Weinshilboum and Axelrod, 1971; Weinshilboum and Axelrod, 1971; Goldstein, Freedman and Bonnay, 1971).* The assay uses either phenylethylamine or tyramine as a substrate and is based on the sequential conversion of the product of the dopamine-β-hydroxylase reaction to a radioactively labeled N-methyl derivative by reaction with partially purified bovine adrenal phenylethanolamine-N-methyltransferase in the presence of S-adenosyl-L-methionine-methyl-C^{14}. The N-methyl derivatives are separated by solvent extraction and their radioactivity is determined.

$$\text{phenylethylamine} \xrightarrow{\text{dopamine-}\beta\text{-hydroxylase}} \text{phenylethanolamine}$$

$$\xrightarrow[S\text{-adenosylmethionine-methyl-}C^{14}]{\text{phenylethanolamine-}N\text{-methyltransferase}} C^{14}\text{-}N\text{-methylphenylethanolamine}$$

Endogenous inhibitors are inactivated either by copper or N-ethylmaleimide.

Tissues were homogenized in 25 to 400 volumes of 0.005 M Tris buffer, pH 7.5, containing 0.1 % Triton X-100. Homogenates were centrifuged at 10,000 × g for 10 min. Two hundred μl of the supernatant fluid was added to a 15 ml glass-stoppered centrifuge tube containing a reaction mixture of 25 μl of 0.048M ascorbic acid, pH 6; 25 μl of 0.05 M sodium fumarate, pH 6; 20μl of 0.006M pargyline (a monoamine oxidase inhibitor); 1,500 units of catalase in 10μl of 1.0 M Tris buffer, pH 7.4; 10μl of 0.03 M phenylethylamine; 10 μl of 1.0 M Tris buffer at pH 6; and 10μl of $CuSO_4$ in appropriate concentration (final concentration 10–100 μM) to give an optimal

---

* The author is grateful to Dr. Julius Axelrod (National Institute of Mental Health, Bethesda, Maryland, U.S.A.) for his personal communication about his method.

activity for the tissue being assayed. The optimum concentration of CuSO$_4$ should be preliminarily examined with various amounts of the homogenate. The reaction mixture (total volume 310 μl) was incubated at 37°C for 20 min. The dopamine-β-hydroxylase portion of the assay was then stopped and the phenylethanolamine-N-methyltransferase reaction initiated by adding to each tube a mixture of 10 μl of PNMT, 10 μl of EDTA equivalent to Cu in the first incubation, 10 μl of S-adenosylmethionine-methyl-C^{14} (1 nmole) and 80 μl of 1.0 M Tris buffer at pH 8.6. At pH 8.6 dopamine-β-hydroxylase has less than 5 % of the activity which it has at pH 6. The phenylethanolamine-N-methyltransferase reaction was stopped by the addition of 0.5 ml of 0.5 M borate buffer at pH 10. The C^{14}-N-methylphenylethanolamine was extracted into 6 ml of toluene containing 3 % isoamyl alcohol by vigorous shaking on a Vortex mixer for 15 sec. After centrifugation at low speed, 4 ml of the organic phase was transferred to a counting vial with 10 ml of phosphor for radioactive determination. Blanks consisting of tissue homogenates heated at 95°C for 5 min were run in all experiments, as were internal standards consisting of 100 ng of phenylethanolamine added to the entire reaction mixture. The internal standard was used in the calculation of absolute amounts of dopamine-β-hydroxylase activity and corrected for any inhibition of phenylethanolamine-N-methyltransferase.

Tyramine also can be used as a substrate. The assay was carried out in a similar way except that 10 μl of 0.03 M tyramine was used as a substrate and 40 ng of octopamine HCl was used as the internal standard. After the reaction was stopped with borate buffer, the C^{14}-N-methyloctopamine formed was extracted into a mixture of toluene and isoamyl alcohol, 3/2 (v/v). After centrifugation, 4 ml of the organic phase was transferred to counting vials containing an additional 2 ml of toluene/isoamyl alcohol (3/2). The samples were then dried in a chromatography oven at 80 °C. This drying step was necessary to remove volatile radioactive contaminants which were extracted into the toluene isoamyl alcohol. After drying, the residue was dissolved in 1 ml ethanol, and the radioactivity determined after the addition of 10 ml of phosphor. Although the use of tyramine could increase the sensitivity of the assay, the drawbacks were the high blank values and the possible interference from endogenous tissue stores of octopamine. Phenylethylamine was routinely used as substrate in this assay procedure by Molinoff, Weinshilboum and Axelrod (1971).

III. 4. 4. REPORTED ACTIVITIES

The activities of dopamine-β-hydroxylase with various enzyme prepara-

178

TABLE VII. Distribution of Dopamine-β-Hydroxylase.

Tissue	Enzyme preparation	Substrate	Cofactor	Enzyme activity (nmoles/min)	Reference
Beef adrenal medulla	Slices	Tyramine	(−)	4.3 (per g tissue)	1)
Beef adrenal medulla	Homogenate (with N-ethylmaleimide)	Tyramine	Ascorbate	12,500 (per g tissue)	2)
Beef adrenal medulla	$(NH_4)_2SO_4$ stage	Dopamine	Ascorbate	59.2 (per mg protein)	3)
Human pheochromocytoma				18.5	
Human neuroblastoma				10	
Beef adrenal (whole gland)	A homogeneous enzyme	Dopamine	Ascorbate	3,250 (per mg protein)[a]	4)
Rat vas deferens	$100,000 \times g$ particles	Dopamine	Ascorbate	0.026 (per mg protein)	5)
	DEAE-cellulose stage			12.3	
Bull vas deferens	$100,000 \times g$ particles			0.000	
	DEAE-cellulose stage			3.7	
Rat heart	$100,000 \times g$ particles			0.000	
	DEAE-cellulose stage			32.2	
Dog splenic nerve	Homogenate (with Triton X-100)	Tyramine	Ascorbate	13.2 (per g tissue)	6)
Dog coeliac ganglion				24.9	

[a] 25°C.

1) Pisano, Creveling and Udenfriend, 1960.
2) Kuzuya and Nagatsu, 1969b.
3) Bohuon and Guerinot, 1968.
4) Friedman and Kaufman, 1965b.
5) Austin, Livett and Chubb, 1967.
6) Laduron and Belpaire, 1968a.

tions are shown in Table VII and are expressed as nmoles/min by calculating the reported values. The activities of minces or homogenates are extremely low because of the presence of endogenous inhibitors. The activity in adrenal homogenate was measured by adding N-ethylmaleimide to block the endogenous inhibitors (Nagatsu, Kuzuya and Hidaka, 1967; Kuzuya and Nagatsu, 1969b). A sensitive radioassay using phenylethanolamine-N-methyltransferase and S-adenosylmethionine-methyl-C¹⁴ together with copper or N-ethylmaleimide during the incubation (Molinoff, Weinshilboum and Axelrod, 1971; Weinshilboum and Axelrod, 1971; Goldstein, Freedman and Bonnay, 1971) permitted the assay of the enzyme activity in tissue homogenates and serum.

III. 5. Assay of Phenylethanolamine-N-methyltransferase Activity

A. *Principle*
The assay method originally developed by Axelrod (1962b) is based on the fluorometric or radiometric measurement of metanephrine after the incubation of normetanephrine and S-adenosylmethionine with an enzyme preparation. The radiometric method using (S-methyl-C¹⁴)-S-adenosyl-L-methionine is the most sensitive and convenient. The following procedure, which can be used for assaying the activity of crude adrenal tissue, was described by Fuller and Hunt (1965).

B. *Enzyme preparation*
One part of the adrenal tissue was homogenized with 15 parts of 0.25 M sucrose at 0°C. The homogenate was centrifuged at 50,000 × g for 20 min, and the supernatant was dialyzed against 5 mM phosphate buffer, pH 6.8.

C. *Reagents*
1. *Phosphate buffer* (1.0 M, pH 7.9).
2. *Normetanephrine solution* (4.6 mM). 10.0 mg of (±)-normetanephrine·HCl was dissolved in water to 10 ml.
3. *S-Adenosyl-L-methionine (S-methyl-C¹⁴) solution.* S-Adenosyl-L-methionine (mol wt 398.5) is most stable when stored frozen in dilute sulfuric acid solution at a pH of 2.0–6.0. It is unstable at a higher pH. The isotope stock solution was diluted with dilute sulfuric acid (pH 2.5) to provide a more convenient concentration. Specific radioactivity was usually 50 mCi/mmole.
4. *Toluene-isoamyl alcohol mixture.* 3:2, v/v.
5. *Borate buffer* (0.5 M, pH 10.). 30.9 g of boric acid (mol wt 61.84) was

dissolved in about 900 ml of water. NaOH, 10 N (about 40 ml) was added to pH 10.0. Then water was added to make 1l.

6. *Bray's scintillation solution.* See section III. 2.

D. *Procedure*

An example of the preparation of the incubation mixture (0.3 ml) in a 10 ml glass-stoppered centrifuge tube in an ice bath is shown in the following table:

	Volume (μl)	Amount (μmoles)	Final concentration (M)	
Phosphate buffer (1.0 M, pH 7.9)	25	25	8.3×10^{-2}	
($\pm$)-Normetanephrine (4.6 mM)	25	0.133	3.8×10^{-4}	
(S-Methyl-C^{14})-S-adenosyl-	10	0.002	6.6×10^{-6}	total
L-methionine (50 mCi/mmole)		(0.1 μCi)		1.1×10^{-4}
S-Adenosyl-L-methionine	30	0.03	1.0×10^{-4}	
(1 mM)				
Enzyme	10–20			
Water (total volume)	to 300			

The enzyme concentration was adjusted so that less than 10 % utilization of the labeled substrate occurred (Connett and Kirshner, 1970). Incubation was carried out at 37°C for 30–60 min. For a blank, normetanephrine (substrate) was omitted from the incubation mixture and added after incubation. The reaction was stopped by adding 0.5 ml of borate buffer, 0.5 M, pH 10 and then 5.0 ml of the toluene-isoamyl alcohol mixture was added. The solution was mixed for 30 sec with a mixer and centrifuged at 1,500 rpm for 5 min and 2.0 ml of the supernatant layer was transferred into a counting vial to which 5 ml of Bray's scintillation solution was added. Radioactivity was measured in a liquid scintillation spectrometer. Efficiency was obtained by counting C^{14}-toluene in 2.0 ml of toluene-isoamyl alcohol with the Bray's solution.

E. *Calculation*

$$\frac{(SAM)^* \text{ nmoles}}{(SAM) \text{ cpm}} \times [(\text{Experiment}) \text{ cpm} - (\text{Blank}) \text{ cpm}] = \text{Product (nmoles)}$$

(SAM) cpm: radioactivity of S-adenosylmethionine-methyl-C^{14} counted in the Bray's scintillator.

(SAM) nmoles: total S-adenosylmethionine concentration.

---

* This includes the endogenous tissue [SAM] in a crude enzyme preparation, which is negligibly small.

(Experiment) cpm and (Blank) cpm: radioactivities of experiment and blank counted in the toluene extract plus Bray's scintillator.

F. *Reported activities*
The tissue distribution of phenylethanolamine-*N*-methyltransferase is shown in Table VIII. The reported values of enzyme activity are calculated and expressed as nmoles/min.

TABLE VIII. Distribution of Phenylethanolamine-*N*-Methyltransferase (PNMT).

Enzyme preparation	PNMT activity (nmoles/min) (37°C)	Reference
Rabbit adrenal homogenate	47 (per g tissue)	Axelrod, 1962 b
Rat adrenal homogenate	33	
Monkey adrenal (whole gland) homogenate	28	
Cow adrenal homogenate	13	
Guinea pig adrenal homogenate	8	
Cat adrenal homogenate	5	
Bovine adrenal medulla homogenate	0.67 (per mg protein)	Connett and Kirshner, 1970
A homogeneous enzyme from bovine adrenal medulla	40	
Human adrenal homogenate	0.015 (per mg protein)	Kitabchi and Williams, 1969

III. 6. Assay of Catechol-*O*-methyltransferase Activity

A. *Principle*
Catechol-*O*-methyltransferase activity can be measured either by fluorometry (Axelrod and Tomchick, 1958) or by radioassay (Axelrod, 1962a). The enzyme activity is determined by measuring metanephrine formed from epinephrine and *S*-adenosyl-L-methionine in the presence of Mg^{++}.

A colorimetric enzyme assay based on the reaction of catecholamines with hydroxylamine was reported by Abdel-Latif (1969).

B. *Enzyme preparation*
Since the enzyme is soluble, a high-speed supernatant fraction from isotonic KCl or sucrose homogenate is used as a crude enzyme preparation. One part of tissue was homogenized with 3 parts of 0.25 *M* sucrose or 0.15 *M* KCl at 0°C. The homogenate was centrifuged at 48,000 × *g* for 20 min and 20 *μl* of the supernatant was used for the assay.

C. *Reagents*

1. *Phosphate buffer* (1 M, pH 7.6).

2. *(−)-Epinephrine-*D-*bitartrate* (3 mM). 9.99 mg of (−)-epinephrine-D-bitartrate was dissolved in 0.01 N HCl to 10 ml, and kept in deep freeze.

3. *MgCl₂* (0.1 M). 203 mg of MgCl₂·6H₂O (mol wt 203.33) was dissolved in water to 10 ml.

4. *S-Adenosyl-*L-*methionine (SAM)* (for fluorometry) (3 mM). S-Adenosyl-L-methionine (mol wt 398.5) is most stable when stored frozen in dilute sulfuric acid solution at a pH of 2.0–6.0, therefore, 1.20 mg was dissolved in dilute sulfuric acid to 1.0 ml.

5. *S-Adenosyl-*L-*methionine (S-methyl-*C^{14}*) solution (for radioassay).* The commercially available isotope stock solution (usually about 50 mCi/mmole), was diluted with dilute sulfuric acid (pH 2.5) to give a convenient concentration (10 μCi/ml).

6. *Toluene-isoamyl alcohol mixture.* 3:2, v/v.

7. *Borate buffer* (0.5 M, pH 10). 30.9 g of boric acid (mol wt 61.84) was dissolved in about 900 ml of water. NaOH, 10 N (about 40 ml) was added to make pH 10.0. Then water was added to make 1l.

8. *Bray's scintillation solution.* See section III. 2.

D. *Procedure*

1. *Fluorometry.* An example of the preparation of the incubation mixture (1.0 ml) in a 15 ml glass-stoppered centrifuge tube in an ice bath is shown in the following table:

	Volume (μl)	Amount (μmoles)	Final concentration (M)
Enzyme	500–700		
Phosphate buffer (1 M, pH 7.6)	50	50	5×10^{-2}
MgCl₂ (0.1 M)	100	10	1×10^{-2}
(−)-Epinephrine-D-bitartrate (3 mM)	100	0.3	3×10^{-4}
S-Adenosyl-L-methionine (SAM) (3 mM)	50	0.15	1.5×10^{-4}
Water (total volume)	to 1,000		

The incubation volume can be reduced to one-tenth of that in the original method by Axelrod (1962). When higher sensitivity was required, the total volume 1.0 ml system should be used as in the original method. Incubation was carried out at 37°C for 20 min. For a blank, S-adenosyl-L-methionine was omitted from the incubation mixture and added after incubation. The reaction was stopped by adding 0.5 ml of borate buffer, 0.5 M, pH 10. Then 10.0 ml of toluene-isoamyl alcohol mixture was added and the solution was mixed for 30 sec with a mixer, and centrifuged at 1,500 rpm for 5 min. An 8.0 ml-aliquot of the extract was transferred to another 10-ml glass-stoppered centrifuge tube containing 1.5 ml of 0.1 N HCl and shaken for 5 min. After light centrifugation, the solvent layer was removed by aspiration and 1 ml of the acid extract was transferred to a quartz cuvette for fluorometry. Metanephrine formed was measured at 335 nm after activation at 285 nm. To correct the recovery (about 60 %), a known amount of metanephrine was carried through the extraction procedure and used as a standard.

2. *Radioassay*. An example of the preparation of the incubation mixture (50 μl) in a 15 ml glass-stoppered centrifuge tube in an ice bath is shown in the following table.

	Volume (μl)	Amount (μmoles)	Final concentration (M)	
Enzyme	10			
Phosphate buffer (1M, pH 7.6)	5	5	1×10^{-1}	
MgCl$_2$ (0.1 M)	5	0.5	1×10^{-2}	
(−)-Epinephrine-D-bitartrate (3 mM)	5	0.015	3×10^{-4}	
S-Adenosyl-L-methionine (S-methyl-C^{14}) (SAM) (50 mCi/mmole)	0.002 10	(0.1 μCi)	4×10^{-5}	} total
S-Adenosyl-L-methionine (1 mM)	10	0.01	2×10^{-4}	} 2.4×10^{-4}
Water (total volume)	to 50			

Incubation was carried out at 37°C for 20 min. For a blank, either epinephrine or S-adenosylmethionine was omitted during the incubation and added after incubation. The reaction was stopped by adding 0.5 ml of 0.5 M borate buffer, pH 10. Then 5.0 ml of toluene-isoamyl alcohol mixture was added and the solution was mixed for 30 sec with a mixer, and centrifuged at 1,500 rpm for 5 min. Two ml of the supernatant layer was transferred to a counting vial, and 10 ml of Bray's scintillation solution was added and radioactivity was measured in a liquid scintillation spectrometer. Efficiency was obtained by counting toluene-C^{14} in 2.0 ml of toluene-isoamyl alcohol with the Bray's solution.

E.   *Calculation*
Same as III. 5-E (p. 180).

F.   *Reported activities*
The tissue distribution of catechol-O-methyltransferase is shown in Table IX. The enzyme activity is expressed in nmoles/min by calculating the reported values.

TABLE IX. Distribution of Catechol-O-Methyltransferase (COMT).

Enzyme preparation	COMT activity (nmoles/min) (37°C)	Reference
Rat liver		
Soluble fraction	0.47 (per mg protein)	Axelrod and
Calcium phosphate gel eluate	14	Thomchick,
Soluble fraction	120 (per g tissue)	1958
Rat kidney	35 (per g tissue)	
Spleen	8	
Small intestine	5	
Lung	5	
Brain	3	
Heart muscle	3	
Cow liver	55	
Pig liver	48	
Mouse liver	38	
Guinea pig liver	17	
Man liver ($-10°C$, 3 months)	7	
Cat liver	5	
Rabbit liver	2	
Monkey		
Neurohypophysis	16	Axelrod, Albers
Pons	9	and Clemente,
Caudate nucleus	9	1959
Occipital cortex	8	
Hypothalamus	8	
Dorsal hypocampus	8	
Ventral hypocampus	5	
Amygdala	4	
Superior cervical ganglion	11	
Splanchnic nerve	7	
Sciatic nerve	7	
Splenic nerve	5	
Liver	140	
Submaxillary gland	70	
Parotid gland	60	
Pancreas	58	
Adenohypophysis	35	
Thyroid	10	
Aorta	10	
Dog kidney		
Cortex	0.019 ± 0.002 (per mg protein)	Nagatsu, Rust
Medulla	0.037 ± 0.005	and DeQuattro,
Denervated cortex	0.025 ± 0.001	1969
Denervated medulla	0.035 ± 0.004	

III. 7. Assay of Monoamine Oxidase Activity

Various methods for the assay of monoamine oxidase have been described based on the enzymatic reaction :

$$\boxed{R\text{-}CH_2\text{-}NH_2} + H_2O + \boxed{O_2} \xrightarrow{\text{MAO}} \boxed{RCHO} + \boxed{NH_3} + \boxed{H_2O_2}$$

$$RCHO + H_2O + NAD \xrightarrow[\text{dehydrogenase}]{\text{aldehyde}} \boxed{RCOOH} + NADH_2$$

The assay principles are :
(1) Disappearance of substrate ($R\text{-}CH_2\text{-}NH_2$)
(2) Consumption of oxygen
(3) Formation of the aldehyde
(4) Formation of ammonia
(5) Formation of hydrogen peroxide
(6) Formation of the acid after conversion of the aldehyde
Reliable methods based upon my experience are described in this section. A survey of various assay methods is shown in Table X.

TABLE X.   Assays of Monoamine Oxidase Activity.

Principle	Procedure	Reference
Serotonin disappearance	Colorimetry (Vis)	Udenfriend, Weissbach and Clark, 1955
Kynuramine disappearance	Colorimetry (UV)	Weissbach, Smith, Daly, Witkop and Udenfriend, 1960
Oxygen consumption	Manometry or oxygen electrode	Creasey, 1956; Tipton, 1969
Indoleacetic acid formation from tryptamine	Fluorometry	Lovenberg, Levine and Sjoerdsma, 1962
5-Hydroxyindoleacetic acid formation from serotonin	Fluorometry	Hidaka, Nagatsu and Yagi, 1967
4-Hydroxyquinoline formation from kynuramine	Fluorometry	Kraml, 1965
Benzaldehyde formation from benzylamine	Colorimetry (UV)	Tabor, C., Tabor, H. and Rosenthal, 1954; McEwen and Cohen, 1963
p-Dimethylaminobenzaldehyde formation from p-dimethyl-aminobenzylamine	Colorimetry (Vis)	Deitrich and Erwin, 1969
Ammonia formation	Colorimetry (Vis)	Nagatsu and Yagi, 1966
Hydrogen peroxide formation	Fluorometry	Guilbault, Brignac and Juneau, 1968; Snyder and Hendley, 1968
	Amperometry	Mason and Olson, 1970
Indoleacetaldehyde-C^{14} or indoleacetic acid-C^{14} formation from tryptamine-C^{14}	Radioassay	Wurtman and Axelrod, 1963b

III. 7. 1. Assay Based on the Disappearance of Serotonin (colorimetry) (Udenfriend, Weissbach and Clark, 1955; Udenfriend, Weissbach and Brodie, 1958; Ozaki, M., Weissbach, Ozaki, A., Witkop and Udenfriend, 1960)

A. *Principle*
Serotonin is used as substrate, and after incubation with a monoamine oxidase preparation, the remainder of the serotonin is assayed colorimetrically. This method is highly reproducible.

B. *Enzyme preparation*
Crude or purified enzyme preparations can be used for the assay. Tissue was homogenized with 2 volumes of 0.15 M KCl, 0.25 M sucrose, or water. Usually, 0.5 ml of the rat liver homogenate was used for the assay. The amount of enzyme employed should be such that no more than 60 % will be oxidized during the period of incubation.

C. *Reagents*
 1. *Phosphate buffer* (1 M, pH 7.4).
 2. *Serotonin* (5.69 mM). 23.0 mg of serotonin creatinine sulfate hydrate (mol wt 405.4) [free serotonin (mol wt 176.21), 10.0 mg] was dissolved in water to 10 ml.
 3. *Borate buffer* (0.5 M, pH 10). 94.2 g boric acid was dissolved in 3l H_2O and 165 ml of 10 N NaOH was added. The buffer solution was then saturated with purified n-butanol and NaCl.
 4. *n-Butanol.* n-Butanol was washed with an equal volume of 0.1 N NaOH, then with equal volume of 0.1 N HCl, and finally twice with distilled water.
 5. *Heptane.* Heptane was treated in the same manner as the n-butanol.
 6. *1-Nitroso-2-naphthol solution* (0.1 %). 1-Nitroso-2-naphthol in 95 % ethyl alcohol.
 7. *Nitrous acid reagent.* 0.2 ml of 2.5 % $NaNO_2$ was added to 5 ml of 2 N H_2SO_4. This reagent should be prepared fresh daily.

D. *Procedure*
The incubation mixture (1.75 ml) was prepared in a 10-ml test tube in an ice bath as shown in the table on next page.

At zero time, 0.25 ml of the incubation mixture was transferred to a glass-stoppered centrifuge tube containing 15.0 ml of n-butanol, 2.0 ml of borate buffer (0.5 M, pH 10) and 3 g of NaCl. The reaction mixture was incubated

	Volume (ml)	Amount (μmoles)	Final concentration (M)
Enzyme	0.50	—	—
Phosphate buffer (1.0 M, pH 7.4)	0.25	250	1.4×10^{-1}
Serotonin (5.69 mM)	0.50	2.84	1.6×10^{-3}
Water	to 1.75		

at 37°C for 40 min in air with shaking. Two 0.25-ml aliquots were removed at 20 min and 40 min, respectively, and each aliquot was transferred to a glass-stoppered centrifuge tube containing n-butanol, borate buffer, and NaCl. The mixture in the centrifuge tube was shaken for 10 min and centrifuged. Ten ml of the supernatant n-butanol layer was transferred to another glass-stoppered centrifuge tube containing 10 ml of n-heptane and 2.5 ml of 0.1 N HCl. The mixture was shaken and centrifuged. The supernatant solvent was removed by aspiration, and 2.0 ml of the HCl layer was transferred to another centrifuge tube. One ml of nitrosonaphthol reagent and then 1.0 ml of nitrous acid reagent was added. The mixture was heated at 55°C for 5 min. Five ml of ethylene dichloride was added, and the tube was shaken to extract the unchanged nitrosonaphthol. Thirty five μg (free) (0.199 μmole) of serotonin in 2.0 ml of 0.1 N HCl with nitrosonaphthol was used as a standard. The blank was composed of 2.0 ml of 0.1 N HCl. The tube was then centrifuged, and the supernatant was transferred to a cuvette. The absorbance (purple color) was measured at 540 nm. Recovery of serotonin in the entire extraction procedure was about 90 %. The zero-time value gave an absorbance of about 0.6.

III. 7. 2. ASSAY BASED ON THE FORMATION OF 5-HYDROXYINDOLE-ACETIC ACID FROM SEROTONIN (fluorometry) (Hidaka, Nagatsu and Yagi, 1967)

A. *Principle*
Serotonin is used as substrate and incubated with monoamine oxidase and aldehyde dehydrogenase to convert 5-hydroxyindoleacetaldehyde to 5-hydroxyindoleacetic acid. The acid is separated from serotonin by a cation exchange column and assayed fluorometrically.

Serotonin   5-Hydroxyindoleaceto-
                                    aldehyde

5-Hydroxyindoleacetic acid

B. Reagents

1. *Serotonin-NAD-nicotinamide mixture in phosphate buffer.* For 10 incubation tubes, 11.5 mg (28.4 μmoles) of serotonin creatinine sulfate hydrate (mol wt 405.4), 53 mg (80 μmoles) of NAD (mol wt 663.4), and 61 mg (50 μmoles) of nicotinamide (mol wt 122.2) were dissolved in water to 12.0 ml, and 2.5 ml of phosphate buffer (1 M, pH 7.4) were added.

2. *5-Hydroxyindoleacetic acid.* A solution containing 9.6 mg of 5-hydroxyindoleacetic acid (mol wt 191.2) dissolved in water to 50 ml was prepared and diluted 50-fold. The standard was composed of 0.5 ml containing 10 nmoles.

3. *Aldehyde dehydrogenase preparation* (Lovenberg, Levin and Sjoerdsma, 1962). Guinea pigs were pretreated intraperitoneally with 5–10 mg/kg of β-phenylisopropylhydrazine (JB-516, Catron, Lakeside Laboratories). A twenty percent kidney homogenate was prepared in 0.25 M sucrose, and centrifuged at 100,000 × g for 1 hr. The supernatant obtained had high aldehyde dehydrogenase activity with negligible monoamine oxidase activity, and could be stored at −20°C. The activity of this preparation was checked by measuring the rate of NADH formation during incubation with acetaldehyde (Racker, 1955).

4. *Dowex-50-W-X2* 100–200 mesh, H+-form, 0.5 × 5 cm.

C. Procedure

The incubation mixture (1.75 ml) was prepared in a 10-ml test tube in an ice bath as shown in the following table :

		Volume (ml)	Amount (μmoles)	Final concentration (M)
Serotonin			2.84	1.6×10^{-3}
NAD	Mixture		8.0	4.6×10^{-3}
Nicotinamide	solution	1.45	50	2.9×10^{-2}
Phosphate buffer			250	1.4×10^{-1}
Aldehyde dehydrogenase		0.10		
Enzyme		0.20		
Water		to 1.75		

Incubation was carried out at 37°C for 40 min. At 0, 20 and 40 min, three 0.5 ml-aliquots were removed and placed in boiling water for 2 min. After the addition of 3 ml of chilled distilled water, the denatured protein was centrifuged off. The supernatant was passed through a Dowex-50 column to remove unreacted serotonin. The column was washed with 10 ml of water and both the effluent and the washing were collected in a 30-ml test tube. To the solution 0.5 ml of 1 M phosphate buffer (pH 7.4) and one drop of 2 N NaOH were added to adjust the pH to 7.4. The native fluorescence of 5-hydroxyindoleacetic acid in the neutralized column effluent was measured in an Aminco-Bowman spectrophotofluorometer at 295 nm excitation and 350 nm fluorescence (uncorrected wave length). A blank, to which the monoamine oxidase preparation was omitted during the incubation and added after the incubation, and an internal standard (5-hydroxyindoleacetic acid, 10 nmoles in 0.5 ml water plus 3.0 ml water) were carried out to permit direct calculation of results. In this procedure the recovery of 5-hydroxyindoleacetic acid was 90–95 %.

III. 7. 3. ASSAY BASED ON KYNURAMINE DISAPPEARANCE (colorimetry) (Weissbach, Smith, Daly, Witkop and Udenfriend, 1960)

A. *Principle*
This method is based on the oxidation of kynuramine to 4-hydroxyquinoline by monoamine oxidase. Since kynuramine has an absorption peak at 360 nm, the disappearance of kynuramine can be followed conveniently in a spectrophotometer. This method is one of the most simple and reproducible assays in my experience. By means of spontaneous cyclization of the intermediate aldehyde formed by the oxidative deamination of kynuramine, 4-hydroxyquinoline is formed.

Kynuramine   4-Hydroxyquinoline

B. *Enzyme preparation*
Crude enzyme preparation such as an homogenate or mitochondrial sus-

pension can be used. Kynuramine disappearance was linear with time until the absorbance at 360 nm fell below 0.150. Therefore, a suitable amount of enzyme should be used to obtain the linearity of the absorbance decrease with time. Tissues were homogenized in 5 volumes of distilled water, 0.25 M sucrose or 0.15 M KCl at 0°C. The homogenate was centrifuged at 1,000 × g for 10 min to remove cell debris, and 0.1–1.0 ml of the supernatant was usually used for the assay. For example, the suitable amounts of tissues for rat brain, liver, and kidney were 30, 10 and 40 mg of tissues, respectively.

C. *Reagents*
    1. *Phosphate buffer* (0.3 M, pH 7.4).
    2. *Kynuramine* (1 mM). 16.3 mg of kynuramine dihydrobromide (mol wt 326.1) was dissolved in water to 50 ml.
    3. $ZnSO_4 \cdot 7H_2O$, 10 % aqueous solution.
    4. *NaOH* (1 N).

D. *Procedure*
The kynuramine disappearance can be measured either by continuous recording of the absorbance at 360 nm in the thermostatically controlled cell containing the reaction mixture while in the instrument, or by incubating the samples in a centrifuge tube to measure the absorbance after stopping the reaction.
    1. *Continuous recording of absorbance at 360 nm.* The incubation mixtures (3.0 ml) were prepared in 3-ml silica cuvettes. The procedure is shown in the table below.

	Experimental cuvette (ml)	Blank cuvette (ml)	Amount (μmoles)	Final concentration (M)
Enzyme	0.1–1.0	0.1–1.0	—	—
Phosphate buffer (0.3 M, pH 7.4)	0.50	0.50	150	5×10^{-2}
Water (total volume)	to 3.0	3.0	—	—
Kynuramine (1 mM)	0.50	—	0.50	1.67×10^{-4}

The incubation mixture was preincubated in the cell thermostatically controlled at 37°C while in a self-recording spectrophotometer. The reaction was started by adding kynuramine. In the blank cuvette, kynuramine was replaced with water. After the final addition, mixing was achieved by inversion and an initial reading was made at 360 nm. The initial absorbance at 360 nm was approximately 0.5. The decrease in the absorbance at 360 nm was continuouly recorded, and the initial velocity was obtained.

2. *Discontinuous recording of absorbance at 360 nm.* Incubation was carried out in a centrifuge tube. The enzymatic reaction was stopped with zinc sulfate for deproteinization. After centrifugation, the absorbance of the supernatant was measured at 360 nm. The incubation mixture was prepared in a 10-ml centrifuge tube in an ice bath as shown in the following table :

	Volume (ml)	Amount (μmoles)	Final concentration (M)
Enzyme	0.1–1.0	—	—
Phosphate buffer (0.3 M, pH 7.4)	0.25	75	5×10^{-2}
Kynuramine (1 mM)	0.25	0.25	1.67×10^{-4}
Water (total volume)	to 1.50	—	—

For a blank, the substrate kynuramine was omitted during and was added after incubation. Incubation was carried out at 37°C for 30 min in air with shaking. The reaction was stopped by adding 0.25 ml of 10 % ZnSO$_4$ and 0.05 ml of 1 N NaOH. The reaction mixture was boiled for 2 min and centrifuged. The absorbance of the supernatant at 360 nm was measured against water. The absorbance difference (A_{360} of blank $-A_{360}$ of experimental) was measured to calculate the amount of kynuramine destroyed.

III. 7. 4. ASSAY BASED ON THE FORMATION OF 4-HYDROXYQUINOLINE FROM KYNURAMINE (fluorometry) (Kraml, 1965)

A. *Principle*
Kynuramine is also used as a substrate in this method. Instead of determining the disappearance of kynuramine, the appearance of 4-hydroxyquinoline, which arises from the spontaneous cyclization of intermediate aldehyde formed by the oxidative deamination of kynuramine, is measured. This method is highly reproducible and sensitive.

B. *Enzyme preparation*
As in the kynuramine disappearance method (section III. 7. 3), any crude enzyme preparations can be used. Since this method is highly sensitive, a variety of tissues with low enzyme activities, such as guinea pig atria and cat ganglia, can be assayed.

C. *Reagents*

　1. *Phosphate buffer* (0.3 M, pH 7.4).

　2. *Kynuramine* (1 mM). 16.3 mg of kynuramine dihydrobromide (mol wt 326.1) was dissolved in water to 50 ml.

　3. $ZnSO_4 \cdot 7H_2O$, 10 % aqueous solution.

　4. *NaOH* (1 N).

　5. *4-Hydroxyquinoline standard solution, Stock solution*. 100 nmoles/ml. 19.92 mg of 4-hydroxyquinoline trihydrate (mol wt 199.21) was dissolved in water to 1.0 l. A working solution (1 nmoles/ml) was made by diluting the stock solution 100-fold with water.

D. *Procedure*

The incubation was carried out in a centrifuge tube. The enzymatic reaction was stopped with zinc sulfate for deproteinization. After centrifugation, the supernatant was made alkaline, and the fluorescence of 4-hydroxyquinoline was measured. The incubation mixture was prepared in a 10-ml centrifuge tube in an ice bath as shown in the following table :

	Volume (ml)	Amount (μmoles)	Final concentration (M)
Enzyme	An appropriate amount	—	—
Phosphate buffer (0.3 M, pH 7.4)	0.25	75	5×10^{-2}
Kynuramine (1 mM)	0.25	0.25	1.67×10^{-4}
Water (total volume)	to 1.50		

For a blank, kynuramine was omitted during and was added after incubation. The incubation was carried out at 37°C for 30 min in air with shaking. The reaction was stopped by adding 0.25 ml of 10 % $ZnSO_4$ solution and 0.05 ml of 1 N NaOH. The reaction mixture was boiled for 2 min and centrifuged, and 1 ml of the supernatant was removed and mixed with 2.0 ml of 1 N NaOH. As a standard, 1.0 nmole of 4-hydroxyquinoline in 1.0 ml of water was mixed with 2.0 ml of 1 N NaOH. Fluorescence was measured at 380 nm with an excitation at 315 nm.

III. 7. 5. ASSAY BASED ON THE OXYGEN CONSUMPTION

A. *Manometric assay* (Creasey, 1956)

　1. *Principle*. Manometric assay was widely used in the study of monoamine oxidase until about 1960. A detailed stoichiometric study was made

by Creasey (1956) using tyramine as substrate and washed rat liver mitochondria as enzyme. Under Creasey's assay conditions, one atom of oxygen
was absorbed for each molecule of substrate oxidized and the oxygen
absorbed at 30 min was proportional to the monoamine oxidase concentration.

2. *Enzyme preparations.* Crude monoamine oxidase preparations also
contain catalase, cytochrome c and cytochrome oxidase, aldehyde oxidase
and peroxidase, which are expected to make the observed oxygen uptake

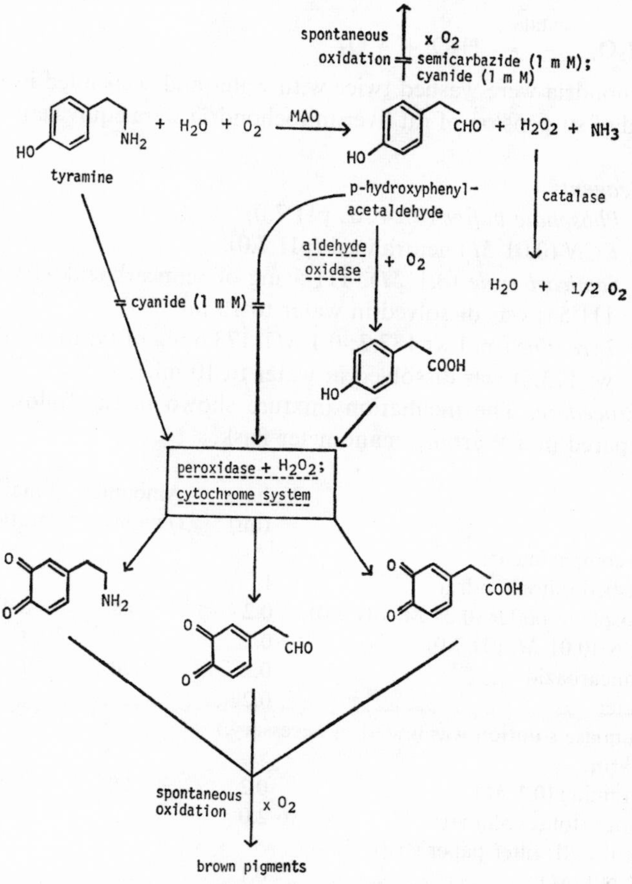

Fig. 29. Reactions likely to occur when tyramine is incubated with crude
monoamine oxidase. ----: reaction absent in washed rat liver mitochondria
(Creasey, 1956).

different from the theoretical value. It was shown that washed rat liver mitochondria contained catalase and peroxidase, but no cytochrome oxidase and aldehyde oxidase activities (Fig. 29). A buffered reaction mixture containing washed mitochondria as enzyme, 10 mM tyramine, 10 mM semicarbazid, 1 mM cyanide was shown to be suitable for measuring monoamine oxidase activity by monometric assay. One atom of oxygen was absorbed for each molecule of substrate oxidized (Creasey, 1956).

$$R\text{-}CH_2\text{-}NH_2 + H_2O + O_2 \xrightarrow{\text{MAO}} R\text{-}CHO + H_2O_2 + NH_3$$

$$H_2O_2 \xrightarrow{\text{catalase}} H_2O + \tfrac{1}{2}O_2$$

Mitochondria were washed twice with water and suspended in water so that 2 ml of suspension of rat liver mitochondria were equivalent to 1 g of tissue.

3. *Reagents*
   a. *Phosphate buffer* (0.24 M, pH 7.0).
   b. *KCN* (0.01 M) neutralized (pH 7.0).
   c. *Semicarbazide* (0.1 M). 111.5 mg of semicarbazide·HCl(mol wt 111.54) was dissolved in water to 10 ml.
   d. *Tyramine* (mol wt 137.2; 0.1 M). 173.6 mg of tyramine·HCl (mol wt 173.6) was dissolved in water to 10 ml.

4. *Procedure.* The incubation mixture shown in the following table was prepared in a Warburg manometer flask.

	Volume (ml)	Amounts (μmoles)	Final concentration (M)
Main compartment:			
Washed mitochondria	1	—	—
Phosphate buffer (0.24 M, pH 7.0)	0.2	48	2.4×10^{-2}
KCN (0.01 M, pH 7.0)	0.2	2	1×10^{-3}
Semicarbazid	0.2	20	1×10^{-2}
Water	0.2		
(Catalase solution was added, if necessary.)			
Side arm:			
Tyramine (0.1 M)	0.2	20	1×10^{-2}
Water (total volume)	to 2.0		
Central well: filter-paper strip			
KCN (2M)	0.1		

The flask was filled with O_2 for 2 min and equilibrated for 10 min before tipping in tyramine from the side arm. A control reaction mixture containing no substrate was also prepared and any O_2 absorbed by it was subtracted from that absorbed in the test reaction mixtures. Oxygen uptake was measured manometrically at 37°C, reading being taken at 0, 10, 20 and 30 min for an activity determination. Calculations were based on the result that one atom of oxygen was absorbed for each molecule of substrate oxidized.

B. *Oxygen electrode method* (Tipton, 1969)
   1. *Principle*. The uptake of oxygen can be measured with an oxygen electrode based on the manometric method of Creasey (1956).
   2. *Enzyme preparations*. See section III. 7. 5. A.
   3. *Reagents*. See section III. 7. 5. A.
   4. *Procedure*. The incubation mixture shown in the following table was in a cell to be used for the oxygen electrode.

	Volume (ml)	Amounts (μmoles)	Final concentration (M)
Phosphate buffer (0.5 M, pH 7.4)	0.10	50	5×10^{-2}
KCN (0.01 M, pH 7.4)	0.10	1	1×10^{-3}
Semicarbazid (0.1 M)	0.10	10	1×10^{-2}
Catalase			
Enzyme			
Water (total volume)	to 1.0		

The mixture was preincubated in air at 30°C for 5 min. The reaction was started by the addition of tyramine.

Tyramine (0.1 M)	0.10	10	1×10^{-2}

The initial velocity of the oxygen uptake was recorded.

III. 7. 6. ASSAY BASED ON THE FORMATION OF BENZALDEHYDE FROM BENZYLAMINE (Spectrophotometry) (Tabor, C.W., Tabor, H. and Rosenthal, 1954; McEwen and Cohen, 1963)

A. *Principle*
The absorption at 250 nm of benzaldehyde formed by the oxidative deamination of benzylamine is measured.

Benzylamine   Benzaldehyde

B. *Enzyme preparations*

Mitochondrial monoamine oxidase in various tissues and plasma amine oxidase can be assayed with this method. Purified plasma amine oxidase can be rapidly assayed simply by measuring the increased absorbance at 250 nm. Even crude tissue preparations can be used for the assay by the extraction procedure (McEwen and Cohen, 1963). Usually, 0.6 ml of 0.25 M sucrose homogenate (tissue : sucrose=1:9) was used for the assay.

C. *Reagents*

1. *Phosphate buffer* (0.3 M, pH 7.4).
2. *Benzylamine* (8 mM). Benzylamine (mol wt 107.16) was purified before use by distillation under reduced pressure in a helium atmosphere and 43 mg of benzylamine was dissolved in phosphate buffer to 50 ml.
3. *Benzaldehyde*. Benzaldehyde (mol wt 106.12) was purified before use by distillation under pressure in a helium atmosphere. The solution was kept in a tightly closed container and was protected from light.
4. *Perchloric acid* (60 %).
5. *Cyclohexane*.

D. *Procedure*

1. *Original method* (Tabor, C.W., Tabor, H. and Rosenthal, 1954). The incubation mixture (total volume, 3.0 ml) contained 200 μM of potassium phosphate buffer (pH 7.2), 10 μM of benzylamine, and enzyme and incubation was carried out at 30°C. One spectrophotometric unit was defined as the amount of enzyme catalyzing an increase of 0.001 per min in the absorbance at 250 nm. The spectrophotometric unit can be converted to μmoles of benzaldehyde formed from the molar absorptivity at 250 nm, $\varepsilon = 1.2 \times 10^4$ M^{-1}cm^{-1}. Four spectrophotometric units in a 3.0-ml incubation mixture are equal to about 1 nmole of benzaldehyde per 3.0 ml.

2. *The modified procedure of McEwen and Cohen* (1963). The original method was modified for the assay of crude enzyme preparations. The reaction was stopped by adding perchloric acid, and the benzaldehyde formed extracted into cyclohexane. The incubation mixture contains (total volume 1.5 ml) : 0.6 ml of serum, plasma or tissue homogenate; 0.75 ml of 0.2 M phosphate buffer (pH 7.2) (150 μmoles, final concentration 0.1 M); 0.15 ml of 8 mM benzylamine (1.2 μmoles, final concentration 0.8 mM) in the same buffer. The blank tube was identical except that the substrate, benzylamine, was not added until the end of the incubation. The reaction mixture was incubated at 37°C for 3 hr in air with shaking. Following incubation (and the addition of the substrate to the blank tube), 0.15 ml of 60

% perchloric acid and then 1.5 ml of cyclohexane were added to each tube. The contents of all tubes were emulsified well with a mixer, allowed to settle at room temperature for 15 min, and then after a second emulsification, centrifuged for 10 min at 2,000 rpm. The absorbance of the cyclohexane extract from the experimental tube against that of the blank extract was measured at 242 nm in cuvettes with a 10 mm light path. One spectrophotometric unit by the original method (Tabor, C.W., Tabor, H. and Rosenthal, 1954) resulted in an absorbance change of 0.0042 per min (McEwen, 1965). Based on the molecular absorptivity of benzaldehyde in water at 250 nm, $\varepsilon = 1.2 \times 10^4 \ M^{-1}cm^{-1}$, 34 spectrophotometric units in the modified procedure were equal to about 1 nmole of benzaldehyde per 1.5 ml.

III. 7. 7. ASSAY BASED ON THE FORMATION OF p-DIMETHYLAMINO-BENZALDEHYDE FROM p-DIMETHYLAMINOBENZYLAMINE (Colorimetry) (Deitrich and Erwin, 1969)

A. *Principle*
The absorption at 335 nm of p-dimethylaminobenzaldehyde formed by the oxidative deamination of p-dimethylaminobenzylamine is measured.

p-Dimethylaminobenzylamine p-Dimethylaminobenzaldehyde

B. *Enzyme preparations*
Any crude enzyme preparation, such as homogenate or mitochondrial suspension, can be used.

C. *Reagents*
  1. *Phosphate buffer* (0.3 M, pH 7.4).
  2. *p-Dimethylaminobenzylamine* (30 mM). 69.6 mg of p-dimethylamino-benzylamine·2HCl·$\frac{1}{2}$H$_2$O (mol wt 232.15) (Cyclo Chemical) was dissolved in water to 10 ml.
  3. *ZnSO$_4$·7H$_2$O*, 10 % aqueous solution
  4. *NaOH* (1N).

D. Procedure

1. *Continuous recording of absorbance at 355 nm.* The incubation mixtures (3.0 ml) were prepared in 3-ml cuvettes as shown in the following table.

	Experimental cuvette (ml)	Blank cuvette (ml)	Amount (μmoles)	Final concentration (M)
Enzyme				
Phosphate buffer (0.3 M, pH 7.4)	0.5	0.5	150	5×10^{-2}
Water (total volume)	to 3.0			
p-Dimethylaminobenzylamine (30 mM)	0.3	—	9	3×10^{-3}

The incubation mixture was preincubated in a cell thermostatically controlled at 30° or 37°C while in a self-recording spectrophotometer. The reaction was started by adding p-dimethylaminobenzylamine. After the final addition, mixing was achieved by inversion and the increase in the absorbance at 355 nm was continuously recorded, and the initial velocity was obtained.

2. *Discontinuous method.* The incubations were carried out in a centrifuge tube. The enzymatic reaction was stopped with zinc sulfate for deproteinization. After centrifugation, the absorbance of the supernatant was measured at 355 nm. The incubation mixture was prepared in a 10-ml centrifuge tube in an ice bath as shown in the following table :

	Volume (ml)	Amount (μmoles)	Final concentration (M)
Enzyme			
Phosphate buffer (0.3 M, pH 7.4)	0.5	150	5×10^{-2}
p-Dimethylaminobenzylamine (30 mM)	0.3	9	3×10^{-3}
Water (total volume)	to 3.0		

For a blank, the substrate p-dimethylaminobenzylamine was omitted during and was added after incubation. The incubation was carried out at 30° or 37°C for 30 min in air with shaking. The reaction was stopped by adding 0.5 ml of 10 % ZnSO$_4$ and 0.1 ml of 1 N NaOH. The reaction mixture was boiled for 2 min and centrifuged. The absorbance of the supernatant at 355 nm was measured against water. The absorbance difference (A_{355} of experimental $-A_{355}$ of blank) was obtained.

E. Calculation

The molar absorptivity of p-dimethylaminobenzaldehyde at 355 nm 2.77 $\times$ 10⁴ $M^{-1}cm^{-1}$ was used for the conversion of the spectrophotometric unit to μmoles of the product.

III. 7. 8. ASSAY BASED ON THE COLORIMETRIC DETERMINATION OF AMMONIA

A. Principle

Ammonia formed from a substrate by the oxidative deamination can be conveniently measured colorimetrically. This method can be generally used for any substrates, however, when a crude enzyme preparation is used, the blank value is high. Consequently, this method is not sensitive.

The amount of ammonia released from the substrate can be measured after isolation by microdiffusion (Baudhuin, Beaufay, Rahman-Li, Sellinger, Wattiaux, Jacques and de Duve, 1964).

An assay method based on the direct measurement of ammonia by the indophenol colorimetry of Yagi and Okuda is described (Nagatsu and Yagi, 1966).

B. Enzyme preparations

When crude tissue preparations such as homogenate or mitochondria are used as enzyme, the material should be dialyzed against water to remove the endogenous ammonia. In case of rat tissue homogenates, the following amounts were used for the assay : liver, 4 % homogenate, 0.5 ml (20 mg tissue); kidney, 20 % homogenate, 0.5 ml (100 mg tissue); and brain, 20 % homogenate, 0.5 ml (100 mg tissue). In case of rat liver mitochondrial suspension, the amount derived from about 100 mg of tissue was used.

C. Reagents

1. Phosphate buffer (0.3 M, pH 7.4).
2. Tyramine (6 mM). 10.4 mg of tyramine·HCl (mol wt 173.6) was dissolved in 0.01 N HCl to 10.0 ml.
3. Sodium tungstate ($Na_2WO_4 \cdot 2H_2O$). 10 g/dl.
4. H_2SO_4 (2 N).
5. $NaOH$ (0.4 N).

6. *(NH$_4$)$_2$SO$_4$ standard, N* = 5.0 μg/ml. 23.6 mg of (NH$_4$)$_2$SO$_4$ were diluted in water to 1.0 *l.*

7. *Phenol reagent.* 5 g of phenol and 2 g of NaOH were dissolved in water to 100 ml. The solution was kept in the dark and refrigerated, and was prepared fresh once a week.

8. *Phosphate buffer* (pH 9.8). 200 ml of 0.1*M* Na$_2$HPO$_4$ (89.5 g/*l*) and 1 ml of 1 *N* NaOH were mixed.

9. *Sodium nitroprusside.* 0.05 % aqueous solution.

10. *Sodium hypochlorite solution* (Antiformin). Cl about 5 % solution.

D. *Procedure*

The following incubation mixture was prepared in a 10-ml centrifuge tube according to the following table.

Centrifuge tube No.	Volume (ml) Experimental 1) (0 time)	2)	3) (0 time)	Blank 4)	Amount (μmoles)	Final concentration (*M*)
Enzyme	0.5	0.5	0.5	0.5	—	—
Phosphate buffer (0.3 *M*, pH 7.4)	0.25	0.25	0.25	0.25	75	5×10^{-2}
Tyramine (6 m*M*)	0.50	0.50	—	—	3	2×10^{-3}
Water (total volume)	to 1.5					

At zero-time, 0.2 ml of sodium tungstate (10 g/d*l*) and 0.2 ml of sulfuric acid (2*N*) were added to tubes 1) and 3), respectively. After mixing, these two tubes were left at room temperature. The reaction mixtures in tubes 2) and 4) were incubated at 37°C for 60 min. The reaction was stopped by adding sodium tungstate and H$_2$SO$_4$. The mixtures were left at room

Test tubes	Blank Water	Standard Ammonia standard	Samples 1)	2)	3)	4)
	1.0	1.0 (5.0 μg, 0.357 μmoles)	1.0	1.0	1.0	1.0
Phenol reagent	1.0	1.0	1.0	1.0	1.0	1.0
Na$_2$HPO$_4$ buffer (pH 9.8)	7.0	7.0	7.0	7.0	7.0	7.0
Nitroprussid, 0.05%	0.5	0.5	0.5	0.5	0.5	0.5
Antiformin (Cl, 5%)	0.5	0.5	0.5	0.5	0.5	0.5

temperature for 15 min. The mixtures in the tubes 1), 2), 3) and 4) were centrifuged at 3,000 rpm for 10 min. Each 0.8 ml of the supernatants was transferred to another 20 ml-test tube and neutralized by adding 0.2 ml of 1.0 N NaOH (total volume, 1.0 ml)

Besides the 4 test tubes, a reagent blank and an ammonia standard solution were prepared as shown in the above table.

After the addition of all the reagents, the total volume is 10.0 ml and the pH should be about 12. The mixture was incubated at 37°C for 10 min. The blue color of indophenol formed from ammonia was measured at 660 nm, taking the blank as reference.

A_{660nm} reading	Standard S	1) E_0	2) E_{60}	3) B_0	4) B_{60}

E. *Calculation*

Ammonia formed (μmoles/min)

$$=\frac{(E_{60}-E_0)-(B_{60}-B_0)}{S} \times 5.0 \times \frac{1}{14} \times \frac{1.9}{0.8} \times \frac{1}{60}$$

III. 7. 9. ASSAY BASED ON THE FLUOROMETRIC DETERMINATION OF HYDROGEN PEROXIDE (Guilbault, Brignac and Juneau, 1968; Snyder and Hendley, 1968, 1971; Tipton, 1969)

A. *Principle*

Hydrogen peroxide formed in the monoamine oxidase reaction can be measured fluorometrically by the conversion of 3-methoxy-4-hydroxy-phenylacetic acid (homovanillic acid) or p-hydroxyphenylacetic acid to highly fluorescent compounds in the presence of peroxidase (Guilbault, Brignac and Juneau, 1968).

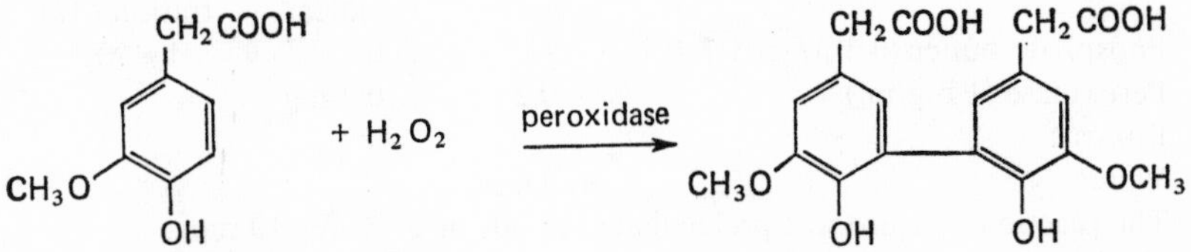

Homovanillic acid (HVA) $\lambda_{ex}=315$ nm, $\lambda_{em}=425$ nm

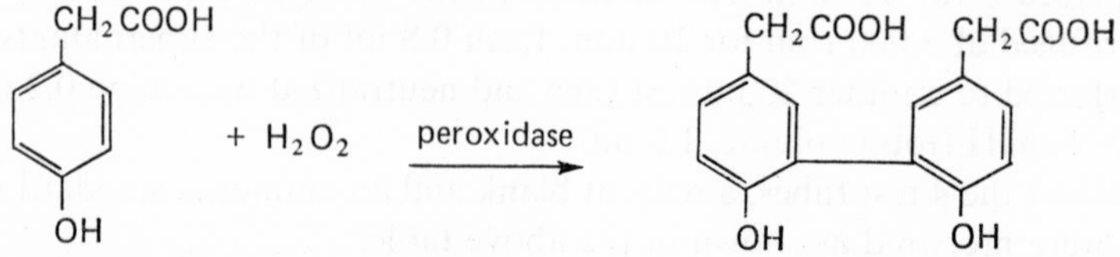

p-Hydroxyphenylacetic acid (HPAA) $\lambda_{ex}=317$ nm, $\lambda_{em}=414$ nm

This method is highly sensitive and reproducible, and can be applicable to any substrates except catecholamines and serotonin. The appearance of the hydrogen peroxide can be continuously monitored by recording the fluorescence in a cuvette with a spectrophotofluorometer.

B. *Enzyme preparations*

Since this fluorometric method is highly sensitive and requires only a small amount of enzymes, crude tissue preparations, such as an homogenate, can be used for the assay.

C. *Reagents*

1. *Phosphate buffer* (0.3 M, pH 7.4).
2. *Homovanillic acid* (HVA), or *p-hydroxyphenylacetic acid* (HPAA). 2.5 mg/ml H_2O.
3. *Horseradish peroxidase.* 1 mg/ml H_2O.
4. *H_2O_2 standard solution* (0.1 mM). The exact molarity of the stock H_2O_2 solution was determined by titration with $KMnO_4$; 0.1 ml containing 10 nmoles of H_2O_2 was used as standard.

D. *Procedure*

The incubation mixture (3.0 ml) shown in the following table was prepared either in a spectrofluorometer cuvette for continuous monitoring or in a centrifuge tube for discontinuous measurement.

	Volume (ml)	Amounts (μmoles)	Final concentration (M)
Phosphate buffer (0.3 M, pH 7.4)	1.0	300	1×10^{-1}
Peroxidase (1 mg/ml)	0.2	0.2 mg	—
Enzyme			
Water	to 2.6		

The reaction mixture was preincubated at 30° or 37°C for 10 min.

HVA or HPAA (2.5 mg/ml)	0.1	0.25 mg	—
Substrate (1 mM)	0.3	0.3	1×10^{-4}
Water (total volume)	to 3.0		

The reaction was started by adding HVA (or HPAA) and the substrate. The increase in the fluorescence at 315 nm excitation and 425 nm fluorescence (HVA), or 317 nm and 414 nm (HPAA) was measured by constant monitoring in a cuvette.

When the discontinuous assay method was used, incubation was carried out at 30° or 37°C for 60 min with shaking. The reaction was stopped by chilling the tube to 0°–3°C. When crude enzyme was used, the mixture was centrifuged at 12,000 × g for 20 min at 0°–3°C to precipitate the mitochondria containing monoamine oxidase and the supernatant was used for the fluorescence assay. Results for blanks containing tissue enzyme but no added substrate were subtracted for calculation of enzyme activity. A calibration curve was determined in each experiment by adding increasing amounts of freshly prepared standard hydrogen peroxide solution (10–40 nmoles) to 3.0 ml of the incubation mixture containing : 0.1 M phosphate buffer, pH 7.4; horseradish peroxidase 0.2 mg; and HVA (or HPAA) 0.25 mg.

III. 7. 10. Assay Based on the Formation of C^{14}-metabolites from Tryptamine-C^{14} (Wurtman and Axelrod, 1963b; Otsuka and Kobayashi, 1964)

A. *Principle*

The deaminated C^{14}-metabolites from tryptamine-C^{14} is measured. This radioassay is simple, very sensitive and highly reproducible. In tissues which lack an excess of aldehyde dehydrogenase, both acid and aldehyde are generated. However, since indoleacetaldehyde has solubility characteristics similar to indoleacetic acid in an acid-toluene system, this assay can be used whether or not aldehyde dehydrogenase is present.

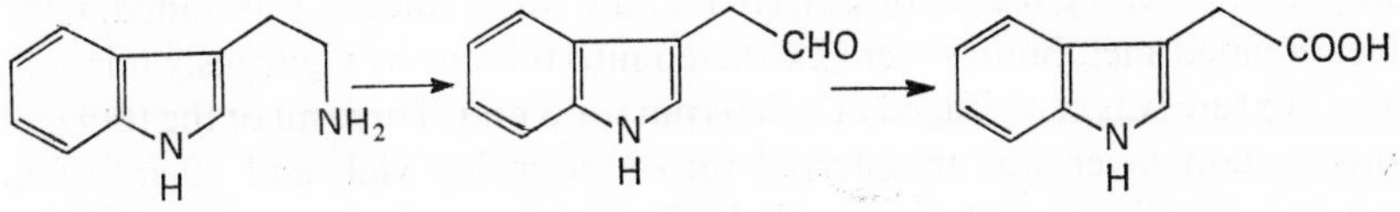

Tryptamine   Indoleacetaldehyde   Indoleacetic acid

B. *Enzyme preparations*

Tissues were homogenized in 0.25 M sucrose or in 0.15 M KCl. The homogenate was diluted to make 10 mg (wet weight) tissue in 1.0 ml and 0.1 ml containing 1 mg tissue was used for one tube.

C. *Reagents*

1. *Phosphate buffer* (0.5 M, pH 7.4).

2. *Tryptamine* (1 mM). 19.7 mg of tryptamine·HCl (mol wt 196.5) was dissolved in 0.01 N HCl to 100 ml.

3. *Tryptamine-C^{14}*. (a) *Stock solution*: Tryptamine-2-C^{14}-bisuccinate (side chain label) $C_8H_6NC^{14}H_2CH_2NH_2$-HOOCCH$_2$CH$_2$COOH (mol wt 276) (specific activity 10.3 mCi/mmole; 0.10 mCi; 2.7 mg) was dissolved in 1.0 ml of 0.01 N HCl. (b) *Working solution*: To 100 μl of the stock solution, 4.9 ml of 0.01 N HCl was added.

4. *HCl* (2N).

5. *Toluene scintillation solution*. PPO (2,5-diphenyloxazole) 4 g and POPOP (1,4-di-2-(5-phenyloxazolyl)benzene) 0.05 g were dissolved in toluene to 1l.

6. *Toluene-C^{14} standard*.

D. *Procedure*

The incubation mixture (0.3 ml) shown in the following table was prepared in a 10-ml glass-stoppered centrifuge tube in an ice bath.

	Volume (μl)	Amount	Final concentration (M)
Enzyme (10 mg tissue/ml)	100	(1 mg tissue)	
Phosphate buffer (0.5 M, pH 7.4)	100	50 μmoles	1.7×10^{-1}
Tryptamine (1 mM)	50	50 nmoles	
Tryptamine-C^{14} (working solution)	50	1 nmole	1.7×10^{-4}
Water (total volume)	to 300	(0.1 μCi)	

Two kinds of blank incubation were used : 1) boiled enzyme (90°C, 3 min); 2) A zero-time blank to which 0.2 ml of 2 N HCl was added at zero-time. Incubation was carried out at 37°C for 20 min. The reaction was stopped by adding 0.2 ml of 2 N HCl, and 6 ml of toluene was added. C^{14}-Deaminated metabolites were extracted into toluene by vigorously mixing. The mixture was centrifuged at 1,500 rpm for 5 min. Three ml of the toluene supernatant layer was transferred into a counting vial, and 10 ml of a toluene scintillator solution added. Counting was made with a liquid scintillation spectrometer.

E. *Calculation*

To 0.1 ml of standard toluene-C^{14} in a counting vial, 2.9 ml of toluene and 10 ml of the scintillator solution were added, and it was counted to get the counting efficiency (%).

$$\text{nmoles } C^{14}\text{-metabolites/min} = \frac{(\exp - \text{blank})\text{cpm} \times \dfrac{100}{\text{efficiency } \%}}{\text{tryptamine-}C^{14} \text{ added, dpm}} \times \frac{6 \text{ ml}}{3 \text{ ml}}$$

$$\times \text{ [tryptamine] nmoles } \times \frac{1}{20}$$

III. 7. 11. SPECTROPHOTOMETRIC ASSAY USING 2,4,6-TRINITROBENZENE-1-SULFONIC ACID (TNBS) (Obata, Ushiwata and Nakamura, 1971).

This method is based on the measurement of substrate disappearance by the reaction of substrate primary amines with 2,4,6-trinitrobenzene-1-sulfonic acid. Any primary amine substrates such as dopamine, serotonin, tyramine or benzylamine can be used. This method is fairly sensitive and simple. A slightly modified procedure is described below.

The following incubation mixture (1.0 ml) shown in the following table was prepared in a centrifuge tube in an ice bath.

	Volume (ml)	Amount (μmoles)	Final concentration (M)
Enzyme (1–10 mg dry weight of bovine liver mitochondria)	0.25		
Substrate (tyramine, serotonin or dopamine) (8 mM)	0.25	2	2×10^{-3}
0.25 M sucrose in 10 mM		sucrose 125	1.25×10^{-1}
Tris-HCl buffer, pH 7.6	0.5	buffer 5	5×10^{-3}

Incubation was carried out at 30°C for 30 to 60 min. The reaction was stopped by adding 0.25 ml of 20 % trichloroacetic acid, and the mixture was centrifuged. To an aliquot (0.25 ml) of the clear supernatant, 3 ml of phosphate buffer (0.5 M, pH 8.0), 0.75 ml of deionized water and 1 ml of 16 mM (in methanol) 2,4,6-trinitrobenzene-1-sulfonic acid solution were added. The mixture was left for 1 hr at 25°C in the dark. Absorbance at 422 nm was measured against a reference mixture without monoamine.

III. 7. 12. REPORTED ACTIVITIES

The tissue distribution of monoamine oxidase is shown in Table XI. The enzyme activities are expressed as nmoles/min by calculating the reported values.

TABLE XI. Distribution of Monoamine Oxidase (MAO).

Enzyme preparation (homogenate)	Substrate	Temperature (°C)	MAO activity (nmoles/min)	Method	Reference
Rat liver (mitochondria)	Tyramine	38	About 30 (per g tissue)	Manometry	1)
Rat liver	Kynuramine	30	1.3 (per mg protein)	Spectrophotometry	2)
	Serotonin	37	8.7		
brain	Kynuramine	30	0.5		
	Serotonin	37	3.3		
Guinea pig liver	Kynuramine	30	3.0		
	Serotonin	37	22		
brain	Kynuramine	30	1.2		
	Serotonin	37	2.7		
Rabbit liver	Kynuramine	30	3.3		
	Serotonin	37	1.2		
brain	Kynuramine	30	0.2		
	Serotonin	37	0.9		
Rat liver	Tryptamine	37	About 20 (per g tissue)	Radioassay	3)
brain	Kynuramine	37	24 (per g tissue)	Fluorometry	4)
Guinea pig atrium			48		
Cat vagal ganglia			23		
sympathetic ganglia			52		

Rat brain liver kidney	Kynuramine	37	69 (per g tissue) 347 28	Spectrophotometry	5)
Rat brain	Tyramine Tryptamine Metanephrine	30	0.70 (per mg protein) 0.47 0.17	Fluorometry	6)
Rat liver brain	p-Dimethyl- aminobenzyl- amine	25	0.23 (per mg protein) 0.18	Spectrophotometry	7)
Bovine caudate nucleus (homogenate) (mitochondria)	Kynuramine	37	0.76 (per mg protein) 3.03	Spectrophotometry	8)

1) Creasey, 1956.
2) Weissbach, Smith, Daly, Witkop and Udenfriend, 1960.
3) Wurtman and Axelrod, 1963b.
4) Kraml, 1965.
5) Kuzuya and Nagatsu, 1969a.
6) Tipton, 1969.
7) Deitrich and Erwin, 1969.
8) Nagatsu, T. and Nagatsu, I., 1970.

Chapter IV

Methods for the Estimation of Catecholamines and Related Compounds

IV. 1. Assay of Catecholamines and DOPA

IV. 1. 1. GENERAL CONSIDERATIONS OF THE CATECHOLAMINE ASSAY

Catecholamines can be assayed by bioassay, colorimetry, spectrofluorometry, or radioassay, depending upon the amount in a sample. The sensitivity and specificity of various methods are shown in Table XII. Bioassay is highly specific and very sensitive, but is also laborious and not as reproducible as the chemical assays. Chemical assays only are described in this chapter.

TABLE XII. Comparison of Various Norepinephrine and Epinephrine Assays.

Method	Limit of sensitivity	Specificity
Bioassay	1 ng	Specific
Spectrophotometry		
UV (279 nm)	10 μg	Non-specific
Visible (after oxidation, 529 nm)	10 μg	Non-specific
Spectrofluorometry		
UV (285 nm/325 nm)	6 ng	Non-specific
Visible		
THI[a] (410 nm/540 nm)	1 ng	Relatively specific
ED[b] (420 nm/520 nm)	1 ng	Specific for catechols
Gas chromatography	1 pg	Specific
Radioassay	1 pg	Specific

[a] THI: Trihydroxyindole method
[b] ED: Ethylenediamine method

Catecholamines (dopamine, norepinephrine, and epinephrine) and DOPA can be assayed simultaneously by similar fluorometric methods because of the presence of a characteristic catechol group. Since the amount of these catechol compounds in tissues is very low (ng order/g tissue), only sensitive methods such as fluorometry, gas chromatography or radioassay are suitable. A detailed description of the fluorometry of catecholamines and related compounds is described by Udenfriend (1962b; 1969).

Procedure for the assay of catecholamines is given in the following outline: *a.* Extraction (precipitation of protein); *b.* Purification and concentration; *c.* Final estimation: fluorometry, gas chromatography or radioassay.

209

A. *Post-mortem loss of catecholamines*

The tissue samples should be taken as soon as possible after death and homogenized immediately in an acid medium. If the analysis must be done after a certain period of time, the tissues should be frozen immediately with dry ice or, preferably, in a mixture of dry ice and acetone ($-78°C$). The frozen sample should be stored at $-20° - -30°C$. For example, the norepinephrine content in mice or rat brain decreased markedly after death. In mice brain the decrease 5, 15, 30 and 60 min, and 4 hr at 25°C after decapitation was 10, 21, 30, 44 and 69%, respectively, and in rat brain the decrease 30 min, 1 hr and 4 hr at 25°C after decapitation was 15, 28 and 53%, respectively (Grabartis, Chessick and Lal, 1966). The frozen tissue should not be thawed before extraction (Euler, 1956).

B. *Extraction*

Catecholamines are very unstable at alkaline pH, therefore, the extraction and purification of catecholamines should be carried out at acidic pH.

1. *Tissues.* The following solvents are generally used for the extraction of catecholamines in tissues.

   a. *Trichloroacetic acid*, 10 %. If necessary, trichloroacetic acid in the extract is removed by extraction with water-saturated diethyl ether.

   b. *Perchloric acid* ($HClO_4$, mol wt 100.47), 0.4 N (about 4 g/dl). Perchloric acid in the extract can be removed by neutralizing with 2.5 M K_2CO_3 to pH 4–6, cooling to 0°C and then removing the precipitate of potassium perchlorate ($KClO_4$) at 0°C in a refrigerated centrifuge.

   c. *Acid alcohol.* For example, ethanol containing 2.5 % of 1 N H_2SO_4.

   d. *Dry n-butanol* (Hogans, 1968).

The most widely used medium for the homogenization, deproteinization, and extraction of catecholamines from tissues may be perchloric acid or trichloroacetic acid. Trichloroacetic acid is the most conveniently used, and subsequent isolation of catecholamines is carried out by alumina. The advantage of perchloric acid for the extraction of catecholamines is that it can be removed as potassium perchlorate at 0°C. This allows the purification of the catecholamines by various ion-exchange columns without prior isolation by alumina.

2. *Urine.* For the catecholamine (free form) assay of urine, an aliquot of a 24-hr urine specimen collected in a glass bottle containing 15 ml of 6 N HCl (Crout, 1961) is generally used. The final pH should be adjusted to about 3 as the content of free catecholamines in urine at this pH shows insignificant changes over a period of more than 2 weeks. Considerable increases in free norepinephrine were observed at pH values below 1 due

to the release of the amine from readily hydrolyzable conjugates (Euler and Lishajko, 1961b). The 24-hr specimen is filtered, and usually 10 % of the total 24-hr urine is used for the assay (Crout, 1961).

3. *Blood.* The accurate fluorometric determination of catecholamines in blood is extremely difficult because of the low concentration (less than 1 $\mu g/l$), however, Weil-Malherbe (1960b) described a procedure for the preparation of plasma. Twenty ml of blood was run through plastic tubing from an anticubital vein into a glass-stoppered 25-ml graduated cylinder containing 5 ml anticoagulant solution (1 g EDTA$\cdot$2Na and 2 g sodium thiosulfate ($Na_2S_2O_3\cdot5H_2O$) dissolved in about 80 ml H_2O with the pH adjusted to 7.4 by the dropwise addition of 1 N NaOH, and the solution made up to 100 ml). The cylinder was inverted gently, the total volume was noted (V_B) and a sample was removed for the hematocrit (H) determination. The remainder was centrifuged for 20 min at 1,000 rpm (250 $\times$ g). Plasma was separated and its volume measured (V_P). After adding an equal volume of sodium acetate solution (0.2 M, purified by passing through a 2 $\times$ 25 cm of Dowex A-1, 50–100 mesh, Na form, and adjusted to pH 8.4 with 0.5 N Na_2CO_3), the pH was adjusted to 8.4 by carefully adding 0.5 N Na_2CO_3. Catecholamines in plasma were subsequently purified with alumina and Amberlite CG-50 columns, and finally measured by the ethylenediamine method. The plasma volume was calculated by the following equation :

Total volume of plasma contained in V_P
(volume of plasma + anticoagulant, separated by centrifugation)

$$= \frac{\text{total vol plasma}}{\text{total vol plasma + anticoagulant}} \times V_P$$

$$= \frac{(V_B - V_BH/100 - 5) V_P}{V_B - V_BH/100}$$

Following the method of Anton and Sayre (1962), plasma was prepared as follows. Heparinized blood was collected in the presence of about 0.5 mg/ml of sodium metabisulfite ($Na_2S_2O_5$), immediately centrifuged in the cold and the plasma frozen until used (stable for several weeks under these conditions). The use of sodium thiosulfate as preservatives markedly interfered with the trihydroxyindole procedure. Up to 30 ml of plasma was placed in a polyethylene centrifuge tube and adjusted to 0.4 N with concentrated $HClO_4$. The tube was stoppered and vigorously shaken for 5 min and then centrifuged at 30,000 $\times$ g at 10°C for 10 min. The clear supernatant was made up to 25 ml with 0.4 N HClO$_4$ and transferred to a 50-ml beaker containing 400 mg alumina and 200 mg EDTA. The catecholamines were purified with alumina by batch adsorption, eluted with 0.05 N perchloric acid, and measured by the trihydroxyindole procedure.

The Weil-Malherbe method (1960b) does not include deproteinization of the plasma, whereas that by Anton and Sayre (1962) does. It was indicated that unless the plasma is diluted at least 1 to 10, the common deproteinizing agents will cause the loss of epinephrine (Weil-Malherbe, 1960). EDTA prevented the clumping of blood platelets with which a proportion of plasma catecholamines seems to be associated. The use of heparin resulted in extensive clumping, particularly when the blood was cooled in ice before centrifuging (Weil-Malherbe, 1960).

C.   *Purification and concentration* (1). *Chromatography*

1.   *Alumina* (aluminum oxide, Al$_2$O$_3$). Alumina can adsorb catechol compounds specifically and is very effective for the isolation and elution of catecholamines. The adsorption does not occur at pH 4 and becomes maximal at pH 8–8.5 (Shaw, 1938). The adsorption of catecholamines at pH 8–8.5 is very rapid. The adsorbed catecholamines can be eluted from alumina by some acids, such as acetic acid (0.2–0.3 N), oxalic acid (0.6 N), HCl (0.1 N), and H$_2$SO$_4$ (0.25 N). Since HCl or H$_2$SO$_4$ dissolves alumina and gives a low recovery, acetic acid (0.2 N) is widely used.

Alumina should be washed with acid and heated before use. The following procedure was described by Crout (1961). Alumina (200–300 g) was boiled in 1l of 2N HCl for 30 min in a reflux condenser and the resulting cloudy supernatant was poured off. The alumina was stirred in 1l of water, allowed to settle for 5 min, and the supernatant was decanted. This washing and decanting process was repeated with water 12–15 times until the wash water became clear after 5 min of settling and was pH 4–5. The alumina was collected in a large suction funnel, allowed to dry overnight in an open pan at room temperature, and then heated in an oven at 100°C for 2 hr. The acid-washed alumina should be kept tightly closed so as not to be exposed to moisture.

The column procedure requires the prior adjustment of the tissue extract to pH 8.0–8.5. Since catecholamines are very unstable at alkaline pH, the titration is carried out rapidly in the presence of 2 % (g/dl) solution of the disodium salt of ethylene diamine tetraacetate. For titration, 3 N then 1 N NH$_4$OH, 5 N then 0.5 N HaOH, or 0.5 N Na$_2$CO$_3$ is generally used.

Batchwise adsorption is recommended because of the stability of catecholamines adsorbed on alumina even at pH 8.5. In the procedure by

Crout (1961), catecholamines were adsorbed on alumina by the batch method and eluted from a column. Details of the Crout's procedure is described in Section IV. 1.3. C.

2. *A strong cation exchange resin column.* A strong cation exchange resin, such as Dowex-50, Amberlite CG-120, Zeokarb-225 or Doulite C-25, can be used for adsorption.

Dowex-50, X-4 (or X-8), 200–400 mesh, Na$^+$, pH 6.0, (buffered with acetate buffer) is generally used. DOPA or acid catechols cannot be adsorbed on this column, and only catecholamines are adsorbed. Norepinephrine and epinephrine are eluted with 0.4 N HCl, and dopamine with 2 N HCl (Bertler, Carlsson and Rosengren, 1958).

Amberlite CG-120, Type 2, 200–400 mesh, Na$^+$, pH 6.0 (buffered with acetate buffer) can also be used.

Duolite C-25, H$^+$ form, 200–300 mesh can completely separate DOPA, norepinephrine plus epinephrine, and dopamine. DOPA was eluted with 0.35 M sodium acetate buffer (pH 5.0), norepinephrine and epinephrine with 7 % ethanol, 3.0 M, pH 6.0 sodium acetate buffer, and dopamine with 25 % ethanol, 3.0 M, pH 6.0 sodium acetate buffer (pH 6.0) (Itoh, Matsuoka, Nakajima, Tagawa and Imaizumi, 1962).

3. *Weak cation exchange resin.* A weak cation exchange resin, such as Amberlite IRC-50, can remove DOPA and catechol acids from catecholamines. When a long column (0.9 × 30 cm) was used, epinephrine, norepinephrine, and dopamine were completely separated (Kirshner and Goodall, 1957a).

Amberlite IRC-50 (XE-64) was washed and cycled with 6 N HCl, water, 10 N NaOH, water, 6 N HCl, and water. The resin was buffered at pH 6.1 by suspending the acid form in 3 volumes of 0.2 M acetic acid and adding concentrated ammonium hydroxide until a stable pH of 6.1 was reached. The resin was filtered and resuspended in 0.2 M ammonium acetate buffer at pH 6.1. The resin kept either in the buffer as suspension or as a powder after filtration and washing with the fresh buffer. The dried resin was suspended in 0.2 M ammonium acetate buffer, pH 6.1, and packed on a column (0.9 × 30 cm). The sample extract was adjusted to pH 6.1 and applied on the column. Elution was carried out with 0.4 M ammonium acetate buffer at pH 5.0. The flow rate was 3.5–4.0 ml/hr, and 1.5 ml fractions were collected.

A short column of (packed volume, 1 ml) Amberlite CG-50, Type 2 resin, buffered with 1 M sodium phosphate buffer at pH 6.0 or 6.5 and washed with water was also used for the isolation of catecholamines (Weil-Malherbe and Bone, 1959; Weil-Malherbe, 1960).

A trichloroacetic acid extract should be extracted with diethyl ether to remove the acid before applying it on the column. The purified solution, an acid eluate from an alumina column, can be applied directly on the Amberlite column. The eluate was mixed with 1 ml of 0.2 M disodium ethylenediamine tetraacetate and 20 mg of ascorbic acid, and titrated to pH 6.0–6.5 and applied on the Amberlite column. Elution of catecholamines was carried out with 5 ml of 1 N acetic acid, or 5 ml of 0.5 N HCl.

4. *Sephadex G-25*. The use of a Sephadex G-25 column for the separation of catecholamines from plasma (2 × 25 cm in 0.01 M acetic acid for 20 ml of plasma) was described by Marshall (1963).

D. *Purification and concentration (2). Extraction method*

Catecholamines can be extracted with butanol. Norepinephrine and epinephrine have a high *n*-butanol-aqueous acid partition ratio when the aqueous phase is salt-saturated. Upon extraction with 10 volumes of *n*-butanol, about 65 % of the catecholamines was removed from salt-saturated, acidified tissue homogenates. The amines were quantitatively returned to an aqueous phase by the addition of *n*-heptane to the butanol and shaking with dilute HCl (Shore and Olin, 1958; Shore, 1959). A good recovery was achieved by extraction of the amines by homogenization with dry butanol. The amines were reextracted with phosphate buffer, pH 6.5 (Hogans, 1968).

A method was described for a single solvent extraction and the simultaneous determination of dopamine, norepinephrine and serotonin (Fleming, Clark, Fenster and Towne, 1965). The method involved extraction of amines with acetone (acetone : tissue = 20 : 1), removal of the acetone by evaporation *in vacuo*, extraction of the residue with butanol saturated with 0.01 N HCl, addition of heptane to return the amines to an aqueous phase, passage of the aqueous phase through an ion exchange (Amberlite CG-50, Type 2, 200–400 mesh, 0.6 × 1 cm, pH 6.1 with phosphate buffer) column which retains the amines but not the amino acids, and elution with 4 ml of 0.1 M sodium acetate buffer, pH 5.2 and fluorometric analysis of the amines.

Another butanol extraction method which permits the simultaneous determination of norepinephrine, dopamine, serotonin, and 5-hydroxyindoleacetic acid was described by Welch, A.S. and Welch, B.L. (1969).

Norepinephrine, dopamine, and serotonin were extracted from the brain using 15 % 1 N formic acid plus 85 % acetone (v/v). The amines were subsequently separated from the amino acids (DOPA) with an Amberlite CG-50 column and measured fluorometrically (Kariya and Aprison, 1969).

IV. 1. 2. COLORIMETRY OF CATECHOLAMINES

A solution containing only a single catecholamine in a concentration higher than 10 μg, can be easily assayed either with UV absorption at 279 nm or visible absorption after oxidation to a chrome (Euler, 1956).

Colorimetric determination of norepinephrine and epinephrine in a mixture is based on the formation of the chromes and iodochromes with iodine oxidation at pH 4 and 6 (Euler and Hamberg, 1949b).

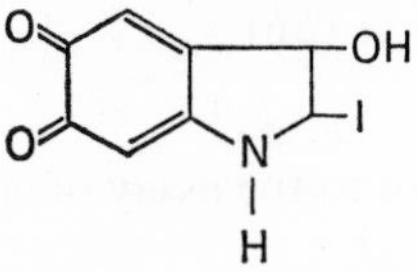

Iodonoradrenochrome

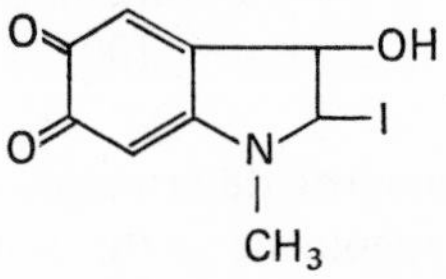

Iodoadrenochrome

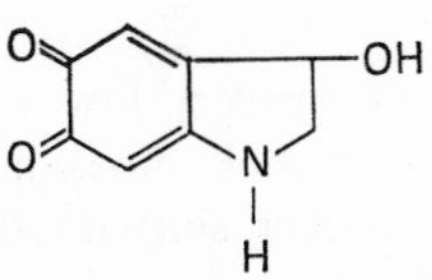

Noradrenochrome

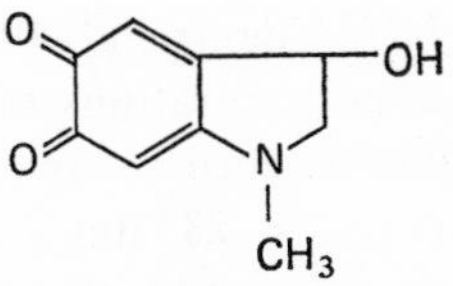

Adrenochrome

The reaction was carried out in two 10-ml glass-stoppered test tubes. To 0.2–2 ml of a sample solution containing 10–100 μg of norepinephrine and epinephrine was added 1 ml of 1 M acetate buffer of pH 4 and 6, respectively, and 0.2 ml of 0.1 N iodine solution. After 1.5 min for the pH 4 reaction and 3 min for the pH 6 reaction, respectively, the equivalent amount of 0.05 N thiosulfate was added. The solution was diluted with water to 5.0 or 10.0 ml and a reading was taken within 5 min at 529 nm. If the color reaction in a mixture of norepinephrine and epinephrine is performed at pH 4 for 1.5 min, the resulting figure shows all of the epinephrine but only some 10 % of the norepinephrine. If the determination is repeated at pH 6, the figure gives the sum of epinephrine and norepinephrine. The amount of norepinephrine and epinephrine was calculated by the following equations.

Epinephrine in the sample $= E$
Norepinephrine in the sample $= N$
Absorbance of the sample oxidized at pH 4 $= A(S4)$
Absorbance of the sample oxidized at pH 6 $= A(S6)$
Absorbance of epinephrine standard (100 μg) oxidized at pH 4 $= A(E4)$

Absorbance of epinephrine standard (100 μg) oxidized at pH 6 = $A(E6)$
Absorbance of norepinephrine standard (100 μg) oxidized at pH 4 = $A(N4)$
Absorbance of norepinephrine standard (100 μg) oxidized at pH 6 = $A(N6)$

$$\frac{A(E4)}{100} E + \frac{A(N4)}{100} N = A \ (S4)$$

$$\frac{A(E6)}{100} E + \frac{A(N6)}{100} N = A \ (S6)$$

This colorimetric determination can be applied to the assay of epinephrine and norepinephrine in the adrenal medulla.

IV. 1. 3. FLUOROMETRY OF CATECHOLAMINES AND DOPA

A. *Principle* (Udenfriend, 1962b, 1969)
Since tissue concentrations of catecholamines are very low, only highly sensitive fluorescence assays are suitable. Catecholamines have native fluorescence (λ_{ex} = 285 nm, λ_{ex} = 325 nm), however, since it is due to their phenolic structure and is therefore not specific, the conversion of catecholamines to the derivatives which have specific fluorescence in the visible wavelength is necessary. Two methods for accomplishing this have been developed : (1) the trihydroxyindole method and (2) the ethylenediamine condensation method.

1. *Trihydroxyindole (THI) method* (Euler and Floding, 1955a, b)
   a. *Principle*. This method is based on the conversion of catecholamines to the highly fluorescent trihydroxyindoles (lutins). The fluorescent trihydroxyindole from epinephrine was isolated and identified to be 3,5,6-trihydroxy-1-methylindole (Ehrlén, 1948; Lund, 1949a, b; Harley-Mason, 1949, 1950; Fischer, 1949) (Fig. 30). The fluorescent lutin from norepinephrine was identified as 3,5,6-trihydroxyindole (Bu'Lock and Harley-Mason, 1951).

Dopamine is not so easily converted to the fluorescent indoles as epinephrine and norepinephrine, but a highly fluorescent compound can be produced by a modification of the procedure (Carlsson and Waldeck, 1958; Carlsson, 1959a).

As shown in Fig. 30, the reaction proceeds in two stages, oxidation and intramolecular rearrangement. It is possible to adjust the reaction condition to produce the fluorescent indoles only from norepinephrine and epi-

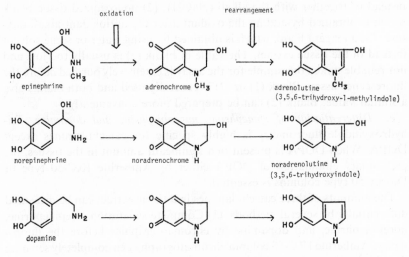

Fig. 30.   Oxidation and rearrangement of catecholamines to fluorescent
trihydroxy- or dihydroxyindole.

nephrine and not from dopamine. Alternatively, it is also possible to
produce the fluorescent compound only from dopamine, and not from
norepinephrine or epinephrine. However DOPA yields a compound with
fluorescence characteristics indistinguishable from those of the fluorophore
of dopamine (Carlsson, 1959a).

An extensive study on the hydroxyindole technique was described by
Laverty and Taylor (1968).

b.   *Oxidation.* The oxidation step of catecholamines is carried out by
potassium ferricyanide, iodine or manganase dioxide. Manganase dioxide
can be removed by centrifugation after the oxidation reaction.

c.   *Stabilization of the trihydroxyindole fluorophore.* The trihydroxyindole procedure is highly specific for catecholamines, but a drawback of
the procedure is the unstability of the fluorophore. Various antioxidants
can stabilize the fluorophore and an ascorbic acid-NaOH mixture is the
most widely used (Euler and Floding, 1955a, b). Ascorbic acid is unstable
in alkaline, but the addition of ethylenediamine or propylene diamine can
increase the stability of the fluorophore (Euler and Lishajko, 1961b).

d.   *Blank in trihydroxyindole procedure.* Since the trihydroxyindole
fluorophores are unstable, a difficult problem is how to prepare a proper
blank. Three kinds of the blank are used : (1) the faded tissue blank which
is obtained by adding the antioxidant (for example, ascorbate) after,

instead of together with the alkali (NaOH); (2) nonoxidized tissue blank which is obtained by adding the oxidant after the antioxidant-alkali mixture; (3) a reagent blank which is obtained by using water or some solvent instead of the tissue extract. The value of blank (3) is usually too low and not reliable unless the sample for the assay is extensively purified before the fluorescence assay. Blank (1) or (2) is generally used and both blanks give a similar value. Blank (2) can be prepared more conveniently.

e. *Differentiation of epinephrine, norepinephrine and dopamine.* Trihydroxyindole fluorometry is highly specific for catecholamines except DOPA. When DOPA is present in a significant amount in the tissues, the preliminary elimination of DOPA either by Amberlite IRC-50 type or Dowex-50 type columns is essential.

The amounts of three catecholamines in a tissue extract can be measured differentially by several methods. (1) Complete separation of epinephrine, norepinephrine, and dopamine by chromatographies before the fluorometry. Amberlite IRC-50 column chromatography can completely separate the three types of catecholamines (Kirshner and Goodall, 1957a). (2) Dopamine can be assayed specifically under specific reaction conditions (Carlsson and Waldeck, 1958; Carlsson, 1959a). DOPA should be removed before the assay. (3) Norepinephrine and epinephrine can be assayed specifically under specific reaction condition. DOPA should be removed before the assay.

Norepinephrine and epinephrine can be differentially measured either by using the oxidation reaction at different pHs (Euler and Floding, 1955a) or by making use of the differences in the activation and fluorescence spectra of the trihydroxyindole fluorophores (Euler and Lishajko, 1959, 1961b). When thioglycolic acid is substituted for ascorbic acid in the alkali-antioxidant mixture, only the fluorescent product of norepinephrine is stabilized (Merrills, 1962, 1963). This was used with an automated trihydroxyindole procedure for the differential analysis of catecholamines (Robinson and Watts, 1965).

Oxidation at pH		3.5 (or 2.0)	6.0 (or 6.5, 7.0)
		Only epinephrine is oxidized. The oxidation of norepinephrine is about 5%.	Both epinephrine and norepinephrine are oxidized.
Fluorescence intensity	Standard	E 0.1 μg	F $(E3.5)$	F $(E6.0)$
after the rearrangement		N 0.1 μg	F $(N3.5)$	F $(N6.0)$
reaction	Sample		F $(S3.5)$	F $(S6.0)$

The differential estimation of epinephrine (E) and norepinephrine (N) by the oxidation at different pHs is carried out as shown in the above table (Euler and Floding, 1955a; Crout, 1961).

The amount of epinephrine (E) and norepinephrine (N) in the sample can be calculated from the following equations:

$$\frac{F(E3.5)}{0.1} E + \frac{F(N3.5)}{0.1} N = F(S3.5)$$

$$\frac{F(E6.0)}{0.1} E + \frac{F(N6.0)}{0.1} N = F(S6.0)$$

If $F(N3.5)$ is neglected,

$$\frac{F(E3.5)}{0.1} E = F(S3.5)$$

$$\frac{F(E6.0)}{0.1} E + \frac{F(N6.0)}{0.1} N = F(S6.0)$$

The differential estimation of epinephrine (E) and norepinephrine (N) by making use of the differences in the activation and fluorescence spectra (multiple-filter technique) of the lutins (Euler and Lishajko, 1959, 1961b) is carried out as shown in the following table.

Measurement of fluorescence	Filter set a	Filter set b
Activation/emission	395 nm/505 nm	410 nm/520 nm
Fluorometer readings		
Standard E 0.1 μg	$F(Ea)$	$F(Eb)$
N 0.1 μg	$F(Na)$	$F(Nb)$
Sample	$F(Sa)$	$F(Sb)$

The amount of epinephrine (E) and norepinephrine (N) in the sample can be calculated from the following equations:

$$\frac{F(Ea)}{0.1} E + \frac{F(Na)}{0.1} N = F(Sa)$$

$$\frac{F(Eb)}{0.1} E + \frac{F(Nb)}{0.1} N = F(Sb)$$

2. *Ethylenediamine (ED) method* (Weil-Malherbe, 1959, 1960b)

Catechol compounds can be converted to highly fluorescent and fairly stable compounds by condensation with ethylenediamine (Natelson,

Lugovoy and Pincus, 1949). Based on this reaction, a fluorometric assay which is well-known as the ethylenediamine method was established (Weil-Malherbe and Bone, 1952, 1957a, b; Weil-Malherbe, 1959, 1960b). The reaction mechanism was established as shown in Fig. 31 (Weil-Malherbe, 1959, 1960a; Harley-Mason and Laird, 1959). The condensation product of norepinephrine or 3,4-dihydroxymandelic acid was identical with that of catechol, thus confirming the fact that the side chains of norepinephrine and dihydroxymandelic acid are cleaved during the condensation reaction (Harley-Mason and Laird, 1959; Yagi, Nagatsu, T. and Nagatsu, I., 1960; Nagatsu and Yagi, 1962a, b). The structure of the main ethylenediamine condensate of epinephrine with ethylenediamine was identified as 2,3-dihydro-3-hydroxy-1-methylpyrrolo-[4,5:g]-quinoxaline, and that of norepinephrine as 1,2,3,4-tetrahydro-1,4,5,8-tetra-azaanthracene (Harley-Mason and Laird, 1959).

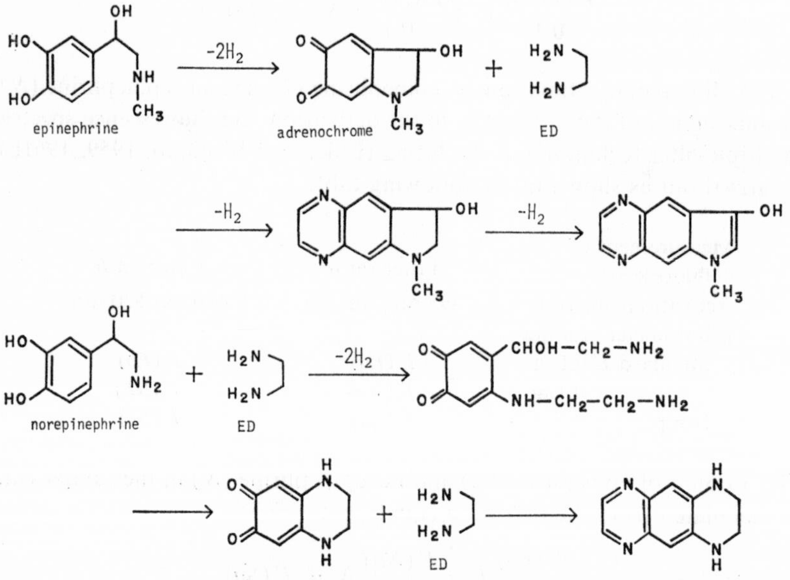

Fig. 31.   Reaction of ethylenediamine (ED) with epinephrine and norepinephrine (Weil-Malherbe, 1959).

Since this ethylenediamine condensate of a catecholamine is specific only to catechol, previous purification and separation of each catecholamine, i.e., dopamine, norepinephrine, and epinephrine, is essential. The advantages of the ethylenediamine method are high sensitivity and stability of the condensates. The condensate of norepinephrine with ethylenediamine is easily decomposed by light. It was recommended that the tubes be left exposed to daylight for at least 30 min before fluorometry (Weil-Malherbe, 1959).

The original ethylenediamine method (Weil-Malherbe and Bone, 1952) is as follows. To a solution (10 ml) containing catecholamines in a 20-ml glass-stoppered centrifuge tube, 0.5 ml of ethylenediamine dihydrochloride (2 M) and 0.7 ml of ethylenediamine were added and the solution was heated at 50°C for 20 min. For norepinephrine, heating at 50°C for 2 hr gave a higher fluorescence (Yagi and Nagatsu, 1960). The fluorescence spectra of the reaction mixture of DOPA and ethylenediamine changed from blue to yellow at 90 min at 50°C (λem 465 nm to 555 nm by excitation at 365 nm) (Yagi, Nagatsu and Nagatsu-Ishibashi, 1960). After cooling, the mixture was saturated with solid sodium chloride and extracted with 6 ml of isobutanol. The butanol layer was separated by light centrifugation and transferred into a fluorometer cuvette. The condensation products of acid catechols such as DOPA are extracted by isobutanol to only a slight extent. The condensate of 3,4-dihydroxymandelic acid is extracted with isobutanol, since the condensate is the same as that of catechol.

Various fluorometric procedures of catecholamines have been proposed. A summary of such procedures is shown in Table XIII. In this section, detailed descriptions of the typical fluorometric procedures which have been tried in our laboratory are provided. The methods for norepinephrine and epinephrine most frequently reported may be the trihydroxyindole procedures by Euler and Floding (1955a) or Euler and Lishajko (1961b), by Crout (1961), by Shore and Olin (1958) and by Anton and Sayre (1962). These procedures use alumina or butanol extraction for isolating catecholamines. For the measurement of dopamine the method of Carlsson and Waldeck (1958) or a modification by Drujan, Sourkes, Layne and Murphy (1959) is most frequently used. To my knowledge, the separation of DOPA, norepinephrine plus epinephrine, and dopamine by Duolite C-25-H$^+$, and subsequent fluorometry is also an excellent procedure (Itoh, Matsuoka, Nakazima, Tagawa and Imaizumi, 1962). A sensitive method for the simultaneous estimation of norepinephrine (epinephrine) and dopamine in tissue was also developed by Hogans (personal communication, 1968), and although this method is not yet published, it is simple and reproducible (Nagatsu, T., Yamamoto and Nagatsu, I., 1970).

TABLE XIII. Fluorescence Assays of Catecholamines (CA).

Reference	CA measured	Principle	Protein precipitant	Isolation procedure	Fluorescence development	Fluorescence measurement (activation → emission)	Sample
Euler and Floding, 1955b	NE, EN	THI	None	Alumina column, 0.3 N oxalic acid elution	Ferricyanide oxidation, pH 3.5 and 6.0; rearrangement with ascorbate-NaOH	filters: Schott BG12 → Chance OY4	Human urine
Euler and Lishajko, 1961b	NE, EN	THI	None (pH 3 for storage)	Alumina column, 0.25 N acetic acid elution	Ferricyanide oxidation, pH 6.2–6.3; rearrangement with ascorbate-NaOH-ED	filters: A, 395 nm → 495 nm; B, 436 nm → 540 nm	Human urine
Crout, 1961	NE, EN	THI	None for urine (15 ml, 6 N HCl in a bottle); TCA (5%) for tissues	Alumina batch adsorption, 0.2 N acetic acid elution	Iodine oxidation, pH 3.5 and 6.5; rearrangement with ascorbate-NaOH and photoactivation	pH 3.5, 410 nm → 520 nm; pH 6.5, 395 nm → 505 nm	Human urine, Tissues
Shore and Olin, 1958	NE	THI	0.01 N HCl	n-Butanol extraction → 0.01 N HCl reextraction	Iodine oxidation, pH 5.0	400 nm → 520 nm	Tissues
Bertler, Carlsson and Rosengren, 1958	NE, EN	THI		Dowex-50-X4-Na+ (acetate buffer, pH 6.0), 0.4 N HCl (for NE) and 2 N HCl (for DA) elution	Ferricyanide oxidation, pH 6.5	A, 410 nm → 540 nm; B, 455 nm → 540 nm	Tissues
Carlsson and Waldeck, 1958	DA	HI	0.4 N PCA		Iodine oxidation, pH 6.5	345 nm → 410 nm	Tissues

Reference	Amines	Method	Deproteinization	Purification	Oxidation	Wavelengths	Source
Weil-Malherbe, 1960b	NE, EN	ED	None	Alumina column, 0.2 N acetic acid elution; Amberlite CG-50-Type 2 column (pH 6.0), 1 N acetic acid elution	ED	A, 420 nm → 510 nm; B, 420 nm → 580 nm	Plasma
Anton and Sayre, 1962	NE, EN	THI	0.4 N PCA	Alumina batch adsorption, 0.05 N PCA elution	Ferricyanide oxidation, pH 7.0 and 2.0	A (pH 7.0), 409 nm → 519 nm; B (pH 2.0), 422 nm → 529 nm	Urine Tissues Blood
Anton and Sayre, 1964	DM, DOPA	HI	0.4 N PCA	Alumina batch adsorption, 0.05 N PCA or 0.05 N HCl elution	Periodate oxidation, pH 7.0	333 nm → 390 nm	Urine Tissues Blood
Itoh, Matsuoka, Nakazima, Tagawa and Imaizumi, 1962	NE, EN, DM	THI ED	0.5 N PCA	Duolite C-25-H⁺ (200–300 mesh), 0.35 M, pH 5.0, sodium acetate for DOPA; 7% ethanol, 3.0 M, pH 6.0, sodium acetate for NE and EN; 25% ethanol, 3.0 M, pH 6.0, sodium acetate for DM	THI for NE and EN, ED for DM		Tissues

EN = epinephrine; NE = norepinephrine; DM = dopamine; (T)HI = (tri)hydroxyindole method; ED = ethylenediamine method TCA = trichloroacetic acid; PCA = perchloric acid.

B. *Trihydroxyindole (THI) fluorometry using ferricyanide oxidation*
   1. *The method by Euler and Floding* (1955a)

Norepinephrine and epinephrine were isolated from urine or trichloro-acetic acid extract of tissues by an alumina column at pH 8.5 and subsequently eluted with 2–10 ml of 0.3 N oxalic acid. In a calibrated 10 ml glass-stoppered cylinder, 1 ml of 1 M acetate buffer of pH 6.0 was added to 0.1–1.0 ml of the eluate. To this was added 0.1 ml of 0.25 % potassium ferricyanide for oxidation which was allowed to act for 2 min. After this, 1 ml of a freshly prepared mixture of 9 ml 20 % NaOH and 1 ml 2 % ascorbic acid was added (rearrangement to trihydroxyindoles). The volume was then brought to 10 ml with water. On addition of ascorbic acid the ferricyanide was reduced and the solution became colourless. The rearrangement to the fluorescent compounds was completed in less than 5 min and the fluorescence was determined. When a slight cloudiness caused by traces of aluminum hydroxide was observed, the sample was centrifuged at 2,000 rpm for 5 min. At pH 6.0 both norepinephrine and epinephrine were completely oxidized and converted to trihydroxyindoles.

The second estimation was made at pH 3.5. To the eluate sample (0.1–1.0 ml) were added 1 ml of 1 M acetate buffer, pH 3.5 and 0.1 ml of 0.25 % potassium ferricyanide solution and 0.1 ml of 0.5 % zinc sulfate solution. Only epinephrine was oxidized to adrenochrome in 3 min, while only about 4 % of the norepinephrine was oxidized.

As a blank, the fluorescent product was allowed to develop and faded by adding all reagents except the stabilizing ascorbic acid. Usually 0.9 ml of 20 % NaOH was added first, and after 2 min, 0.1 ml of 2 % ascorbic acid was added. In another way, first the mixture of NaOH-ascorbic acid was added and then potassium ferricyanide.

Standards were composed of 0.1 μg of norepinephrine and epinephrine each, used in the whole procedure at pH 6.0 and 3.5.

Calculations were made by the following equations:

$$\frac{F(E3.5)}{0.1} E + \frac{F(N3.5)}{0.1} N = F(S3.5)$$

$$\frac{F(E6.0)}{0.1} E + \frac{F(N6.0)}{0.1} N = F(S6.0)$$

where the amount of epinephrine $= E$
   the amount of norepinephrine $= N$
   fluorescence reading at pH 3.5 : for the sample $= F(S3.5)$,
                                    for 0.1 μg epinephrine $= F(E3.5)$,

and for 0.1 μg norepinephrine =
F (N3.5)

fluorescence reading at pH 6.0 : for the sample = F (S6.0),

for 0.1 μg epinephrine = F (E6.0),
and for 0.1 μg norepinephrine =
F (N6.0).

2. *The improved method by Euler and Lishajko* (1961)

By adding small amounts of ethylenediamine (ED) to the alkali-
ascorbic-acid mixture used in the trihydroxyindole method, the fluorescence was greatly stabilized. The fluorescence of the trihydroxyindole
products was read with two filter sets and the amounts of epinephrine and
norepinephrine computed. This method was highly reproducible.

Norepinephrine and epinephrine were isolated from urine (25 ml, stocked
at pH 3) or tissues by alumina column. Tissues were first extracted with 2–
5 volumes of 10 % trichloroacetic acid for 30 min. To the extract or urine
0.5 g of EDTA·2Na was added, and the pH adjusted to 8.2–8.5. The sample
was passed through an alumina column (1 g), and catechols were eluted
with 10 ml of 0.25 N acetic acid. The eluate was centrifuged at 600–1,000
× g for a few min. The eluate was adjusted to pH 6.2–6.3.

The following procedure was the same as the Euler and Floding procedure (1955a) (1), except that oxidation was carried out only at pH 6.0–6.5.
To n ml of the sample, pH 6.2–6.3, in a graduated cylinder, 0.1 ml of 0.25
% potassium ferricyanide was added. Oxidation was carried out for 3 min.
After this n+1 ml of alkali-ascorbic acid containing 0.2 ml of ethylenediamine per 10 ml was added and glass-distilled water added up to 10 ml.
After thorough mixing, the fluorescence was read in a fluorometer with
filter set a (λ_{ex} = 395 nm, λ_{em} = 495 nm) and b (λ_{ex} = 436 nm, λ_{em} = 540
nm). The blank was prepared by adding alkali-ascorbic acid-ethylenedi-
amine to the sample and then ferricyanide. Standards composed of 0.1 μg
of norepinephrine and epinephrine each, were used throughout the reaction.

Calculations were made by the following equations:

$$\frac{F(Ea)}{0.1} E + \frac{F(Na)}{0.1} N = F(Sa)$$

$$\frac{F(Eb)}{0.1} E + \frac{F(Nb)}{0.1} N = F(Sb)$$

where the amount of epinephrine = E
the amount of norepinephrine = N
fluorescence reading at filter set a : for the sample = F (Sa),

for 0.1 µg epinephrine =
F (Ea),
for 0.1 µg norepinephrine =
F (Na)
fluorescence reading at filter set b :   for the sample = F (Sb),
for 0.1 µg epinephrine =
F (Eb),
for 0.1 µg norepinephrine =
F (Nb).

C. *Trihydroxyindole (THI) fluorometry using iodine oxidation* (Crout, 1961)
This method is based on the oxidation of norepinephrine and epinephrine with iodine and the subsequent rearrangement by an alkali-ascorbic mixture under light irradiation. The arrangement reaction was slow (30 min), but the fluorescent products were fairly stable. This method is also widely used and is reproducible.

A 24-hr urine specimen was collected in a glass bottle containing 15ml 6 N HCl, the final pH of which should be about 3. An aliquot of urine equivalent to 10 % of the 24-hr volume (50–250 ml) was used for the assay. Tissues were homogenized in 5–10 volumes of 5 % trichloroacetic acid and centrifuged, and the supernatant was used for the assay. The urine sample was transferred into a 400-ml beaker and diluted to approximately 200 ml with water, and 5 ml of 0.2 M EDTA·2Na(Na₂C₁₀H₁₄O₈N₂·2H₂O, 37.2 g to 500 ml with water) was added. The tissue extracts were transferred to a 30-ml beaker containing 10 ml of 0.2 M sodium acetate (1M, CH₃COONa· 3H₂O, 68 g to 500 ml with water) and 0.5 ml of 0.2 M EDTA·2Na. Alumina (acid-washed and heated), 3 g for urine and 0.5 g for tissue extracts, was added. The mixture was brought to pH 8.4–8.5 by constant stirring with a magnetic stirrer and constant monitoring using a glass electrode and a pH meter and the dropwise addition of 5N NaOH (or 3 N NH₄OH) initially and then 0.5 N NaOH (or 1 N NH₄OH). The mixture was stirred for 5 min at pH 8.4–8.5. To minimize the grinding of alumina by the stirring bar, the stirrer should be run just fast enough to keep the alumina suspended. After 5 min of stirring, the electrode and stirring bar were rinsed with a few ml of deionized water. The alumina was allowed to settle for 3–5 min. The slightly turbid supernatant was carefully decanted and discarded. The alumina precipitate was transferred quantitatively with deionized water to a glass column (1.2 cm (in diameter) × 20 cm with a 100-ml reservoir for urine, and 0.5 cm (in diameter) × 15 cm with a 2.2 × 4.0 cm reservoir for tissue extract) with a small wad of glass wool over the constriction. The water was allowed to drain through, and the column was washed with two 10-ml portions of water. Elution was made with 0.2 N acetic acid. In the column for the tissue extracts, 2–5 ml of 0.2 N acetic acid was used. For urine column, 3 ml of 0.2 N acetic acid eluate was discarded, and then 9.4 ml of 0.2 N acetic acid was added for elution, and it was collected in a calibrated centrifuge tube, diluted to 9.5 ml, and finally made up to 10 ml by adding 0.5 ml of 0.2 M EDTA. The eluate was centrifuged to remove occasional granules of alumina. The catecholamines in the eluate were stable for several weeks at 2°C.

Norepinephrine (mol wt 169.2) and epinephrine (mol wt 183.2) standard solutions were prepared as follows : stock norepinephrine standard (1,000 μg/ml), 19.9 mg of (−)-norepinephrine bitartrate monohydrate (mol wt 337.2) in 10.0 ml of 0.01 N HCl; working norepinephrine standard (1.0 μg/ml), 0.100 ml of the stock norepinephrine standard was diluted with 0.01 N HCl to 100 ml; stock epinephrine standard (1,000 μg/ml), 18.2 mg of (−)-epinephrine bitartrate (mol wt 333.3) in 10.0 ml of 0.01 N HCl; working epinephrine standard (1.0 μg/ml), 0.100 ml of the stock epinephrine standard was diluted with 0.01 N HCl to 100 ml.

The trihydroxyindole reaction was carried out at pH 6.5 and 3.5. The following series of test tubes were prepared. Sample volume of the eluate used for the assay was 0.1–0.2 ml for urine and 0.1–1.0 ml for tissues. For accurate determination of epinephrine in urine or of norepinephrine in tissues, larger aliquots of the eluate (up to 1.0 ml) can be taken for the assay. However, when aliquots of this size are used, more attention must be given to accurate pH adjustment and to the problem of quenching.

Tube	Aliquot	Content
For pH 6.5 oxidation		
1.	0.20 μg norepinephrine (N)	N external standard
2.	0.20 μg epinephrine (E)	E external standard
3.	0.20 ml of water	Reagent blank
4.	0.20 ml eluate	Sample
5.	0.20 ml eluate	Sample blank
6.	0.10 ml eluate+0.10 μg N	Internal standard
For pH 3.5 oxidation		
7.	0.20 μg norepinephrine	N external standard
8.	0.20 μg epinephrine	E external standard
9.	0.20 ml water	Reagent blank
10.	0.20 ml eluate	Sample
11.	0.20 ml eluate	Sample blank
12.	0.10 ml eluate+0.10 μg E	Internal standard

To each tube were added 1.0 ml of 1 M acetate buffer (pH 6.5 or 3.5), and then 0.10 ml of 0.1 N iodine solution (0.635 g iodine and 2.5 g sodium iodide were dissolved in 50 ml water). The solutions were allowed to stand for 4 min. During this waiting period a 1 % ascorbic acid solution was prepared. Then 0.50 ml of 0.05 N sodium thiosulfate (2.48 g sodium thiosulfate ($Na_2S_2O_3 \cdot 5H_2O$) was dissolved in water to 200 ml) was added to each tube to destroy the excess iodine. The iodochromes and chromes were formed at this stage. 1.0 ml of a freshly mixed 5 N NaOH-1 % ascorbic acid solution (7 : 3, v/v) was added to each tube except the sample blanks (tubes 5 and 11). To the latter two tubes 0.70 ml of 5 N NaOH was added and 15 min were allowed to pass to allow for any fluorescent hydroxyindoles to deteriorate, and then 0.30 ml of 1 % ascorbic acid was added to complete the blank. All the tubes were diluted to 5.0 ml with water and allowed to stand under irradiation by a fluorescent lamp for 30–45 min before reading.

When ferricyanide is used as the oxidizing agent, the isomerization of chromes to trihydroxyindoles occurs rapidly (1–2 min). With iodine, this process requires 40–60 min and is activated by light. At pH 3.5, epinephrine is oxidized quantitatively, but norepinephrine remains almost unchanged.

The pH 6.5 series were read at 395 nm activation and 505 nm fluorescence, and the pH 3.5 series at 410 nm activation and 520 nm fluorescence. For the pH 6.5 series, the galvanometer reading for the 0.20 μg of norepinephrine was adjusted to about 80, while for the pH 3.5 series the reading for the 0.20 μg of epinephrine was about 80.

The reading for each tube was recorded, and the appropriate blank value was subtracted. The reading for 0.20 μg of each standard and 0.20 ml of eluate at each pH was calculated. If any sample tubes read off the scale, the eluate was diluted appropriately with water and reassayed. The reading of the external standard of epinephrine at pH 6.5 oxidation was corrected for same degree of quenching as that for norepinephrine.

The reading of 0.2 μg of norepinephrine at pH 3.5 oxidation is very low. It assumes significance in the calculation only when the concentration of norepinephrine is quite high as compared to epinephrine. In most cases, the entire reading at pH 3.5 may be taken as due to epinephrine alone.

The concentration of norepinephrine and epinephrine in the alumina eluate was estimated by solving the following simultaneous equations:

$$\frac{F\,(E6.5)}{0.2}\,E + \frac{F\,(N6.5)}{0.2}\,N = F\,(S6.5)$$

$$\frac{F\,(E3.5)}{0.2}\,E + \frac{F\,(N3.5)}{0.2}\,N = F\,(S3.5)$$

where E = concentration of epinephrine in eluate, $\mu g/0.2$ ml

N = concentration of norepinephrine in eluate, $\mu g/0.2$ ml

$F\,(E6.5)$ = reading of 0.2 μg epinephrine at pH 6.5 calculated from the norepinephrine internal standard

$F\,(N6.5)$ = reading of 0.2 μg norepinephrine at pH 6.5 measured from the internal standard

$F\,(S6.5)$ = reading of 0.2 ml of the sample (the reading of the sample blank was subtracted)

$F\,(E3.5)$ = reading of 0.2 μg epinephrine at pH 3.5 calculated from the internal standard

$F\,(N3.5)$ = reading of 0.2 μg norepinephrine at pH 3.5 calculated from the internal standard (this value may be neglected)

$F\,(S3.5)$ = reading of 0.2 ml of the eluate (the reading of the sample blank was subtracted)

For 24-hr norepinephrine (or epinephrine), excretion in μg was calculated as follows:

$$[N \text{ (or } E) \text{ in 0.2 ml eluate]} \times \frac{10}{0.2} \times \frac{\text{24-hr-urine volume}}{\text{Volume of aliquot analyzed}}$$

D. *Fluorometry of dopamine* (Carlsson and Waldeck, 1958)
Dopamine can be measured fluorometrically by the ethylenediamine condensation method, but since the fluorophores of dopamine and epinephrine have almost the same fluorescence characteristics, complete separation of dopamine from other catechol compounds is necessary before the assay.

Dopamine cannot be converted to a hydroxyindole under the oxidation condition generally used for the assay of norepinephrine and epinephrine. However, with certain modifications in the technique, a highly fluorescent hydroxyindole, which differs markedly from those of adrenolutine and noradrenolutine, can be produced. This original method by Carlsson and Waldeck (1958) was modified by Drujan, Sourkes, Layne and Murphy (1959).

Dopamine was isolated either with alumina or Dowex-50-Na$^+$ columns. The pH of the eluate was adjusted to about 6.5. To a test tube were added 1–3 ml of sample (0.2–2 μg dopamine), 0.5 ml of 0.1 M phosphate buffer, pH 6.5, water to give a total volume of 3.8 ml, and 0.05 ml of iodine solution (0.02 N; 0.254 g of iodine and 5 g of KI were dissolved in 5 ml of water and diluted to 100 ml). After 5 min, 0.5 ml of alkaline sulfite solution (5.04

g $Na_2SO_3 \cdot 7H_2O$ was dissolved in 10 ml water and diluted with 5 N NaOH to 100 ml) was added. After another 5 min 0.6 ml of 5 N acetic acid (the pH dropped to about 5.3) was added. The sample was heated at 45°C under standard laboratory lighting conditions for 30 min. (In the original method of Carlsson and Waldeck (1958), the samples, in silica test tubes, were irradiated by means of a mercury lamp (peak emission 254 nm) for 10 min.) The fluorescence was read in a spectrophotofluorometer. Activation and fluorescence peaks were at 345 nm and 410 nm, respectively (uncorrected values).

A standard and a reagent blank were run together with the sample. When tissue extracts were analyzed, a tissue blank and an internal standard were also run together with the sample. The tissue blank was a sample treated as above, except that 5 N sodium hydroxide instead of the alkaline sulfite solution had been added. The internal standard was a sample treated as above, except that known amount of dopamine had been added. Epinephrine, norepinephrine, and epinine added in amounts equal to that of dopamine did not interfere with the assay. DOPA yielded a compound with fluorescence characteristics indistinguishable from those of the fluorophore of dopamine. The concentrations of DOPA in tissues are generally considered to be low. However, when the presence of DOPA is expected, preliminary separation of DOPA from dopamine by Dowex-50-Na^+ is necessary.

E.   *Simultaneous fluorescence assay of dopamine, norepinephrine and epinephrine by a modified hydroxyindole method*

When dopamine, norepinephrine, and epinephrine are treated on the basis of ferricyanide oxidation (Euler and Floding, 1955a) or iodine oxidation (Crout, 1961), only norepinephrine and epinephrine yield highly fluorescent trihydroxyindole compounds. On the other hand, when the three catecholamines are treated on the basis of iodine oxidation and subsequent photochemical or heat activation, only dopamine yields a highly fluorescent compound. This is due partly to the differences in fluorescence characteristics, partly to low yields of adrenolutine and noradrenolutine under the experimental conditions by Carlsson and Waldeck (1958).

By slightly modifying the reaction conditions by Carlsson and Waldeck (1958), it is possible to increase the yields of adrenolutine and noradrenolutine together with the formation of the fluorophore of dopamine. Hogans* developed a sensitive method for the simultaneous estimation of norepine-

---

* Merck Institute for Therapeutic Research, West Point, Pennsylvania, U.S.A.

phrine and dopamine in tissue. She developed a method to extract catecholamines from tissues by using dry butanol and, subsequently, measuring dopamine and norepinephrine simultaneously in the same solution based on
the fact that the fluorescence characteristics of the fluorophores derived
from norepinephrine and dopamine following oxidation with iodine are
sufficiently different. The characteristic features of the procedure are the
inclusions of a metal chelating agent (EDTA), the use of heat following
oxidation, and the use of an acid final pH.* This method has not yet been
published by Hogans, but appears to be widely sued in many laboratories.
Some modifications of this method have been made in our laboratory,
which permit the differential estimation of epinephrine together with dopamine and norepinephrine in the same solution (Nagatsu, T., Yamamoto
and Nagatsu, I., 1970).

The reaction conditions of the hydroxyindole procedure for the assay of
catecholamines have been extensively studied by Laverty and Taylor (1968),
and the use of an acid final pH for norepinephrine was also proposed.

1.   *The original method*

Animal tissue (brain, heart, kidney, and spleen) was thoroughly homogenized with dry n-butanol, keeping a ratio of 1 ml of butanol per 150 mg
tissue. After centrifugation, 4 ml aliquots of the clear supernatant solution
were extracted for 15 sec with 3 ml of 0.1 M phosphate buffer, pH 6.5.
Aliquots of this extract containing from 0.02 to 2.0 μg of catecholamines
(usually 1–2 ml) were diluted to 2 ml with phosphate buffer and 1.0 ml of
4 % EDTA·2Na. Exactly 2 min after the addition of 0.2 ml of iodine solution (4.8 g KI and 0.25 g sublimed iodine in 100 ml water), 0.5 ml of alkaline
sulfite (5 ml of 12.6 % anhydrous sodium sulfite made up to 25 ml with 5
N NaOH) was added. Exactly 2 min later 0.6 ml of 5 N acetic acid was
added. The solutions were heated in a boiling water bath for 5 min, then
cooled rapidly by immersion in cold water.

Standard solutions containing 0.1 μg of dopamine and norepinephrine
and a water blank were treated similarly. The fluorescence reading of the
water blank was subtracted from all other readings. In our laboratory, a
tissue blank and an internal standard were also run together with the
sample. The tissue blank was prepared by adding alkaline sulfite first and
then iodine solution. The internal standard was a sample treated as above,
except that a known amount of dopamine or norepinephrine had been
added to the tissue.

---

* I am grateful to Dr. Alice F. Hogans for the detailed information on the method,
and to Dr. Morton Levitt for introducing the method to me.

The intensities of fluorescence in the resulting solutions were determined in a spectrophotofluorometer at the following wavelengths (excitation (nm)/fluorescence (nm)) : 310/365 for dopamine and 385/480 for norepinephrine.

The recovery for dopamine or norepinephrine added to the tissue were about 50 %. The use of an internal standard of dopamine or norepinephrine can correct the recovery.

DOPA yields a fluorescent compound indistinguishable from dopamine by this method. Preliminary treatment to remove DOPA is necessary, if the sample is expected to contain DOPA.

2. *A modified method*

The original method by Hogans is slightly modified in our laboratory (Nagatsu, T., Yamamoto and Nagatsu, I., 1970). The modification permits the measuring of dopamine, norepinephrine, and epinephrine, simultaneously. Catecholamines were isolated from tissues either by the dry *n*-butanol extraction method (Hogans) or by alumina (Crout, 1961). Catecholamines were eluted from alumina with 2 ml of 0.2 N HCl. The eluate was adjusted to pH 6.5 or 3.5 and used for the assay. This method was applied to the determination of catecholamines in dental pulp (Nakano, Kuzuya and Nagatsu, 1970).

If DOPA is present in the sample, this should be separated first. A modified Duolite C-25 column procedure (Itoh, Matsuoka, Nakazima, Tagawa and Imaizumi, 1962) can be used to eliminate DOPA from dopamine, norepinephrine and epinephrine (Nagatsu, unpublished results). The tissue was homogenized with about 10 volumes of 0.4 N perchloric acid. The homogenate was centrifuged at 10,000 $\times$ g for 10 min at 0°C. The supernatant was neutralized with 2.5 M K_2CO_3 to pH 4 with a pH meter. The $KClO_4$ precipitate was removed by centrifugation at 10,000 $\times$ g for 10 min at 0°C. The supernatant was passed through a column of Dowex-50-W-X2 (200–400 mesh), Na^+ form (buffered at pH 6.0 with potassium phosphate buffer) 0.5 cm diameter, packed volume 2.0 ml. The column was washed with 10 ml of water and then with 10 ml of 0.2 M sodium acetate buffer, pH 6.0, and DOPA came through the column. If the assay of DOPA is desired, the effluent and washings with water and acetate buffer are retained. Epinephrine, norepinephrine, and dopamine were subsequently eluted in the dark with 8 ml of 25 % ethanol-3 M sodium acetate buffer, pH 6.0. Two 2.0-ml aliquots of the effluent, one for the assay and the other for the sample blank, were used for the assay.

The tissue extracts containing catecholamines were pipetted into 4 tubes (tubes 5, 6, 9, 10). The pH of each two samples was adjusted either to 6.5

(tubes 5, 6) with phosphate buffer or 3.5 (tubes 9, 10) with acetic acid. The following series of test tubes were prepared.

Tube	Aliquot	Content	Reading (nm)		
For pH 6.5 oxidation (room temperature)					
1.	0.10 μg dopamine (DM)	DM external standard	310/365		
2.	0.10 μg norepinephrine (NE)	NE external standard		385/480	
3.	0.10 μg epinephrine (EN)	EN external standard		385/480	
4.	0.1 ml, 0.01 N HCl	Reagent blank	310/365	385/480	
5.	2.0 ml sample	Sample	310/365	385/480	
6.	2.0 ml sample	Sample blank	310/365	385/480	
For pH 3.5 oxidation (in ice bath)					
7.	0.10 μg epinephrine	EN external standard			410/500
8.	0.1 ml, 0.01 N HCl	Reagent blank			410/500
9.	2.0 ml sample	Sample			410/500
10.	2.0 ml sample	Sample blank			410/500

The pH 6.5 series (tubes, 1–6) reaction was carried out at room temperature, and the pH 3.5 series (tubes, 7–10) reaction in an ice bath. To each tube either 0.1 M phosphate buffer, pH 6.5, or the phosphate buffer adjusted to pH 3.5 with glacial acetic acid to a total volume of 2.0 ml, then 1.0 ml of 4 % EDTA, and 0.2 ml of the iodine solution were added. Exactly 2 min later, 0.5 ml of alkaline sulfite was added. For the blanks, the additions of iodine and alkaline sulfite were made in reverse. Exactly 2 min later, 0.6 ml of 5 N acetic acid was added. The solutions were heated in a boiling water bath for 5 min, then cooled rapidly by immersion in cold water. The fluorescence intensity in the resulting solution were determined in a spectrophotofluorometer at the following wavelengths (excitation (nm)/fluorescence (nm)) : for the pH 6.5 series at the dopamine peak (310/365), and the norepinephrine peak (385/480); for the pH 3.5 series at the epinephrine peak (410/500), as shown in the above table. The blank values were subtracted from the readings. The concentrations of dopamine (D), norepinephrine (N) and epinephrine (E) in the sample were estimated differentially by solving the following equations :

$$\frac{F(D365)}{0.1} D = F(S365)$$

$$\frac{F(E500)}{0.1} E = F(S500)$$

$$\frac{F(E480)}{0.1} E + \frac{F(N480)}{0.1} N = F(S480)$$

where (blank values were subtracted from all values)

$F(D365)$ = reading of 0.1 μg dopamine at 365 nm (sample oxidized at pH 6.5)

$F(N480)$ = reading of 0.1 μg norepinephrine at 480 nm (sample oxidized at pH 6.5)

$F(E500)$ = reading of 0.1 μg epinephrine at 500 nm (sample oxidized at pH 3.5)

$F(S365)$ = reading of sample at 365 nm (sample oxidized at pH 6.5)

$F(S480)$ = reading of sample at 480 nm (sample oxidized at pH 6.5)

$F(S500)$ = reading of sample at 500 nm (sample oxidized at pH 3.5)

When the oxidation was carried out at pH 3.5 in an ice bath, only epinephrine was converted to a fluorescent compound, and the fluorescence intensities of norepinephrine or dopamine at 500 nm were negligibly small.

DOPA can be assayed by this procedure as its sensitivity for DOPA is very high. Oxidation was carried out at pH 6.5 at room temperature, and fluorescence was measured at 365 nm by excitation at 310 nm.

F. *Fluorometry of DOPA*

DOPA can be isolated, first by alumina together with other catechols, and then further by Amberlite IRC-50 or Dowex-50-Na$^+$ columns. DOPA can be converted to a highly fluorescent hydroxyindole compound by ferricyanide oxidation (Euler and Floding, 1955a) or by iodine oxidation in the dopamine assay (Carlsson and Waldeck, 1958). The iodine oxidation procedure by Crout (1961) does not yield significant fluorescence of DOPA. DOPA forms a fluorescent compound by the ethylenediamine condensation (Weil-Malherbe and Bone, 1952). This condensate is not extractable with isobutanol.

The tissue concentrations of DOPA are very low. However, its assay is often required after the administration of DOPA. Usually DOPA is isolated by column procedures and is measured by a hydroxyindole reaction (for example, that used by Anton and Sayre, 1964).

G. *Automated fluorometric method for the determination of catecholamines*

An automated procedure for assay of norepinephrine and epinephrine is described here. After a initial purification of catecholamines by adsorption

TABLE XIV: Fluorometric and Radiometric Determination of Catecholamines in Human Plasma.

Reference	Volume	Preservatives	Deproteinization	Isolation and fluorometry	Normal value ($\mu g/l$)	
					NE	EN
1)	blood 30 ml	heparin	(—)	alumina THI	0.30 ± 0.07	0.06 ± 0.05
2)	blood 20 ml	EDTA-sodium thiosulfate sol. 5 ml	(—)	alumina Amberlite CG-50 ED	0.58 ± 0.108 (0–3.10)	0.22 ± 0.044 (0–1.17)
3)	plasma 30 ml	heparin, sodium metabisulfite (0.5 mg/ml)	perchloric acid, 0.4 N	alumina THI	0.97	0.48
4)	blood 18 ml	EDTA sol. (1% in 0.9% NaCl) 2 ml	(—) or perchloric acid, 0.4 N	Dowex-50 THI	0.3 ± 0.11	0.0
5)	plasma 10 ml	sodium citrate (4 mg/ml), ascorbic acid (2 mg/ml)	(—)	Amberlite IRC-50 Radiometry	0.20 ± 0.08 male: 0.20 ± 0.08 female: 0.21 ± 0.09	0.05 ± 0.03 0.06 ± 0.04 0.04 ± 0.03

EN = epinephrine; NE = norepinephrine; THI = trihydroxyindole method; ED = ethylenediamine method.

1) Cohen and Goldenberg, 1957.
2) Weil-Malherbe, 1960b.
3) Anton and Sayre, 1962.
4) Häggendal, 1963.
5) Engelman and Portnoy, 1970.

TABLE XV. Excretion of Catecholamines and Their Metabolites in Human Urine.

Compound		Value	Unit	Reference
EN-free	day	0.34	μg/25 mg creatinine	Anton and Sayre, 1966
	night	0.18		
free		0–15	μg/24 hr	Crout, 1968
conjugated		8.69 ± 0.68	μg/24 hr	Hoeldtke and Sloan, 1970
NE-free	day	0.73	μg/25 mg creatinine	Anton and Sayre, 1966
	night	0.36		
free		20–70	μg/24 hr	Crout, 1968
conjugated		77.5 ± 11.0	μg/24 hr	Hoeldtke and Sloan, 1970
DM-free	day	3.35	μg/25 mg creatinine	Anton and Sayre, 1966
	night	2.56		
free		100–350	μg/24 hr	Crout, 1968
conjugated		615±40	μg/24 hr	Hoeldtke and Sloan, 1970
MN-conjugated	day	4.69	μg/25 mg creatinine	Anton and Sayre, 1966
	night	4.16		
		50–200	μg/24 hr	Crout, 1968
		72.1±5.74	μg/24 hr	Smith and Weil-Malherbe, 1962
		(28.3–113)		
NMN-conjugated	day	5.07	μg/25 mg creatinine	Anton and Sayre, 1966
	night	4.57		
		100–500	μg/24 hr	Crout, 1968
		158.6±17.5	μg/24 hr	Smith and Weil-Malherbe, 1962
		(78.0–369)		
MT-free	children	37	μg/24 hr	Käser, 1970
	(2–13 years)	0.10	μg/mg creatinine	

				Reference
VMA-free	adult (25–105 years)	88	μg/24 hr	Anton and Sayre, 1966
		0.067	μg/mg creatinine	
	day	141.4	μg/25 mg creatinine	
	night	102.8		
		1.6 (0.3–3.4)	μg/mg creatinine	Wilk, Gitlow, Mendlowitz, Franklin, Carr and Clarke, 1965
HVA-free		3.7±1.1	mg/24 hr	Pisano, Crout and Abraham, 1962
		5.7±1.3	mg/24 hr	Karoum, Anah, Ruthven and Sandler, 1969
		2–6	mg/24 hr	Crout, 1968
		5.4±1.4 (3.7–7.5)	mg/24 hr	Sato, 1965
DOMA-free		4.2±1.5	mg/24 hr	Karoum, Anah, Ruthven and Sandler, 1969
		720±320	μg/24 hr	Miyake, Yoshida and Imaizumi, 1962
		920±310	μg/24 hr	Drujan, Alvarez and Diaz Borges, 1966
		91	μg/24 hr	Sato and DeQuattro, 1969
DOPAC-free		1200±420	μg/24 hr	Drujan, Alvaroz and Diaz Borges, 1966
MHPG-free		2.4±0.8	mg/24 hr	Karoum, Anah, Ruthven and Sandler, 1969
	free	0.208	μg/mg creatinine	Shimizu and LaBrosse, 1969
	glucuronide	1.21		
	sulfate	1.304		
	total	2.72		

EN=epinephrine; NE=norepinephrine; DM=dopamine; MN=metanephrine; NMN=normetanephrine; MT=methoxytyramine; VMA=vanillylmandelic acid; HVA=homovanillic acid; DOMA=dihydroxymandelic acid; DOPAC=dihydroxyphenylacetic acid; MHPG=3-methoxy-4-hydroxyphenylglycol.

TABLE XVI. Distribution of Catecholamines and Their Metabolites in Tissues.

Substance	Species	Tissue	Value	Unit	Reference
EN	Rat	Brain	0	μg/g	Crawford and Yates, 1970
	Rat	Heart	0.05±0.02	μg/g	Robinson and Watts, 1965
		Adrenals	657.6±52.2		
	Rat	Brain	0.04	μg/g	Anton and Sayre, 1962
		Heart	0.05		
		Spleen	0.07		
		Adrenals	600.0		
	Human	Adrenals	1173.2		
NE	Rat	Brain	0.17	μg/g	Crawford and Yates, 1970
	Rat	Heart	1.01±0.06	μg/g	Robinson and Watts, 1965
		Adrenals	133.4±13.3		
	Rat	Brain	0.15	μg/g	Anton and Sayre, 1962
		Heart	0.27		
		Spleen	0.47		
		Adrenals	172.00		
	Human	Adrenals	86.79		
DM	Rat	Brain	0.70	μg/g	Crawford and Yates, 1970
	Rat	Brain	0.68	μg/g	Anton and Sayre, 1964
		Heart	0.03		
MN	Rat	Brain	0	μg/g	Crawford and Yates, 1970
	Frog	Brain	0.15	μg/g	Anton and Sayre, 1966
	Rat	Adrenals	4.4		
	Rabbit	Adrenals	3.2		
	Dog	Adrenals	12.3		

NMN	Rat	Brain	0.02	$\mu g/g$	Crawford and Yates, 1970
	Rat	Brain	0.07	$\mu g/g$	Anton and Sayre, 1966
	Frog	Brain	0.08		
MT	Rat	Brain	0.06	$\mu g/g$	Crawford and Yates, 1970
DOMA	Human	Plasma	1.4±0.2	$\mu g/l$	Sato and DeQuattro, 1969
	Rat	Heart	0.02	$\mu g/g$	
	Human	Adrenals	1.2		
		Pheochromocytoma	0.3		
MHPG	Rabbit	Hypothalamus	0.045–0.159	$\mu g/g$	Sharman, 1969
	Mouse		0.040–0.077		
	Cat		0.018		
DHPG	Rabbit	Hypothalamus	0.030–0.126	$\mu g/g$	Sharman, 1969
	Mouse		0.029–0.054		
	Cat		0.018, 0.022		
Octopamine	Rat	Adrenals	491±49	ng/g	Molinoff and Axelrod, 1969
		Brain	4.7±0.93		
		Heart	49.6±2.8		
		Salivary Glands	95.7±8.8		

EN = epinephrine;   NE = norepinephrine;   DM = dopamine;   MN = metanephrine;   NMN = normetanephrine;
MT = methoxytyramine;   DOMA = dihydroxymandelic acid;   MHPG = 3-methoxy-4-hydroxyphenylglycol;
DHPG = dihydroxyphenylglycol.

on alumina, the neutralized eluates were subjected to automatic analysis, in which potassium ferricyanide and an alkaline stabilizing agent were automatically mixed sequentially with the dialyzed catecholamines. The fluorescent trihydroxy derivatives formed were then delivered to a flow cell in a fluorometer and the fluorescence recorded. A differential estimation was obtained by running samples through the system, first with ascorbic acid stabilization to obtain the combined fluorescence of both amines and then with thioglycolic acid stabilization to obtain the fluorescence of nor-epinephrine alone (Robinson and Watts, 1965). This procedure was successfully applied to tissues, urine and blood.

In another automated procedure, catecholamines were isolated with Dowex-50W-X8 column, and then oxidation was carried out with iodine. The catecholamines were converted to trihydroxyindoles, and the concentration of norepinephrine and epinephrine present in the sample was determined by the differential spectrum technique. Tracer amounts of tritium-labeled norepinephrine or epinephrine were added to the samples, and the efficiency of the isolation process was calculated from radiochemical analysis of the ion-exchange column eluate (Martin and Harrison, 1968).

The ethylenediamine method was also used for the automated assay of epinephrine and norepinephrine. An amberlite IRC-50 column was used for the isolation of the catecholamines (Viktora, Baukal and Wolff, 1968).

An automated fluorometric method for the determination of dopamine was also described (Craig, Azzaro, Frame and Hunt, 1970).

H. *Assay of conjugated catecholamines*

A large portion of catecholamines and catecholamine metabolites are excreted in urine in a conjugated form (Euler and Orwén, 1955; Weil-Malherbe, 1961). The free forms can be liberated either by hydrolyzing at an acid pH or by incubation with the sulfatase. Acid hydrolysis is carried out at pH 1.0–1.5. Total (free plus conjugated) catecholamines were determined by hydrolyzing the urine aliquot (100°C for 20 min at pH 0.5–1.0) prior to assay (Crout, 1960b). The use of the alumina filtrate and the subsequent hydrolysis at pH 1.0 were recommended (Hoeldtke and Sloan, 1970).

I. *Concentration of catecholamines and their metabolites in plasma, urine and tissues*

The concentrations of catecholamines and their metabolites in plasma, urine and tissues are summarized in Tables XIV, XV and XVI.

IV. 1. 4. IDENTIFICATION OF CATECHOLAMINES

Catecholamines can be identified by paper or thin-layer chromatography, or by high-voltage electrophoresis. Catecholamines isolated by alumina or other chromatographic procedures were evaporated to dryness under nitrogen and reextracted with a small volume (0.2 ml) of ethanol/0.5 N HCl (100/1, v/v).

Gas chromatography is useful not only for the identification but also for the assays (see section IV. 1. 5).

The R_f values of catecholamines in the presence of various solvents either in paper chromatography or in thin-layer chromatography are shown in Table XVII; n-butanol/acetic acid/water (4/1/1) was most frequently used as solvent.

Catecholamines can also be separated by high-voltage electrophoresis in 4 % formic acid or in pyridine/acetic acid/water (1/10/89) at 2.5–5 kV for 1–1.5 hr (Nagatsu, Levitt and Udenfriend, 1964b).

Chromatograms and electrophoretograms can be developed in the following ways :

1) $K_3Fe(CN)_6$. The chromatograms were sprayed with 0.25% potassium ferricyanide aqueous solution and then exposed to ammonia vapor. With low concentrations, the spots were located by fluorescence under ultraviolet light (max. at 360 nm).

2) Ethylenediamine. Ethylenediamine was predistilled and mixed with equal volume of water. The sprayed chromatograms were dried for 20 min at 50–60°C and the spots revealed under ultraviolet light (max. at 360 nm).

3) p-Nitroaniline. A 1 : 1 : 2 mixture of the following solutions was made immediately prior to using and kept at 2°C: (a) 0.1 g of p-nitroaniline dissolved in 2 ml of conc HCl and made up to 100 ml with distilled water, (b) 0.2 g of $NaNO_2$ dissolved in 100 ml of water, (c) 10 g of K_2CO_3 dissolved in 100 ml of water (de Potter, Vochten and de Schaepdryver, 1965).

Complete separation of catecholamines and their metabolites was possible through a 2-dimensional technique employing electrophoresis and thinlayer chromatography (Schweitzer and Friedhoff, 1969). The following compounds were completely separated:

1) Norepinephrine (NE),
2) Normetanephrine (NMN),
3) 3-Methoxy-4-hydroxymandelic acid (VMA),
4) 3,4-Dihydroxyphenylglycol (DHPG),
5) 3-Methoxy-4-hydroxyphenylglycol (MHPG),
6) 3,4-Dihydroxymandelic acid (DHMA),

TABLE XVII. R_f Values of Catecholamines in Paper Chromatography and Thin-layer Chromatography.

Solvent	R_f								Reference
	DOPA	DM	NE	EN	NMN	MN	DOMA	VMA	
Paper chromatography									
n-Butanol saturated with 0.5 N HCl	0.21	0.24	0.10	0.17					Crawford, 1951
Phenol saturated with H$_2$O and SO$_2$	0.29	0.43	0.28	0.51					
Phenol/0.2 N acetic acid/n-butanol (85/11/4)	0.11	0.28	0.16	0.36	0.46	0.74		0.83	Laasberg and Shimosato, 1966
Dansylated catecholamines									
Benzene/methanol/cyclohexane (88.5/1.5/10)		0.65	0.27	0.50					Diliberto and DiStefano, 1969
Thin-layer chromatography									
Cellulose powder									
n-Butanol saturated with 3 N HCl			0.31	0.38	0.48	0.58	0.80	0.89	de Potter, Vochten and de Schaepdryver, 1965
MN cellulose 300 G (containing approximately 1.5 g CaSO$_4$·$\frac{1}{2}$ H$_2$O)									
Methanol/n-butanol/benzene/water (4/3/2/1)	0.11–0.14	0.46–0.51	0.32–0.37						Schneider and Gillis, 1965
Acetone/t-butanol/formic acid/water (180/180/1/39)	0.06–0.07	0.42–0.49	0.30–0.37						
MN cellulose 300 GF (Brinkman, Inc., New York), activated 30 min at 110°C.									
n-Butanol/ethanol/1 N acetic acid (35/10/10)	0.23	0.50	0.38						Johnson and Boukma, 1967
Silica gel									
N-Dansylated catecholamines									
Benzene/dioxane/acetic acid (90/25/4)		0.30	0.14	0.23					Kitani, Imai and Tamura, 1970

DM = dopamine; NE = norepinephrine; EM = epinephrine; NMN = normetanephrine; MN = metanephrine; DOMA = 3,4-dihydroxymandelic acid; VMA = 3-methoxy-4-hydroxymandelic acid (vanillylmandelic acid).

7) Dopamine (DM),
8) 3-Methoxytyramine (MT),
9) 3-Methoxy-4-hydroxyphenylacetic acid (HVA),
10) 3,4-Dihydroxyphenylethanol (DHPE),
11) 3-Methoxy-4-hydroxyphenylethanol (MHPE),
12) 3,4-Dihydroxyphenylacetic acid (DOPAC), and
13) DOPA.

Catecholamines were also separated as dansyl(DNS)-catecholamines (Diliberto and DiStefano, 1969) and complete dansylation was possible as follows. One milliliter of 0.1 N NaHCO$_3$ and 1 ml dansyl reagent (17.55 mg dansyl Cl/ml acetone) were added to 6.5 μmoles catecholamine. The dansyl reagent was added as soon as possible to avoid decomposition of the catecholamine. The reaction was carried out in the dark at an ambient temperature for 12 hr. When the reaction was complete, the NaHCO$_3$ was precipitated by the addition of 8 ml acetone, and then filtered or centrifuged. The supernatant was used for chromatography. This procedure could be scaled down to 1/100 volume. Benzene/methanol/cyclohexane (88.5/1.5/10) was used as solvent for the development of chromatograms made with a sheet of Whatman SG 81 paper (20 × 20 cm). The development was made in the dark and derivatives were revealed by means of a UV lamp. The dansylated catecholamines emitted a yellow fluorescence.

N-Mono-dansylation of catecholamines was possible by protecting the pyrocatechol with alumina (Kitani, Imai and Tamura, 1970). The catecholamine (6 × 10^{-9} mole) was adsorbed on alumina at pH 8.8. The alumina was washed with 0.25 M triethylamine-carbonate buffer (pH 8.8). Dansylation of the catecholamine on the surface of alumina was carried out with dansyl-Cl (3.7 × 10^{-6} mole in 0.2 ml of dioxane) in 0.25 M triethylamine-carbonate buffer (0.2 ml) at pH 8.8 for 5 min. One drop of pyridine was added for the degradation of the reagent. Alumina was washed with the buffer, methanol and distilled water, successively. DNS-catecholamines were eluted from alumina with 10 ml of 0.2 N acetic acid. The eluate was evaporated under reduced pressure. The residue was chromatographed by silica gel thin-layer chromatography with benzene/dioxane/acetic acid (90/25/4) as solvent.

IV. 1. 5. Gas-Liquid Chromatography of Catecholamines
Gas-liquid chromatography has the advantage of higher resolution, however, its practical application is a problem because of the instability of the derivatives. Metanephrine, epinephrine, dopamine, normetanephrine, and norepinephrine were completely separated as Schiff's base trimethylsilyl

ether derivatives (2-pentanone condensation products) (Kawai, Nagatsu, Imanari and Tamura, 1966). Catecholamines in the bovine adrenal medulla were separated as trimethylsilyl derivatives of epinephrine and Schiff's base-trimethylsilyl derivatives of norepinephrine (Kawai and Tamura, 1966, 1967). The use of the electron capture detection of fluoroacetyl catecholamine derivatives permitted detection in the range of nano- to picograms (Kawai and Tamura, 1968a). This method was successfully applied to the gas-chromatographic assay of catecholamines in urines and pheochromocytoma tissues (Kawai and Tamura, 1968b). The procedures by Kawai and Tamura are as follows. Catecholamines were isolated from urine by alumina. Tumor tissues were extracted with 5 % trichloroacetic acid and catecholamines were isolated by alumina. To 0.5 ml aliquot of the 0.2 N acetic acid eluate (10 ml) from alumina a drop of 0.5 % acetylacetone aqueous solution was added. The solution was evaporated to dryness in a water bath at 50°C under reduced pressure. The residue was treated with 0.05 ml of tetrahydrofuran and one drop of trifluoroacetic anhydride for 10 min at room temperature. The reaction mixture was diluted to an appropriate volume with n-hexane and was injected directly into a gas chromatograph column. A gas chromatograph equipped with an electron capture detector and glass tubes for columns, 2.0 m in length and 4 mm in internal diameter was used. The column packings were 2 % GE-XF 1105 on Gas-Chrome P (80–100 mesh). The column (and injection) temperature and detector temperature were 190° and 200°C, respectively. A similar procedure was described by Clarke, Wilk, Gitlow and Franklin (1967) which permitted the determination of dopamine in urine at a ng level.

IV. 1. 6. RADIOASSAY OF CATECHOLAMINES

The radioassay of catecholamines by the double isotope derivative technique is highly sensitive and suitable for the accurate measurement of low concentrations of the amines, for example in blood. The three types of radioassays covered here are: 1) the formation of norepinephrine-N-methyl-C^{14} from S-adenosylmethionine-methyl-C^{14} by phenylethanolamine-N-methyltransferase (Saelens, Schoen and Kovacsics, 1967); 2) the formation of methoxy-catecholamine-C^{14} from S-adenosylmethionine-methyl-C^{14} by catechol-O-methyltransferase (Engelman, Portnoy and Lovenberg, 1968; Engelman and Portnoy, 1970); and 3) acetylation of catecholamines with acetic-H^3 anhydride (Franklin and Mayer, 1968).

Details of the procedure by Engelman, Portnoy and Lovenberg (1968) and Engelman and Portnoy (1970) are described in a form of a flow sheet on pages 246–249.

The double isotope derivative assay by Engelman, Portnoy and Lovenberg (1968) and Engelman and Portnoy (1970) is based on the conversion of norepinephrine and epinephrine to their metanephrines-C^{14} by incubation with S-adenosylmethionine-methyl-C^{14} and catechol-O-methyltransferase in the presence of tracer quantities of norepinephrine-7-H^3. The radioactive metanephrine and normetanephrine so formed were isolated on an Amberlite IRC-50 column, and separated on thin-layer chromatography and were then oxidized to vanillin by $NaIO_4$. The radioactive vanillin was measured by a liquid scintillation spectrometer. This method measured norepinephrine and epinephrine in urine as well as plasma. Absolute values were obtained for each sample owing to the internal tracer recovery. Using the counting efficiencies of the C^{14} and H^3 isotopes, the absolute dpm in each sample due to C^{14} and H^3 was determined. The quantity of norepinephrine and epinephrine present in the original sample was calculated from the following equation :

$$\frac{\text{vanillin-}C^{14}\text{ dpm} \times 169 \text{ ng NE (or 183 ng EN)/ nmole} \times 100}{\text{spec. act. of SAM-}C^{14}\text{ (dpm/nmole)} \times \% \text{ recovery of NE-}H^3 \text{ (or EN-}H^3)}$$

$$= \frac{\text{ng NE (or EN) equivalents}}{\text{in sample}}$$

Since quantitation of results derived from double isotope derivative assays is absolutely dependent on the specific activities of the isotope reagents, it is necessary to confirm the values for the specific activities claimed by the manufacturer. Resting total catecholamine concentration ($\mu g/l$ plasma) in human plasma samples obtained by this method was: male and female; norepinephrine 0.20 ± 0.08, epinephrine 0.05 ± 0.03; female, norepinephrine 0.21 ± 0.09, epinephrine 0.04 ± 0.03; and male, norepinephrine 0.20 ± 0.08, epinephrine 0.06 ± 0.04.

The other double isotope derivative dilution assay employed acetic-H^3 anhydride to form labeled derivatives (Franklin and Mayer, 1968). C^{14}-labeled tracer catecholamines were added to plasma or urine. Tracer and endogenous catecholamines were extracted by adsorption on alumina. They are then simultaneously acetylated and eluted from the alumina with acetic-H^3 anhydride. Carrier compounds were added and the derivative of each catecholamine was isolated by serial glass fiber-paper chromatography and gas-liquid chromatography. Determination of endogenous quantities was based on H^3/C^{14} ratios of the purified derivatives. The ratio was increased in proportion to the dilution of added tracer-C^{14} catecholamine by endogenous unlabeled compounds.

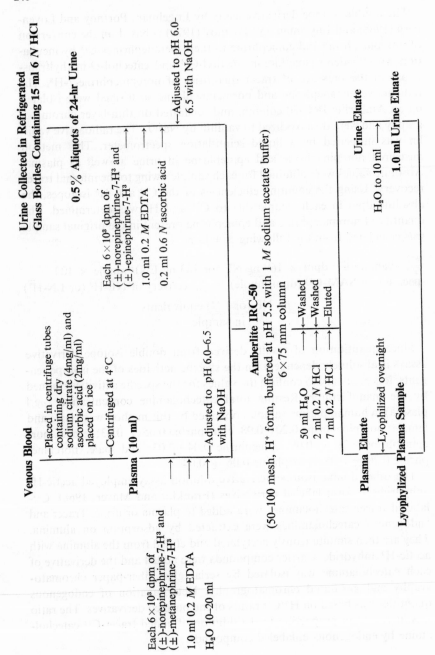

Venous Blood

← Placed in centrifuge tubes containing dry sodium citrate (4mg/ml) and ascorbic acid (2mg/ml) and placed on ice

← Centrifuged at 4°C

Plasma (10 ml)

Each 6 × 10³ dpm of
(±)-norepinephrine-7-H³ and
(±)-metanephrine-7-H³

1.0 ml 0.2 M EDTA

H₂O 10–20 ml

← Adjusted to pH 6.0–6.5 with NaOH

Urine Collected in Refrigerated Glass Bottles Containing 15 ml 6 N HCl

0.5% Aliquots of 24-hr Urine

Each 6 × 10³ dpm of
(±)-norepinephrine-7-H³ and
(±)-epinephrine-7-H³

1.0 ml 0.2 M EDTA

0.2 ml 0.6 N ascorbic acid

← Adjusted to pH 6.0–6.5 with NaOH

Amberlite IRC-50
(50–100 mesh, H⁺ form, buffered at pH 5.5 with 1 M sodium acetate buffer)
6 × 75 mm column

50 ml H₂O → Washed
2 ml 0.2 N HCl → Washed
7 ml 0.2 N HCl → Eluted

Plasma Eluate

← Lyophilized overnight

Lyophylized Plasma Sample

Urine Eluate

H₂O to 10 ml →

1.0 ml Urine Eluate

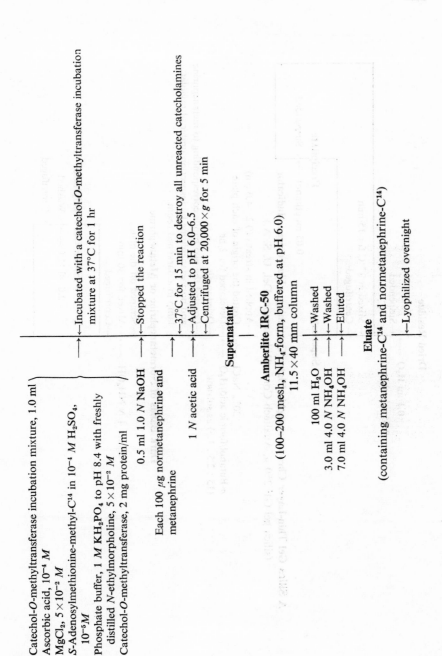

Catechol-O-methyltransferase incubation mixture, 1.0 ml
Ascorbic acid, 10^{-4} M
MgCl$_2$, 5×10^{-2} M
S-Adenosylmethionine-methyl-C^{14} in 10^{-1} M H$_2$SO$_4$, $10^{-5} M$
Phosphate buffer, 1 M KH$_2$PO$_4$ to pH 8.4 with freshly distilled N-ethylmorpholine, 5×10^{-2} M
Catechol-O-methyltransferase, 2 mg protein/ml

→ Incubated with a catechol-O-methyltransferase incubation mixture at 37°C for 1 hr

0.5 ml 1.0 N NaOH → Stopped the reaction

Each 100 μg normetanephrine and metanephrine

1 N acetic acid → 37°C for 15 min to destroy all unreacted catecholamines
→ Adjusted to pH 6.0–6.5
→ Centrifuged at $20,000 \times g$ for 5 min

Supernatant

Amberlite IRC-50
(100–200 mesh, NH$_4$-form, buffered at pH 6.0)
11.5×40 mm column

100 ml H$_2$O → Washed
3.0 ml 4.0 N NH$_4$OH → Washed
7.0 ml 4.0 N NH$_4$OH → Eluted

Eluate
(containing metanephrine-C^{14} and normetanephrine-C^{14})

→ Lyophilized overnight

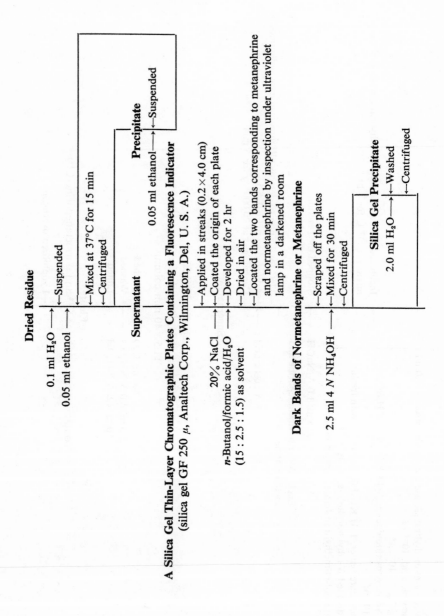

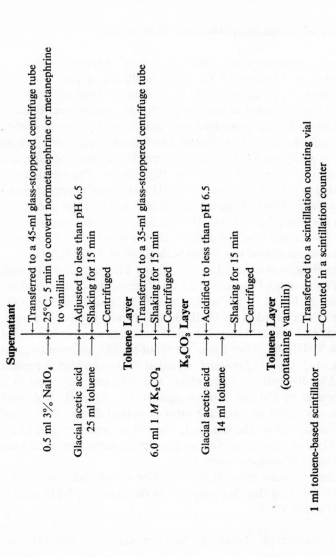

IV. 2.   Assay of Normetanephrine and Metanephrine

IV. 2. 1. SPECTROPHOTOMETRIC ASSAY OF NORMETANEPHRINE AND METANEPHRINE BY CONVERSION TO VANILLIN (Pisano, 1960)

Normetanephrine and metanephrine in urine were adsorbed on Amberlite CG-50, eluted and converted to vanillin which was assayed spectrophotometrically. The following procedure was developed by Pisano (1960).

The urine, collected in acid or toluene, was filtered if necessary. Ten ml was adjusted to pH 0.9 with 6 N HCl, transferred to a capped test tube, and placed in a boiling water bath for 20 min (hydrolysis). The solution was cooled, adjusted to pH 6.0–6.5 with 1 N NaOH and diluted to approximately 20 ml with water. The hydrolyzed sample (pH 6.0–6.5) was allowed to pass through the Amberlite CG-50, pH 6.0–6.5, 1 × 5 cm column at a rate of about 0.5 ml per min. The column was then washed with 15–20 ml of water and the metanephrine was eluted with 10 ml of 4 N NH₄OH.

The column eluate was adjusted to 10.0 ml and 2 aliquots of 4.0 ml each were taken. To one aliquot was added 0.1 ml of periodate solution (sodium metaperiodate, NaIO₄, 2 % in water, stored at 3°C) with mixing. To the other aliquot, which served as the blank, 0.1 ml of water in place of periodate was added. As a reagent blank, 0.1 ml of periodate solution was added to 4.0 ml of 4 N NH₄OH. After 1 min, 0.1 ml of bisulfite solution (sodium metabisulfite, Na₂S₂O₅, 10 % in water, stored at 3°C) was added to prevent the strong U.V. absorption of periodate. The solutions were read in a spectrophotometer at 350 and 360 nm against 4 N NH₄OH. A distinct vanillin peak was indicated when the ratio of optical density at 360 and 350 nm was the same as for the standard. The 360 nm reading was used for calculation. Material absorbing with an absorption maximum at 333 nm indicated evidence of contamination.

The excretions of metanephrines in normal or non-pheochromocytoma urines were 0.6 ± 0.3 mg/day. In pheochromocytoma urines, 3–113 mg/day is described (Pisano, 1960).

IV. 2. 2. FLUORESCENCE ASSAY OF NORMETANEPHRINE AND METANEPHRINE

A. *Principle*

Normetanephrine and metanephrine can be assayed fluorometrically by a reaction similar to the trihydroxyindole reaction. Their excitation and emission fluorescence spectra are identical with those of norepinephrine and epinephrine. It is generally assumed that normetanephrine and metanephrine are converted to noradrenolutine and adrenolutine after oxidative demethylation. The reaction was first demonstrated by Bertler, Carlsson and Rosengren (1958, 1959), and subsequently applied to the determination of normetanephrine in the brain (Carlsson and Lindqvist, 1962). The method was also adapted for the measurement of normetanephrine and metanephrine in urine (Häggendal, 1962; Smith and Weil-Malherbe, 1962; Brunjes, Wybenga and Johns, 1964; Taniguchi, Kakimoto and Armstrong, 1964). A detailed description on the comparison between these procedures was made by Weil-Malherbe and Smith (1966).

The following 5 steps were necessary in the fluorometric assay of normetanephrine and metanephrine (Weil-Malherbe and Smith, 1966).

1. *Removal of catecholamines* using alumina, decomposition in alkaline medium, or oxidation with ferricyanide.

2. *Isolation of normetanephrine and metanephrine* using Amberlite CG-50, Amberlite CG-120, or Dowex-50 columns. Normetanephrine and metanephrine could be fractionated with an Amberlite CG-50 column (Taniguchi, Kakimoto and Armstrong, 1964). A series of reciprocal solvent extractions could also isolate the metanephrines (Anton and Sayre, 1966).

3. *Oxidation* using $Fe(CN)_6^{+++}$ plus Zn^{++}, I_2, or KIO_4 often at different pH levels.

4. *Rearrangement to trihydroxyindoles* using alkaline ascorbate, or alkaline sulfite.

5. *Differential measurement of normetanephrine and metanephrine* by oxidation at different pH levels (Smith and Weil-Malherbe, 1962; Anton and Sayre, 1966), by differential spectrofluorimetry (Häggendal, 1962; Brunjes, Wybenga and Johns, 1964). or by chromatographic separation (Taniguchi, Kakimoto and Armstrong, 1964).

B. *The Smith and Weil-Malherbe method* (1962)

The method included hydrolysis of urine at pH 1.0–1.5 at 100°C for 15 min, an alumina column to remove catecholamines, electrodialysis, incubation with sulfatase at 37°C for 24 hr, isolation of normetanephrine and metanephrine with an Amberlite CG-50 column. Metanephrine alone was measured by oxidation at pH 3.0 by adding potassium ferricyanide and zinc sulfate. Metanephrine plus normetanephrine were measured by oxidation at pH 7.9 by adding iodine. The rat excreted primarily the glucuronide (Axelrod, Senoh and Witkop, 1958), while the main conjugate in the human being appeared to be the sulfate (Weil-Malherbe, 1960b). The combination of acid hydrolysis and incubation with sulfatase yielded results similar to those obtained with the sulfatase preparation alone, but the excess over the results of acid hydrolysis alone was statistically significant for both nor-metanephrine and metanephrine (Smith and Weil-Malherbe, 1962).

C. *The Anton and Sayre method* (1966)

A specific and sensitive method for the determination of metanephrine and normetanephrine in tissue, urine and plasma from man and laboratory animals was described by Anton and Sayre (1966). The amines were selectively extracted by the use of a particular combination of ions, organic solvents and pH and then converted to fluorescent derivatives by periodate oxidation. In this method, water redistilled four times in all glass stills was used. The second distillation was carried out in the presence of EDTA at about 1 g/l.

1. *Preparation of tissue and plasma samples.* Tissue (1.0 g) was homogenized in 3.0 ml of 1.0 N HCl in an ice bath. The homogenate was transferred to a 15-ml polypropylene tube and centrifuged at about 30,000 × g for 20 min in a refrigerated centrifuge. In the case of plasma, 4.0 ml were placed in a 15-ml polypropylene tube and adjusted to 1.0 N using concentrated HCl. The tube was capped, shaken for 5 min, and then centrifuged in the same way as for tissue homogenate. The supernatant was transferred to a 10-ml beaker containing 1.0 ml of 1 M Tris buffer and adjusted to pH 6.8 to 7.2 with 5.0 N and 1.0 N NaOH. Urine was collected in a receptacle containing about 10 ml of 5.0 N HCl per 24-hr sample. Three ml of urine was pipetted into a 10-ml beaker and adjusted to pH 0.90 with 5.0 N HCl. The pH-adjusted urine sample was transferred to a 15-ml round bottom, glass-stoppered centrifuge tube, capped with a marble and placed in a boiling water bath for 20 min. After cooling with running tap water, the sample was poured back into the same 10-ml beaker. One ml of 1 M Tris buffer was added and pH adjusted to 6.8 to 7.2 with HCl or NaOH, depending on the urine sample. The pH-adjusted urine sample was returned to the same glass-stoppered centrifuge tube, and extracted with 5.0 ml of isoamyl alcohol for 3 min. The mixture was centrifuged in a clinical centrifuge for 5 min. The organic phase and all of the thin, pigmented precipitate which had formed between the aqueous and organic phases were removed by aspiration.

2. *Purification of normetanephrine and metanephrine from urine, plasma and tissue samples.* The treated tissue, plasma and urine samples (about 4.0–4.5 ml) were transferred to 50-ml polypropylene centrifuge tubes and 1 ml of borate buffer (1.0 M, pH 10.0; 30.92 g of boric acid was dissolved in 450 ml of water and the pH was adjusted to 10.0 with pellets and 5 N NaOH. The solution was saturated with NaCl and n-butanol, and read-

justed to pH 10.0, made up to 500 ml, and filtered through two sheets of Whatman No. 1 paper) was added. After mixing well, 7.0 ($\pm$ 5 %) g of K_2HPO_4 powder was added. The solution was mixed well to saturate the sample and 15 ml of ether was added. The tube was capped with a tightly fitting plastic cap, then the solution was shaken for 10 min and centrifuged at top speed in a clinical centrifuge for 4 min. The ether layer was transferred to a 40-ml glass-stoppered centrifuge tube containing 4.0 ml of 0.1 N HCl and the solution was shaken for 10 min and centrifuged in a clinical centrifuge for 2 min. The ether layer was discarded. The acid phase was transferred to a 50-ml polypropylene centrifuge tube and 1 ml of the borate buffer was added. After mixing well, 9.0 ($\pm 2\%$) of K_2HPO_4 powder was added. The solution was mixed well for about 20 sec to saturate the solution and 15 ml of ether was added. The tube was capped with a tightly fitting plastic cap and the solution was shaken for 10 min and centrifuged at top speed in a clinical centrifuge for 4 min. The ether layer was transferred to a 40-ml glass-stoppered centrifuge tube containing 1.5 ml of 0.01 N HCl and the solution was shaken for 10 min and centrifuged in a clinical centrifuge. The ether layer was discarded after which the acid phase was transferred to a small test tube.

3. *Fluorophor formation.* To a 0.20-ml aliquot of the acid extract in a small test tube, 0.20 ml of distilled water, 0.10 ml of EDTA (disodium, dihydrate, 50 mg/ml) and 0.05 ml of citric acid-sodium acetate buffer, 0.80 M, pH 5.0 (high pH) (adjust a 2.0 M citric acid solution to pH 5.0 with 2.0 M solution of sodium acetate and then dilute with distilled water to 0.80 M), or citric acid solution, 0.85 M (low pH) were added. Following this, 0.05 ml of the periodate solution ($NaIO_4$, 20 mg/ml) was added. The solution was mixed thoroughly and allowed to stand for exactly 4 min and 0.10 ml of the sulfite solution (Na_2SO_3 anhydrous powder, 100 mg/ml) and 0.30 ml of the alkaline ascorbate reagent (dissolve 10 mg of ascorbic acid in 0.10 ml of distilled water, add 10.0 ml of 10.0 N NaOH and mix throughly) were added quickly. The solution was mixed thoroughly. The solution (total volume, 1.0 ml) was transferred to a quartz cuvette. An Aminco-Bowman spectrophotofluorometer with slit arrangement No. 5 and the RCA IP-28 photomultiplier tube were used to measure relative fluorescence, at 409 nm activation and 519 nm fluorescence for normetanephrine plus metanephrine with the high pH sample and at 422 nm and 531 nm for metanephrine with the low pH sample. The readings were taken within 15 min.

Blanks were prepared by following the same procedure, except that the periodate was replaced by 0.05 ml of water.

External standards of normetanephrine and metanephrine were determined by taking 1.064 μg of normetanephrine/ml in a cuvette to produce a net fluorescence of 100 at a high pH (the blank, 0.20) and 3.5 at low pH; and 0.71 μg of metanephrine/ml in a cuvette to produce a net fluorescence of 107 at high pH and 100 at low pH (the blank, 0.20).

An internal standard containing both normetanephrine and metanephrine was included with each series, and the results were corrected for an average recovery of 50 %.

IV. 3.   Assay of 3-Methoxytyramine (3-*O*-Methyl Dopamine)

3-Methoxytyramine was first identified by paper chromatography in the urine from rats given intraperitoneal injection of dopamine (Axelrod, Senoh and Witkop, 1958). It was also found by fluorometric methods to be present in brain homogenates of various mammals (Carlsson and Waldeck, 1964). In the fluorometric method described here 3-methoxytyramine, normetanephrine, and metanephrine together with dopamine, norepinephrine and epinephrine, can be assayed in the same brain sample (Crawford and Yates, 1970). This method is based on the acetylation of catecholamines and 3-*O*-methylcatecholamines and subsequent isolation of the acetylated amines by paper chromatography (Laverty and Sharman, 1965). The brain tissue was homogenized in perchloric acid which was removed as an insoluble potassium salt. The acid metabolites of the amines were extracted from the acidified extract with ethyl acetate. After extraction, the aqueous extract was treated with acetic anhydride and sodium hydrogen carbonate and the acetylated derivatives of the amines were extracted with dichloromethane. The dichloromethane extract containing the acetylated amines was chromatographed on paper in the organic phase of a mixture of toluene/ethyl acetate/methanol/water (10/1/5/5). The acetylated amines were eluted and estimated fluorometrically. 3-Methoxytyramine, norepinephrine, dopamine and normetanephrine in rat brain as μg/g tissue were: 0.06; 0.17; 0.70; and 0.02, respectively. Epinephrine and metanephrine were not detected in rat brain.

A fluorometric assay of free 3-methoxytyramine in human urine was reported by Käser (1970). To 20 ml of a 24-hr urine specimen, 1 ml of 0.2 *M* EDTA solution, 0.25 ml of a 2 % ascorbic acid solution and 1 ml of 0.1 *M* phosphate buffer, pH 6.5 were added. After titration to pH 6.5, the urine was passed at 25°C through a thermostatized column containing Dowex AG 50-W-X8, 200–400 mesh, in Na form (0.4 × 3.5 cm). The column adsorbed the catecholamines and their methoxy derivatives were washed with a mixture of 10 ml phosphate buffer, 1 ml ascorbic acid solution, and 40 ml water. Norepinephrine and epinephrine were eluted with 7 ml of 1 N HCl (flow rate 7–9 drops/min). Dopamine and 3-methoxy-tyramine were eluted with 25 ml of 5 N HCl at the same flow-rate. To 5 ml of this fraction, 3 ml of 0.5 M citrate-boric acid buffer, pH 6.5 and 3 ml of 10 N NaOH were added. By heating this alkaline solution at 50°C for 20 min dopamine but not 3-methoxytyramine was destroyed. The same solution was then adjusted to pH 6.5 with HCl. Each 3 ml of the solution was put into 2 tubes (sample and blank). To the sample tube, 0.5 ml of saturated NaCl solution and 0.2 ml of 0.02 N iodine solution (oxidation) were added. To the blank tube, 0.5 ml of NaCl solution and 0.45 ml of 5 N NaOH were added. After 4 min of oxidation, 0.5 ml of alkaline sulfite solution (dissolve 5.04 g $Na_2SO_3 \cdot 7H_2O$ in 10 ml water and dilute with 5 N NaOH to 100 ml) was added to the sample tube (Carlsson and Waldeck, 1958). After 5 min, 1.0 ml of 5 N HCl was added. The solution was heated at 80°C for 30 min. At this stage, 0.05 ml of 2 M Na_2SO_3 solution, 1.0 ml of 5 N HCl and 0.2 ml of 0.02 N iodine solution were added to the blank tube. The fluorescence was read at 330 nm activation 385 nm fluorescence. An internal standard of 3-methoxytyramine was carried through the entire procedure and used for the calculation. Urinary excretion of free 3-methoxytyramine by this method was: children (2–13 years), 37.0 μg/24 hr, 0.10 μg/mg creatinine, and adults (25–102 years), 88.4 μg/24 hr, 0.067 μg/mg creatinine.

IV. 4. Assay of 3-Methoxy-4-hydroxymandelic Acid (Vanillylmandelic Acid, Vanilmandelic Acid, VMA)

Since vanillylmandelic acid in urine is a main metabolite of catecholamines and a valuable diagnostic tool for pheochromocytoma, various procedures have been developed for its measurement. A detailed review of the assay procedures was described by Sandler and Ruthven (1966).

The following procedures were used for quantitative and qualitative determination of vanillylmandelic acid.

1) Paper chromatography
2) High-voltage paper electrophoresis
3) Thin-layer chromatography
4) Spectrophotometry
5) Gas chromatography

IV. 4. 1. PAPER CHROMATOGRAPHY AND HIGH-VOLTAGE ELECTRO-
PHORESIS OF VANILLYLMANDELIC ACID

Paper chromatography was first introduced for the isolation and identification of vanillylmandelic acid by Armstrong, Shaw and Wall (1956). One-
dimensional or two-dimensional paper chromatography was extensively
used for the identification of the compound, especially in the urine samples
of pheochromocytoma patients (Robinson, Ratcliffe and Smith, 1959;
Gitlow, Mendlowitz, Khassis, Cohen and Sha, 1960; Jacobs, Sobel and
Henry, 1961; Gödicke and Brosowski, 1964; Coward and Smith, 1966). An
isopropanol/ammonia/water (20/1/2) system was generally used as a first
solvent, and a benzene/propionic acid/water (2/2/1) as a second solvent.

The qualitative and quantitative determination of vanillylmandelic acid
by paper chromatography was also valuable for the diagnosis of neuroblastoma (Gitlow, Bertani, Rausen, Gribetz and Dziedzic, 1970).

The two-dimensional paper chromatographic method (Armstrong,
Shaw and Wall, 1956; Kakimoto and Armstrong, 1962) has been used in
the extensive investigations of functional neural crest tumors by Gjessing
(1968).

High-voltage paper electrophoresis was also valuable for the separation
of normetanephrine, metanephrine and vanillylmandelic acid (Yoshinaga,
Itoh, Ishida, Sato and Wada, 1961).

Paper chromatographic identification of vanillylmandelic acid, normetanephrine and metanephrine in urine has been widely used for the diagnosis of pheochromocytoma. However, for the purpose of screening, even
the development of the paper chromatogram was not necessary. Sato,
Yoshinaga, Ishida, Itoh and Wada (1961, 1962) developed a simple and
rapid screening method of pheochromocytoma (urine, one-drop test) based
on the semi-quantitative identification of the vanillylmandelic acid and
other diazo-reacting catecholamine metabolites in urine by the intensity
of a color reaction with one drop of urine sample on a sheet of filter paper.
Three kinds of stock reagents which should be stored in a refrigerator were
used: reagent 1, 0.1 g of p-nitroaniline dissolved in 2 ml of concentrated
HCl and water added to 100 ml; reagent 2, 0.2 % sodium nitrite; reagent
3, 10 % potassium carbonate. Diazotised p-nitroaniline reagent was prepared by mixing reagent 1, 2 and 3 (1/1/2) in this order just prior to using.
One drop of urine was applied to a sheet of filter paper and dried. The
reagent was sprayed on the paper within 120 sec after mixing. Normal urine
showed a faint orange yellow color, whereas pheochromocytoma urine
showed a distinct purple color.

IV. 4. 2. THIN-LAYER CHROMATOGRAPHY OF VANILLYLMANDELIC ACID

Thin-layer chromatography is a more rapid and sensitive procedure for the identification of vanillylmandelic acids and other catecholamine metabolites, and is especially useful for clinical diagnosis (Zöllner and Wolfram, 1969). Vanillylmandelic acid (Schmid, Zicha, Krautheim and Blumberg, 1962; Schmid and Henning, 1963; Annino, Lipson and Williams, 1964) and homovanillic acid (Sankoff and Sourkes, 1963) were assayed with silica gel as a support. An isopropanol/ethyl acetate/ammonia/water (45/30/17/8) system was used for development, and Gibbs' reagent for location. Using an isobutanol/acetic acid/ cyclohexane (80/7/10) mixture as a solvent, catecholamines, vanillylmandelic acid, and homovanillic acid were completely separated (Segura-Cardona and Soehring, 1964).

Tautz, Voltmer and Schmid (1965) described a procedure for the assay of vanillylmandelic acid, homovanillic acid, and vanillic acid by thin-layer chromatography. Ten to twenty ml of 24-hr urine was adjusted to pH 0 with concentrated HCl, saturated with NaCl and extracted with three 50 ml portions of ether. The ether extract was evaporated to dryness, and the residue dissolved in 1 ml of ethanol. A 0.1 ml sample of the ethanol solution was applied to a thin-layer plate. Thin-layer adsorbent was prepared with 25 g silica gel G, 25 g kieselguhr G, 2.5 g fluorescent pigment ZS super, and 90 ml water. The layer thickness was 250 μm, and the layer was dried at 105°C for 1 hr. Development was carried out by means of chamber saturation with isopropanol/ethyl acetate/ammonia/water (45/30/17/8) to a height of 8 cm. The layer was dried and twice developed with benzene/acetic acid (90/10) in 15 cm runs. The substances were identified under short-wave UV light (254 nm) through their fluorescence quenching. The corresponding zones were scrapped off and eluted with 2.5 ml of alkalised methanol solution (2 % aqueous Na_2CO_3/methanol, 1/3). After centrifuging at 5°C, 2 ml of the supernatant liquid was mixed with 0.2 ml of freshly prepared diazotised Rose reagent (0.25 % p-aminophenyl-β-diethylaminoethyl sulfone in 1% HCl / 0.5% aqueous $NaNO_2$ solution, 3/1, mixed at 0°C immediately before use and kept in the dark) and left for 30–60 min. The absorbance was measured at 490 nm for vanillylmandelic acid and vanillic acid, and at 370 nm for homovanillic acid. Standards as well as reagent and adsorbent blanks were subjected to the same procedure. The limit of detection was about 0.05 μg/ml.

IV. 4. 3. SPECTROPHOTOMETRY OF VANILLYLMANDELIC ACID

Two kinds of simple and rapid spectrophotometric assays are described by Sandler and Ruthven (1961) and Pisano, Crout and Abraham (1962). Vanillylmandelic acid was extracted from urine, converted to vanillin, and subsequently assayed spectrophotometrically. These two methods were extremely useful for the diagnosis of catecholamine-secreting tumours.

Vanillylmandelic acid   Vanillin

A.   *The Sandler and Ruthven method* (1961)

Vanillylmandelic acid was isolated from urine on a Dowex-AG-X2 column, eluted with acetate buffer, acidified, and extracted with ethyl acetate. The ethyl acetate was removed and the vanillylmandelic acid converted to vanillin by autoclaving with sulfuric acid and alumina for 1 hr. After centrifugation, the absorbance of vanillin in the supernatant was measured at 365 and 380 nm both before and after the addition of sodium borohydride, and compared to standards carried through the same procedure. This method was further improved by Miyake, Yoshida and Imaizumi (1962).

B.   *The Pisano, Crout and Abraham method* (1962)

Vanillylmandelic acid was extracted with ethyl acetate from acidified salt-saturated urine, reextracted with potassium carbonate, and oxidized to vanillin with periodate at 50°C for 1 hr. The vanillin was extracted from the mixture with toluene and reextracted into potassium carbonate. Its absorbance was measured at 360 nm. This procedure was simple and most widely used for the assay of vanillylmandelic acid.

A 24-hr urine specimen was collected in a bottle containing 10 ml of 6 N hydrochloric acid and was stored at 3°C. An aliquot equivalent to 0.2 % of the 24-hr volume was placed in a 50-ml glass-stoppered extraction tube, diluted to 5.5 ml with water, and further acidified with 0.5 ml of 6 N HCl. A saturating amount of NaCl (about 3 g) and 30 ml of ethyl acetate were added, and the mixture was placed for 5 min on a mechanical shaker to extract the phenolic acids. After centrifugation, 25 ml of the ethyl acetate layer was transferred to a second extraction tube and the phenolic acids were returned to 1.5 ml of 1 M potassium carbonate by shaking for 3 min. The mixture was centrifuged and 1.0 ml of the carbonate layer was transferred to a third extraction tube. After the addition of 0.1 ml of periodate solution (sodium metaperiodate, $NaIO_4$, 2 % in water), the tube was placed in a 50°C water bath for 30 min to convert vanillylmandelic acid to vanillin. The tube was cooled, and 0.1 ml of bisulfite solution (sodium metabisulfite, Na₂S₂O₅, 10 % in water) was added to reduce residual periodate. The sample was then neutralized with 0.3 ml of 5 N acetic acid and 0.6 ml of 3.0 M potassium phosphate buffer, pH 7.5. Vanillin was extracted from this solution by shaking for 3 min with 20 ml of toluene. After centrifugation, 15 ml of the toluene layer was transferred to a forth extraction tube and the vanillin was recovered by shaking for 3 min with 1 M potassium carbonate. For patients with pheochromocytoma it was convenient to use 4.0 ml of 1 M potassium carbonate for this final step; for normal patients, 1.5 ml was used. The mixture was centrifuged and the carbonate layer, containing vanillin, was transferred to a microcuvette. The absorbance was determined at 360 nm against a reagent blank which was prepared by substituting water for urine. The absorbance of vanillin solution was directly proportional to concentration in the range of 10–100 μg per sample carried through the entire procedure with 1.5 ml carbonate for the final extraction. The overall recovery was about 85 % (after correction for aliquots was made). Urine blanks were prepared by treating urine aliquots exactly as described except that the incubation at 50°C was done without periodate. The preparation of urine blanks is advisable for precise studies, but for other purposes the extra tube may not be needed. Vanillylmandelic acid, 10 mg/ml of 0.01 N HCl, was used as the stock solution. A 40 μg/sample was adequate as an internal standard. Dietary vanillin did not affect the vanillylmandelic method of Pisano, Crout and Abraham (1962) (Green and Walker, 1970). A modification of this method was described by Wisser and Stamm (1970).

C. *The Rosano method* (1964)
A specific method in which vanillylmandelic acid is enzymatically oxidized with the aid of a L-mandelic acid dehydrogenase from specially adapted cells of Pseudomonas fluorescence, was reported.

IV. 4. 4. GAS CHROMATOGRAPHY OF VANILLYLMANDELIC ACID
Gas chromatography seems to be highly sensitive and useful for the assay of catecholamine metabolites, including vanillylmandelic acid (Wilk, Gitlow, Mendlowitz, Franklin, Carr and Clarke, 1965; Karoum, Anah, Ruthven and Sandler, 1969). Pentafluoropropionates and heptafluorobutyrates of normetanephrine, metanephrine, 3-methoxytyramine, 3-methoxy-4-hydroxyphenylethylene glycol, vanillylmandelic acid, and homovanillic acid can be examined by gas chromatography along with electron capture detection and mass spectrometry (Änggård and Sedvall, 1969).

A selective and sensitive method for the determination of vanillylmandelic acid in urine was established by Imai and Tamura (1970). The method consisted of the separation of vanillylmandelic acid by adsorption on Amberlite XAD-2 from urine at pH 1 and gas chromatography of vanillylmandelic acid after methylation in ethanol in a short period and trifluoroacetylation. An aliquot of urine was acidified to pH 2 with 1 N HCl and diluted to 10 volumes with water. Five ml of the solution was passed through an SE-Sephadex column (1.5 ml, H^+ form) to remove the urinary pigments and the column was washed with 4 ml of water. The effluent and the washings were combined and, after adjustment to its pH to 1 with 1 N HCl, passed through an Amberlite XAD-2 column (2 ml, 200–400 mesh, conditioned with 0.1 N HCl), which was washed with 2 ml of 0.1 N HCl. The adsorbed vanillylmandelic acid was eluted with 4 ml of water and the successive 2 ml of 10 % methanol in water. An aliquot of the combined eluate was concentrated under reduced pressure and dried over calcium chloride for 5 min *in vacuo* at room temperature. The residue was dissolved in 0.5 ml of ethanol, and one drop of freshly prepared ethereal diazomethane (28 mg of diazomethane per ml of ether) was added. After 10 sec, the reaction was stopped by adding a few drops of 0.1 N acetic acid. Following this 0.1 ml of tyramine solution in 0.1 N acetic acid (containing 0.723 μg of tyramine hydrochloride) was added to the mixture. The solution was evaporated to dryness under reduced pressure and dried over calcium chloride for 5 min. The residue was trifluoroacetylated with one drop of ethyl acetate and 10 μl of trifluoroacetic anhydride for 5 min, then diluted with 0.5 ml of n-hexane. One μl of the solution was injected to a gas chromatograph equipped with electron capture detector (Shimadzu GC 4APE gas chromatograph, 1.4 m glass column packed with 2 % GE-XF 1105 on Gas Chrom P, column temperature, 120°C). The peak height ratio of vanillylmandelic acid : tyramine (internal standard) was shown to be completely linear to the concentration of vanillylmandelic acid (0–5 $\times$ 0.307 μg).

IV. 5. Assay of 3-Methoxy-4-hydroxyphenylacetic Acid (Homovanillic Acid, HVA) and 3-Methoxy-4-hydroxybenzoic Acid (Vanillic Acid)

3-Methoxy-4-hydroxyphenylacetic acid (homovanillic acid) is the principal urinary metabolite of dopamine and DOPA (Shaw, McMillan and Armstrong, 1957; Goldstein, Friedhoff and Simmons, 1959). The excretion was elevated in the urine of patients with neuroblastoma and malignant pheochromocytoma.

The following procedures were used for the assay of homovanillic acid.

1) Paper chromatography (Armstrong, Shaw and Wall, 1956)
2) Thin-layer chromatography (Sankoff and Sourkes, 1963)
3) High-voltage paper electrophoresis (Studnitz, 1962)
4) Spectrophotometry (Ruthven and Sandler, 1964)
5) Spectrofluorometry (Andén, Ross and Werdinius, 1963; Sharman, 1963; Sato, 1965)
6) Gas chromatography (Williams and Greer, 1962; Karoum, Anah, Ruthven and Sandler, 1969; Änggård and Sedvall, 1969)

Two-dimensional paper chromatography was carried out by using benzene/propionic acid/water (2/2/1) and isopropyl alcohol/ammonia/water (8/1/1) as the first and second solvents. This method was successfully applied to the assay of 3-methoxy-4-hydroxyphenyllactic acid (vanyllactic acid) (Gjessing, 1963a,b).

Thin-layer chromatography was useful for the assay of homovanillic acid, together with vanillylmandelic acid and vanillic acid (Tautz, Voltmer and Schmid, 1965).

The colorimetric method was used for the assay of homovanillic acid in urine (Ruthven and Sandler, 1962).

The most sensitive method is the fluorescence assay and the method by Sato (1965) is simple and specific. Homovanillic acid was adsorbed on Dowex AG-1 (Cl form), eluted, and extracted. The acid was oxidized by potassium ferricyanide in alkali to give the fluorescence product, which was then measured. A 24-hr urine specimen was collected in a bottle containing 10 ml of 6 N HCl and stored at 3°C. One ml of urine was adjusted to pH 4.5 by dropwise addition of 1 N NaOH and using a pH paper and mixed thoroughly with 1 ml of 1 M acetate buffer, pH 4.5. This was applied to a Dowex-1 X4 (chloride form) column (0.6 × 3.0 cm) at a rate of about 0.6 ml per min. The column was then washed with 3 ml of water and eluted with 18 ml of 1.5 M NaCl into a 50 ml glass-stoppered extraction tube. The eluate was acidified with 2 ml of 1 N HCl. A saturating amount of solid NaCl and 20 ml of dichloroethane were added, and the homovanillic acid was extracted for 5 min in a mechanical shaker. After centrifugation, 18 ml of the organic layer was transferred to a second extraction tube. The original sample was then extracted again with 20 ml of the solvent, and the two extracts were combined. The homovanillic acid was returned to 4 ml of 0.05 M Tris buffer, pH 8.5 by shaking for 5 min. The mixture was centrifuged and the organic layer discarded. One ml of the final extract was placed in a test tube for the formation of the fluorophore, while a second

1-ml portion served as a sample blank. To the test sample 1 ml of 5 N ammonia and 0.2 ml of 0.01% potassium ferricyanide was added. After 4 min, 0.2 ml of 0.1% L-cysteine solution was added to stop the reaction. The sample blank was made in the same way as the test sample except that the sequence of the addition of cysteine and potassium ferricyanide was reversed. The fluorescence was measured at 320 nm (activation)/420 nm (fluorescence). The calculation was based on the use of known amounts of an internal standard (5 or 10 μg homovanillic acid added to an aliquot of urine). The urinary excretion of homovanillic acid by this method was 5.4 $\pm$ 1.4 (3.7 − 7.5) mg/day.

3-Methoxy-4-hydroxybenzoic acid (vanillic acid) was found in human urine following an intravenous infusion of norepinephrine-2-C[14] (Goodall, Kirshner and Rosen, 1959). The vanillic acid was isolated and identified by ion exchange and paper chromatography.

IV. 6.   Assay of 3,4-Dihydroxymandelic Acid (DOMA) and 3,4-Dihydroxyphenylacetic Acid (DOPAC)

3,4-Dihydroxymandelic acid (DOMA) and 3,4-dihydroxyphenylacetic acid (DOPAC) are formed from epinephrine or norepinephrine and dopamine by the successive action of monoamine oxidase and aldehyde dehydrogenase.

DOMA   DOPAC

The following principles were applied to the determination of these two acids. 1) Conversion of DOMA to protocatechuic aldehyde (Miyake, Yoshida and Imaizumi, 1962; DeQuattro, Wybenga, Studnitz and Brunjes, 1964; Weil-Malherbe and Smith, 1966); 2) Condensation with ethylenediamine (DOMA : Wada, 1963; DOMA and DOPAC : Drujan, Alvarez and Díaz Borges, 1966; DOPAC : Murphy, Robinson and Sharman, 1969); 3) Enzymatic radioassay (conversion of DOMA to vanillylmandelic acid-C[14] by incubation with S-adenosyl-methionine (methyl-C[14]) and catechol-O-methyltransferase) (Sato and DeQuattro, 1969).

IV. 6. 1. SPECTROPHOTOMETRIC ASSAY OF DOMA BASED ON THE CONVERSION OF DOMA TO PROTOCATECHUIC ALDEHYDE

DOMA   Protocatechuic aldehyde

Miyake, Yoshida and Imaizumi (1962) described an assay procedure of DOMA by the conversion reaction of DOMA to protocatechuic aldehyde analogous to the oxidation of vanillylmandelic acid to vanillin. Conversion was carried out by heating at 100°C in 10 M acetic acid. The mean value by this method was 720 $\pm$ 320 μg/24-hr urine.

DeQuattro, Wybenga, Studnitz and Brunjes (1964) described a method in which DOMA was oxidized by shaking an ethyl acetate extract containing the acid with 4 N ammonia for 3 min.

Weil-Malherbe made a precise examination of the reaction condition of the oxidation of DOMA to protocatechuic aldehyde and found that it depends on the presence of traces of heavy metals, particularly copper. In the presence of cupric ions the reaction rate increased, however, DOPAC formed the same product although at a slower rate (Weil-Malherbe, 1964b; Weil-Malherbe and Smith, 1966). The problem of oxidizing DOMA to protocatechuic aldehyde without interference from DOPAC was solved by an enzymatic method using a L-mandelic acid dehydrogenase from specially adapted cells of Pseudomonas fluorescence. Vanillylmandelic acid and p-hydroxymandelic acid which interfered with the assay were separated by the preliminary adsorption of DOMA on alumina (Weil-Malherbe, 1967). The urinary excretion of DOMA was 98 μg/24-hr.

These spectrophotometric assays are convenient for the assay of DOMA in urine.

IV. 6. 2. FLUOROMETRIC ASSAY OF DOMA AND DOPAC BASED ON THEIR CONDENSATION WITH ETHYLENEDIAMINE

DOPAC and DOMA produces fluorescent condensates with ethylenediamine. The ethylenediamine condensate of DOMA is identical with that of norepinephrine.

Drujan, Alvarez and Díaz Borges (1966) described a method for determination of DOMA and DOPAC. DOMA and DOPAC was extracted from acidified urine with ethyl acetate, and subjected to paper electrophoresis. Areas of the sample strips corresponding to DOMA and DOPAC were cut out and extracted with 0.01 N HCl. Ethylenediamine was added to the extract, and the solution heated at 60°C for 30 min to produce ethylenediamine condensates of DOMA and DOPAC. The reaction mixture was saturated with NaCl and extracted with n-butanol. The organic phase was used for DOMA determination and the aqueous phase for DOPAC determination. The fluorescence intensity was measured at 425 nm/490 nm for DOMA and 420 nm/540 nm for DOPAC (activation/emission). The following mean values were obtained : for DOMA 920 μg $\pm$ 310 (S.D.)/24-hr urine; and for DOPAC 1200 μg $\pm$ 420 (S.D.)/24-hr urine.

DOPAC in the brain was determined by the ethylenediamine method (Murphy, Robinson and Sharman, 1969). A value, 0.17 $\pm$ 0.01 μg/g in the anterior part of the nucleus basalis of pigeon brain was reported (Ahtee, Sharman and Vogt, 1970).

IV. 6. 3. ENZYMATIC RADIOASSAY OF DOMA (Sato and DeQuattro, 1969)

Sato and DeQuattro (1969) developed a sensitive and specific assay for DOMA in human urine, plasma, and tissues. DOMA was isolated by alumina and extracted with ethyl acetate. The extract was incubated with S-adenosyl-L-methionine (methyl-C^{14}) and catechol-O-methyltransferase. The vanillylmandelic acid-C^{14} formed from DOMA was oxidized to vanillin-C^{14} with periodate, and the latter compound counted in a scintillation spectrometer. The internal standard of DOMA was subjected to the entire procedure and served for the calculation. Normal urinary excretion of DOMA by this method was : 3.8 $\pm$ 2.0 (S.E.M.) (1.5–7.4) μg/hr or 91 μg/ 24 hr. The concentration of DOMA in normal adult plasma was : 1.4 $\pm$ 0.2 (S.E.M.) (0.8 − 3.2) μg/l.

IV. 7.   Assay of Alcoholic Metabolites of Catecholamines:
3-methoxy-4-hydroxyphenylglycol (MHPG, or 3-methoxy-4-hydroxyphenylethyleneglycol, MOPEG), 3,4-dihydroxyphenylglycol (DHPG, or 3,4-dihydroxyphenylethyleneglycol, DOPEG), and 3-methoxy-4-hydroxyphenylethanol (MHPE)

These alcoholic metabolites of catecholamines are formed by the successive action of monoamine oxidase and alcohol dehydrogenase on catecholamines or 3-O-methylcatecholamines.

OH OH OH

MHPG (MOPEG)   DHPG (DOPEG)   MHPE

3-Methoxy-4-hydroxyphenylglycol was first discovered as its sulfate conjugate in rat urine (Axelrod, Kopin and Mann, 1959). The glucuronic acid conjugate of 3-methoxy-4-hydroxyphenylglycol was isolated from human urine. This compound is a metabolite of 3-methoxy-4-hydroxyphenylglycol-H[3] and norepinephrine-C[14] (Shimizu and LaBrosse, 1969). A separate spectrophotometric determination of 3-methoxy-4-hydroxyphenylglycol and 3-methoxy-4-hydroxymandelic acid with the same sample of urine was described by Ceasar, Ruthven and Sandler (1969). 3-Methoxy-4-hydroxyphenylglycol was separated from the latter compound with an anion exchange resin, AG1-X2, extracted into ethyl acetate, and finally converted to vanillin. The formed vanillin was measured spectrophotometrically. The glycol metabolites of norepinephrine and epinephrine in tissues and urine were measured by gas chromatography (Karoum, Anah, Ruthven and Sandler, 1969; Änggård and Sedvall, 1969; Sharman, 1969). Trimethylsilyl ether/ester derivatives prepared from ethyl acetate or dichloromethane extract of hydrolyzed urine were measured by the use of argon ionisation detector. The normal urinary output of 3-methoxy-4-hydroxyphenylglycol was 2.4 ± 0.8 mg/24 hr (Karoum, Anah, Ruthven and Sandler, 1969).

Pentafluoropropionate and heptafluorobutyrate derivatives were stable and had higher responses for electron capture detection and mass spectrometry (Änggård and Sedvall, 1969). The formation of acetyl-heptafluorobutyryl derivatives of MHPG or DHPG (Fig. 32) and a subsequent gas chromatographic assay using electron capture detection was successfully applied to the detection and estimation of free MHPG and DHPG in hypothalamic brain tissue by Sharman (1969).

IV. 8.   Assay of Tyramine

Tyramine was reported to be present in various tissues (Spector, Melmon, Lovenberg and Sjoerdsma, 1963). It was extracted with ether and reextracted with dilute HCl. Tyramine in the extract was assayed fluorometrically by reaction with 1-nitro-2-naphthol (Waalkes and Udenfriend, 1957; Spector, Melmon, Lovenberg and Sjoerdsma, 1963).

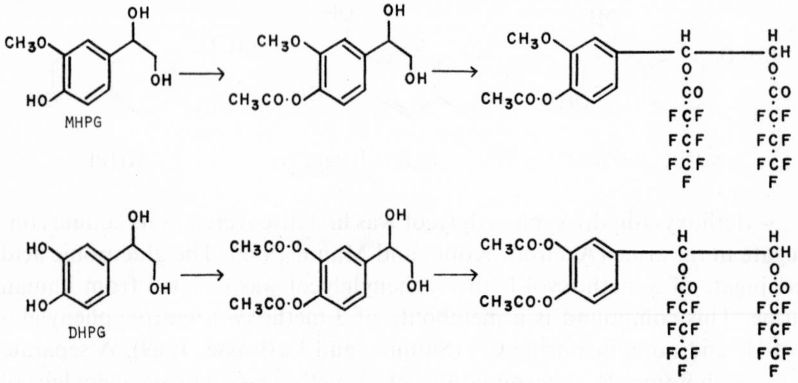

Fig. 32. Formation of acetyl-heptafluorobutyryl derivatives of 3-methoxy-4-hydroxyphenylglycol (MHPG) and 3,4-dihydroxyphenylglycol (DHPG) (Sharman, 1969).

Tissues were weighed and homogenized in 3 volumes of cold 0.01 N HCl. An aliquot of the homogenate containing 0.5 g of tissue was transferred to a 60-ml glass-stoppered bottle containing 1 g solid NaCl. The pH was adjusted to 10.5 by addition of small amounts of anhydrous sodium carbonate and a few drops of 1 N NaOH. Four ml of salt-saturated 0.5 M borate buffer, pH 10.5 and 30 ml of ether were added to each aliquot and the mixture shaken for 10 min. After centrifugation, 25 ml of the organic phase was transferred to a second 60-ml bottle. The alkaline homogenate was again shaken with ether (15 ml) for 10 min and centrifuged. Ten ml of the ether phase was removed and pooled with the first portion. The organic phase was then shaken for about 5 min with 3 ml of ether-equilibrated 0.01 N HCl. After centrifugation and removal of the organic phase, tyramine in the aqueous phase was assayed fluorometrically by the method of Waalkes and Udenfriend (1957). To a 2-ml aliquot of the acid extract, 1 ml 1-nitroso-2-naphthol reagent (0.1 % 1-nitroso-2-naphthol in 95 % ethanol) and 1 ml of nitric acid reagent (24.5 ml of 1 : 5 nitric acid is mixed with 0.5 ml of 2.5 % NaNO$_2$) were added. The mixture was heated for 30 min at 55°C. The mixture was allowed to cool for 10 min and shaken with 5 ml of ethylene dichloride to remove excess reagent. Two ml of the aqueous phase was transferred to a cuvette and the fluorescence was measured in a spectrophotofluorometer at 465 nm/565 nm (activation/emission). Tissue blanks were prepared by first heating the acid extract with the nitric acid reagent at 55°C for 30 min, cooling and then adding 1-nitroso-2-naphthol reagent.

The mixture was then incubated again at 55°C for 30 min and shaken with ethylene dichloride as described above.

Tyramine was identified by paper chromatography, gas chromatography and enzymatic methods. Using this method, 1–6 μg/g of tyramine was found in various parts of the brain of rat, rabbit and dog (Spector, Melmon, Lovenberg and Sjoerdsma, 1963).

Gunne and Jonsson (1965) measured the amounts of tyramine in rabbit brain after chromatographic separation on an Amberlite CG-120 (100 × 4 mm) column. Tyramine concentration by this method was very low, below 10 ng/g of brain.

IV. 9. Assay of Octopamine

Octopamine was present in the posterior salivary glands of *Octopus vulgaris* (Erspamer and Boretti, 1951), in urine from normal animals and in organ extracts from animals treated with monoamine oxidase inhibitors (Kakimoto and Armstrong, 1962a, b). It was found to be contained in the sympathetic nerves of the sympathetically innervated organs of the rat (Molinoff and Axelrod, 1969). This discovery was based on an enzymatic assay which measured 0.5 ng of octopamine in a 0.5-ml tissue extract.

The detailed procedure of the enzymatic assay of octopamine was described by Molinoff, Landsberg and Axelrod (1969).

Frozen organs were weighed and were kept frozen until homogenization. Once samples were allowed to thaw, the octopamine concentration fell rapidly. Tissues were homogenized in 2 to 8 ml of ice-cold Tris-buffer, 0.01 M or 0.1 M, pH 8.6, containing the monoamine oxidase inhibitor, pargyline (50 μg/ml). The homogenates were heated at 95°C for 5 min immediately after homogenization, and the denatured proteins were removed by centrifugation. Duplicate 0.5-ml aliquots of the supernatant from each homogenate were transferred to 15-ml glass-stoppered centrifuge tubes. Twenty-five ng of octopamine were added to one of the aliquots as an internal standard. The enzyme assay was initiated by adding 1 nmole of S-adenosyl-L-methionine (methyl-C^{14}) and 10 μl of partially purified cow adrenal phenylethanolamine-N-methyltransferase to 0.5 ml of homogenate. The mixture was incubated for 30 min at 37°C, and the reaction was then stopped by the addition of 0.5 ml of 0.5 M borate buffer, pH 10. The radioactive synephrine (N-methyloctopamine) was extracted with 6 ml of a mixture of toluene-isoamyl alcohol (3/2) by agitating the incubation tube on a Vortex mixer for about 10 sec. Under these conditions, epinephrine, formed by the N-methylation of norepinephrine, was not extracted. A 4-ml aliquot of the toluene-isoamyl alcohol mixture was transferred to a counting vial containing a 2-ml aliquot of fresh toluene-isoamyl alcohol, and the contents of the vial were evaporated to dryness in a chromatography oven at 70°C. The addition of an aliquot of fresh solvent aided in a volatilization of slightly volatile contaminants, probably S-adenosylmethionine-C^{14}. One ml of ethanol was added to the counting vial, followed by 10 ml of phosphor containing 4 g of 2,5-diphenyloxazole and 50 mg of 1,4-bis-2-(5-phenyloxazolyl) benzene per l of toluene. The radioactivity of the samples was determined in a liquid scintillation spectrometer.

Phenylethanolamine was assayed by the same procedure except that the radioactive product was extracted with 3 % isoamyl alcohol in toluene. Since N-methylphenylethanolamine is volatile, the samples were counted without being dried.

IV. 10.   Assay of Adrenochrome

A sensitive and specific fluorometry of adrenochrome was reported by Szala, Axelrod and Perlin (1958). By this method less than 20 μg/l of a fluorescent material was found in the plasma of both normal and schizophrenic subjects, but this material did not have the characteristic activation and fluorescent spectra of synthetic adrenochrome. On the other hand, adrenochrome added to plasma and treated by the procedure described above had fluorescence characteristics identical with those of untreated adrenochrome. As little as 20 μg of added adrenochrome per liter of plasma could be estimated by this procedure (Szala, Axelrod and Perlin, 1958). The reported presence of adrenochrome in human plasma and cerebrospinal fluid with an abnormally high level in schizophrenic cerebrospinal fluid (Hoffer, 1958a, b) might be due to the lack of specificity of the assay method.

The method by Szala, Axelrod and Perlin (1958) is as follows. Blood was drawn and immediately chilled to 0–5°C and centrifuged in a refrigerated centrifuge. One milliliter of plasma was transferred to a glass-stoppered centrifuge tube containing 0.2 ml of KH_2PO_4 solution (0.5 ml) and 15 ml of n-butanol which had been successively washed with one fifth volume 1 N NaOH, 1 N HCl and three times with water. The tube was shaken and centrifuged. Ten milliliters of the butanol layer was transferred to another tube containing 3 ml of 0.1 N HCl and 25 ml of ethyl acetate which had been washed as in the case of n-butanol. After shaking, the tubes were centrifuged and the upper layer removed by aspiration. A 0.5 ml aliquot of the acid extract was transferred to a test tube and 0.5 ml of a mixture of 2 % ascorbic acid/20 % NaOH (1/9, v/v) added. After 5 min the fluorescence was measured at 525 nm after activation at 410 nm. A known amount of adrenochrome added to KH_2PO_4 solution and run through the above procedure served as a standard. All values were corrected for the small reagent blank.

IV. 11. Assay of Tyrosine

Since tyrosine is the precursor of catecholamines, its assay is frequently encountered in catecholamine research.

The spectrophotometric (Udenfriend and Cooper, 1952b) and fluorometric (Waalkes and Udenfriend, 1957) procedures are the most important assay procedures.

Under appropriate conditions, 1-nitro-2-naphthol reacts with tyrosine, tyramine and many other substituted phenols to yield red colored derivatives. These products rapidly change to stable yellow substances from which the excess reagent is separated by extraction into ethylene dichloride.

A tissue sample was homogenized with 5 % trichloroacetic acid and made up to 5.0 ml with 5 % trichloroacetic acid. After 10 min, the tube was centrifuged, and 2.0 ml of the supernatant was transferred to a 20-ml glass-stoppered centrifuge tube.

In case of plasma, 3.0 ml of water and 1.0 ml of 30 % trichloroacetic acid were added to 1.0 ml of plasma, and the mixture was centrifuged after 10 min. Two ml of the supernatant was transferred to a centrifuge tube.

For spectrophotometric assay a tissue extract containing about 500 nmoles of tyrosine in 2 ml was used, whereas for spectrofluorometric assay an extract with about 2 nmoles was used.

The effluent from an alumina column which adsorbs catecholamines is used for the assay of tyrosine, especially in case of the tyrosine hydroxylase assay using crude tissue preparations; fluorescence assay should be used for this purpose. An aliquot of the effluent sample which contained about 2–4 nmoles of tyrosine was transferred into a centrifuge tube and made up to a final concentration of about 5 % in a total volume of 2.0 ml by adding 30 % trichloroacetic acid.

For blanks, 2.0 ml of 5 % trichloroacetic acid solution was placed in another centrifuge tube.

To 2 ml of the deproteinized tissue extract in a glass-stoppered centrifuge tube, 1 ml each of the 1-nitroso-2-naphthol reagent (0.1 % 1-nitroso-2-naphthol in 95 % ethanol) and the nitric acid reagent (1 : 5 nitric acid containing 0.5 mg per ml of $NaNO_2$) were added. The tube was stoppered, placed in a 55°C water bath for 30 min, and cooled. Ten ml of ethylene dichloride was added, and the tube was shaken to extract the unchanged nitrosonaphthol. The tube was then centrifuged at low speed and the supernatant aqueous layer was transferred to a cuvette.

By means of spectrophotometry, absorbance at 450 nm was determined. Standards were prepared by heating 500 nmoles of tyrosine with nitrosonaphthol in the same manner as the unknown samples.

In a fluorometric assay, the fluorescence intensity was measured at 460 nm/570 nm (activation/emission). Standard solutions containing 2 nmoles of tyrosine were carried through the entire procedure.

Some tissues, such as spleen (Udenfriend, personal communication) and kidney (Nagatsu, Rust and DeQuattro, 1969), contained substances which interfered with the tyrosine assays and gave higher values than those obtained by an amino acid analyzer.

IV. 12. Automated Analysis of Catecholamines and the Amine Derivatives by Condensation of Ninhydrin, Aldehydes and Primary Amines (Samejima, Dairman and Udenfriend, 1971; Samejima, Dairman, Stone and Udenfriend, 1971)*

Samejima, Dairman and Udenfriend (1971) discovered a new reaction involving the condensation of ninhydrin, certain aldehydes, and primary amines (amines, amino acids and peptides) to yield highly fluorescent ternary products. This reaction can be widely applied to the assay of amino acids, peptides and amines.

To a 13 × 100 mm test tube, 2.0 ml of 0.2 M phosphate buffer (pH 6, 7 or 8; 7 for catecholamines), 0.2 ml of an aqueous solution of ninhydrin (50 mM), 0.1 ml of sample solution and 0.1 ml of phenylacetaldehyde in ethanol (10 mM) were added. After mixing thoroughly, the tubes were covered with aluminum foil and transferred to a 60°C water bath for a suitable incubation period; 15 min at pH 8.0, 60 min at pH 7.0 and 120 min at pH 6.0. The tubes were then cooled in an ice bath for a few min, kept at room temperature for 10 min and the fluorescence was measured within 1 hr with excitation at 390 nm and emission at 490 nm. Biologically important amines such as tyramine, norepinephrine, normetanephrine, dopamine, DOPA, tryptamine and serotonin, all produced intense fluorescences. It was also possible to automate the ninhydrin fluorescence proce-

---

* I am grateful to Dr. Sidney Udenfriend for personal information on this assay procedure.

dure for assay of column effluents. It would be possible to measure all the catecholamines and the derivatives by this method.

IV. 13. Fluorescence Histochemistry of Catecholamines

The development of the fluorescence histochemistry of catecholamines (Falck, Hillarp, Thieme and Torp, 1962; Falck, 1962) which can demonstrate the presence of extremely small amount of catecholamines in the tissues resulted in amazing progress in the field of adrenergic mechanisms. The principle is based on the use of formaldehyde condensation reactions to visualize catecholamines, which was first described by Eränko (1955) with the adrenal medulla.

The most important discovery made around 1962 showed that catecholamines in a dry protein matrix can condense with formaldehyde vapors to yield highly fluorescent derivatives by the catalytic action of protein (Falck, Hillarp, Thieme and Torp, 1962; Falck, 1962). The presence of excessive amounts of water inhibited the formaldehyde condensation re-

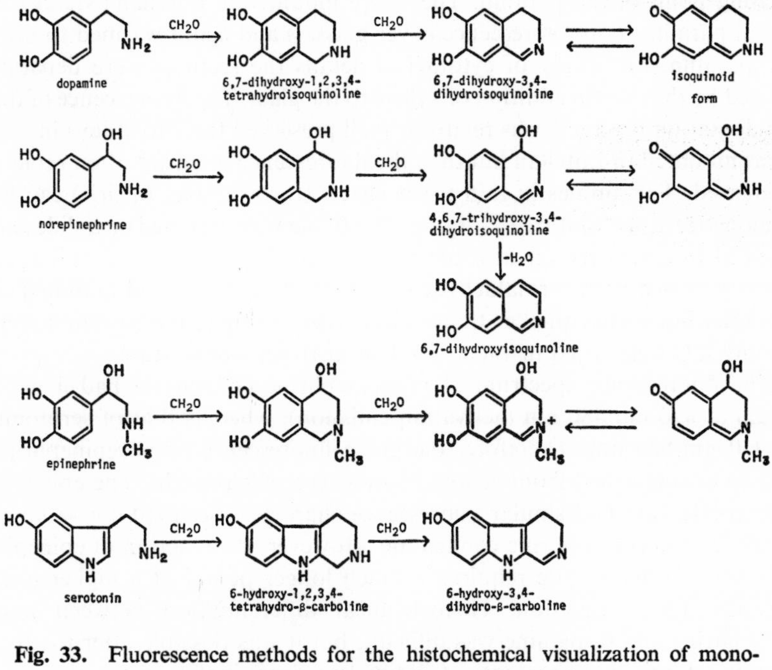

Fig. 33. Fluorescence methods for the histochemical visualization of monoamines (Corrodi and Hillarp, 1963, 1964).

actions of catecholamines. The reaction mechanism is shown in Fig. 33 (Corrodi and Hillarp, 1963, 1964). The fluorescence of the formaldehyde condensation products of catecholamines disappeared almost completely on reduction with sodium borohydride (Corrodi, Hillarp and Jonsson, 1964).

Detailed methodological descriptions of the fluorescence method for the cellular demonstration of biogenic monoamines were made by Dahlström and Fuxe (1964) and by Falck and Owman (1965). The outline of the fluorescence methods was described by Falck (1962) as follows:

Pieces of the tissue to be studied were immediately excised and frozen in propane or isopentane cooled by liquid nitrogen. They were dried in vacuo at $-35°C$ for 8–10 days. After thorough drying the pieces were treated with formaldehyde gas at 80° C for 1 hr in a closed glass vessel containing para-formaldehyde. During this treatment the catecholamines and serotonin condensed with formaldehyde to intensify fluorescent products that were not extracted with hot paraffin or xylene. The preparations were then infiltrated in vacuo with paraffin at 60° C for 10 min. Sections $(3-8\mu)$ were placed on non-fluorescent slides which were warmed just to the melting point of the paraffin. They were mounted in Entellan (Merck) or liquid paraffin (non-fluorescence cover-glasses) and again warmed to melt the paraffin. For study of cytological details the sections were deparaffinized by the careful addition of xylene to the glass. The fluorescence of the condensation products was relatively well preserved for 2 to 3 days in sections mounted in Entellan but then the fluorescence intensity often rapidly decreased. The amines in thin tissue sheets (for example, rat iris) can be demonstrated without freeze-drying. The tissue was stretched on a slide and allowed to dry in the air at room temperature for 5 to 20 min. It is then directly heated with formaldehyde gas, washed in xylene and mounted as a whole. Somewhat thicker tissue sheets (for example, mesenterium containing fat) were dried in vacuo for 1 hr at room temperature.

The fluorescence spectrum of norepinephrine condensate had a maximum at 410 nm/480 nm (activation/emission), whereas that of serotonin at 410 nm/525 nm. Therefore, the green fluorescence of norepinephrine can be distinguished from yellow fluorescence of serotonin. The epinephrine condensate had similar fluorescence characteristics (410 nm/480 nm) to those of norepinephrine condensate. However, the reaction of epinephrine with formaldehyde required a much longer period at a higher temperature for completion. Histochemical differentiation between norepinephrine and dopamine was difficult, but it was possible after the formation of the fully aromatic 6,7-dihydroxyisoquinoline from the norepinephrine condensate, i.e., 4,6,7-trihydroxy-3,4-dihydroisoquinoline (Corrodi and Jonsson, 1965).

Chapter V

Estimation of the Turnover Rate or Synthesis Rate of Catecholamines

The estimation of the turnover rate of catecholamines is frequently required as an indicator of the adrenergic activity. Several methods have been used to estimate the rate of turnover of catecholamines (Table XVIII). Theoretically, the turnover rate values obtained by these various methods should be similar, and the turnover rate should be identical to the synthesis rate in a steady state of a single catecholamine compartment. However, the estimated turnover rate values were considerably different with each method, and the estimated synthesis rate was often higher than the turnover rate. There are still many uncertainties about catecholamine turnover estimations with the present methods (Persson and Waldeck, 1970). However, the estimation of the turnover rate or synthesis rate of catecholamines is quite valuable for comparative studies. The absolute turnover rate or synthesis rate values should be evaluated with some precautions.

The term "turnover" refers to the process of renewal of a substance in the body or in a given tissue. Renewal can take place in two different ways: (1) the substance is synthesized in a given tissue or (2) the substance is synthesized somewhere else and arrives in the tissue cells through the bloodstream (Zilversmit, 1960). In case of catecholamines, the amine is mostly synthesized in a given tissue.

The term "turnover rate" means the rate at which a substance turns over in a given metabolic pool or compartment (amount per unit of time). The meaning of turnover rate is unequivocal only when a steady state exists, i.e., when the rate of synthesis (or transport into a compartment) equals the rate of metabolism (or release). Therefore, the turnover rate should be equal to the synthesis rate.

If two pools of catecholamines, a small functionally active pool with high turnover and a large pool from which the amines are slowly released, exist, only the turnover of the large pool would be reflected in the half-lives (Persson and Waldeck, 1970).

TABLE XVIII. Methods for the Estimation of the Turnover Rate or Synthesis Rate of Catecholamines.

Estimation	Principle	Method		Reference
Turnover rate	The rate of disappearance of labeled catecholamines	Isotopic method	Tyrosine-C^{14} or DOPA-H^3 intraperitoneal injection	1, 2)
			Norepinephrine-H^3 intravenous injection	3–5)
	The rate of disappearance of the endogenous catecholamines after synthesis inhibition	Non-isotopic method	α-Methyl-p-tyrosine intraperitoneal injection	4, 5)
Synthesis rate	The accumulation of labeled amines after infusion or injection of labeled tyrosine	Isotopic method	Perfusion of the isolated organs with tyrosine-C^{14}	6, 7)
			Injection to the animals with tyrosine-C^{14}	8–10)

1) Udenfriend, Cooper, Clark and Baer, 1953.
2) Udenfriend and Zaltzman-Nirenberg, 1963.
3) Costa, Boullin, Hammer, Vogel and Brodie, 1966.
4) Costa and Neff, 1966.
5) Brodie, Costa, Dlabac, Neff and Smookler, 1966.
6) Spector, Sjoerdsma, Zaltzman-Nirenberg, Levitt and Udenfriend, 1963.
7) Levitt, Spector, Sjoerdsma and Udenfriend, 1965.
8) Sedvall, Weise and Kopin, 1968.
9) DeQuattro, Nagatsu, Maronde and Alexander, 1969.
10) Neff, Ngai, Wang and Costa, 1969.

V. 1.   Methods for the Estimation of the Turnover Rate of Catecholamines

V. 1. 1. ISOTOPIC METHODS

A. *Principle*

Labeled norepinephrine is incorporated into a norepinephrine pool in a given sympathetically innervated tissue by the injection of a tracer dose of: either labeled precursor, i.e., L-tyrosine-C^{14}, L-tyrosine-H^3, or L-DOPA-H^3, or the labeled amine itself, i.e., norepinephrine-H^3. The isotopically labeled norepinephrine is constantly rapidly taken up into the norepinephrine pool in the sympathetic neurons, secreted from the sympathetic nerve endings and replaced by the same amount of newly synthesized non-labeled norepinephrine. Consequently, when the specific activities (S) of norepinephrine in a given tissue are plotted against time (t), it decreases exponentially. If log S is plotted against time on semi-logarithmic paper, a straight line can be obtained (Fig. 34). The turnover rate can be calculated from the value of the half life which can be obtained from the graph and the amount (pool size) of norepinephrine, as shown in Fig. 34.

B.   *Labeling of the catecholamine pool by the injection of a labeled precursor* (tyrosine-C^{14} or DOPA-H^3)

1. *Principle.* A precursor of catecholamines (dopamine, norepinephrine, and epinephrine) is injected into the animals in order to label the catecholamines in a given tissue. The turnover rate is estimated from the rate of disappearance of label from the individual catecholamines (Udenfriend, Cooper, Clark and Baer, 1953). Since the amino acid precursor, i.e., tyrosine or DOPA, can cross the blood brain barrier and be incorporated into the brain, this method can be applicable not only to the peripheral sympathetically innervated organs but also to the brain (Udenfriend and Zaltzman-Nirenberg, 1963).

2. *Procedure.* Udenfriend and Zaltzman-Nirenberg (1963) determined the turnover rate of norepinephrine and dopamine in guinea pig brain by this method. 200μCi of DL-DOPA-H^3 (224 μCi/μmole) were administered intraperitoneally to guinea pigs weighing 200 to 250 g. Eight groups of guinea pigs were used, and each group was composed of 5 animals. At 2, 4, 6, 8, 10, 12, 16 and 24 hr after the injection, the animals were killed and decapitated. The brain was removed immediately and homogenized in 10 ml of 5% trichloroacetic acid. The homogenate was centrifuged and ca-

techolamines were isolated by adsorption and elution from alumina by the method of Crout (1961). Aliquots of the alumina eluate were assayed fluorometrically for norepinephrine (Crout, 1961) and dopamine (Drujan, Sourkes, Layne and Murphy, 1959). To the remainder of the eluate 20 μg of each amine as carrier was added. The solution was adjusted to pH 6 and passed through an Amberlite IRC-50 (Na⁺) column (packed volume, 1.5 ml), buffered at pH 6, to remove any traces of DOPA. Norepinephrine and dopamine were eluted with 1 N acetic acid and were again chromatographed on a Dowex-50 (H⁺) column (Bertler, Carlsson and Rosengren, 1958). When 1.5 ml (packed volume) of Dowex-50 column was used, norepinephrine was generally eluted with 15 ml of 1 N HCl, and dopamine subsequently with 15 ml of 2 N HCl (these volumes of HCl should be checked in a preliminary experiment). The eluate containing norepinephrine or dopamine was collected in a scintillation-counter vail, and evaporated to dryness in a draft under the stream of nitrogen in a water bath below 40°C. The residue was dissolved in 1.0 ml of water. An aliquot (0.1 ml) of the solution was used for the determination of norepinephrine or dopamine by measuring the native fluorescence at 285 nm/325 nm (excitation/fluorescence). To the rest (0.9 ml) of the solution in the scintillation-counter vial, 10 ml of Bray's scintillator solution (naphthalene 60 g, PPO 4 g, POPOP 0.2 g, methanol 100 ml, ethyleneglycol 20 ml, p-dioxane to 1.0 l) (Bray, 1960) were added. Radioactivity was counted in a liquid scintillation spectrometer. The specific activity (cpm/nmole) (mean value) of each animal group was plotted (log scale) against time on a semi-logarithmic graph. $T_{\frac{1}{2}}$ (hr) value was determined from the straight line for norepinephrine and dopamine, respectively, and the value of rate constant (K) was calculated as shown in Fig. 34. The rate constant multiplied by the pool size (nmoles/g tissue) of norepinephrine or dopamine which was measured separately, equaled the turnover rate (nmoles/g/hr). Udenfriend and Zaltzman-Nirenberg (1963) reported the following results with guinea pig brain: for norepinephrine, the specific activity at 2 hr = about 2,000 cpm/nmole, $T_{1/2}$ = 4 hr, pool size = 0.25 μg/g, turnover rate = 0.033 μg/g/hr; and for dopamine, the specific activity at 2 hr = about 3,000 cpm/nmole, $T_{1/2}$ = 2.5 hr, pool size = 0.6 μg/g, turnover rate = 0.11 μg/g/hr.

C. *Labeling of the catecholamine pool by the intravenous injection of radioactive amine (norepinephrine-H³)*

1. *Principle.* When radioactive norepinephrine is injected intravenously, it is rapidly taken up by sympathetic neurons and mixes with the

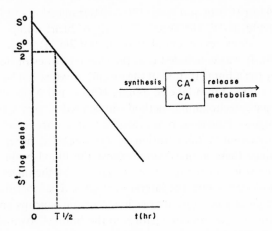

Fig. 34. Estimation of the turnover rate of a catecholamine (CA) by the isotopic method.

If [CA]   = the amount of CA in the CA pool (pool size)

[CA*] = the amount of labeled CA

S^t = the specific activity of CA at time $t = \dfrac{CA^*}{CA}$

S^0 = the specific activity of CA at zero time

$T_{1/2}$ = half-life (the time in which specific activity of CA is halved)

k = rate constant (the percentage of the CA pool that is renewed per unit of time)

then $S^t = S^0 e^{-kt}$

$\log S^t = \log S^0 - 0.4343\ kt$

$$k = \frac{\log S^0 - \log S^t}{0.4343\ t} = \frac{1}{1.44\ T_{1/2}}$$

Turnover rate $= k \cdot [CA]$

endogenous norepinephrine stores. The turnover of the norepinephrine pool in a given sympathetically innervated tissue could be estimated by measuring the change of norepinephrine specific activity with time (Montanari, Beaven, Costa and Brodie, 1963).

After the injection of greater than tracer amounts of ($\pm$)-norepinephrine-H³, the labeled amine taken up by heart produced a diphasic decline of radioactivity (Axelrod, Hertting and Patrick, 1961). If a dose of radio-labeled norepinephrine increased the endogenous pool of norepinephrine by more than 0.02 μg norepinephrine/g heart, a diphasic decline resulted (Costa, Boullin, Hammer, Vogel and Brodie, 1966). After the administration of small tracer amounts of ($\pm$)-norepinephrine (0.1 μg/kg), the norepinephrine specific activity declined as a single exponential over a period of 48 hr (Costa and Neff, 1966). After injection of 0.165 μg/kg of (−)-norepinephrine-H³, the specific activity of heart norepinephrine also declined as a single exponential (Costa, Boullin, Hammer, Vogel and Brodie, 1966). It was concluded that the characteristics of decline are not influenced by the administration of the racemic mixture but by the amounts of the administered radio-labeled amines (Costa and Neff, 1966).

This isotopic catecholamine method can be used for any sympathetically innervated organs. However, brain catecholamine stores cannot be studied after the intravenous administration of radio-labeled norepinephrine or dopamine, since these amines cannot cross the blood-brain barrier. The catecholamine stores in the brain can be labeled by the injection of radio-active catecholamines into the lateral ventricles. The labeled amines given by intraventricular route rapidly reach adrenergic neurons and selectively label endogenous catecholamine stores in the brain (Glowinski and Axelrod, 1965, 1966).

2. *Procedure.* The following procedures were established (Costa and Neff, 1966; Neff and Costa, 1966; Brodie, Costa, Dlabac, Neff and Smookler, 1966).

Six groups of male Sprague-Dawley rats (5 animals for each group), weighing 180–210 g, were used for the experiment. Five μCi/kg of (±)-norepinephrine-7-H³ (6.2 Ci/mmole) was injected intravenously. At 0, 4, 8, 16, 24, 48 hr after the injection, the animals were sacrificed by cervical fracture, and their hearts immediately removed. The hearts were homogenized in 10 ml of 5 % trichloroacetic acid. The homogenate was centrifuged and norepinephrine was isolated by adsorption and elution from alumina by the method of Crout (1961). An aliquot of the alumina eluate was assayed fluorometrically for norepinephrine (Crout, 1961). The rest of the alumina eluate was transferred to a scintillation-counter vial and evaporated to dryness in a draft under the stream of nitrogen in a water bath. The residue was dissolved in 1.0 ml of water, and 10 ml of Bray's scintillator solution was added for the assay of the radioactivity in a liquid scintillation counter. The specific activity of extracted heart norepinephrine was calculated by dividing the radioactivity (dpm) found in the alumina eluate by the μg of norepinephrine found per g of heart, and plotted against time (hr) on a semi-logarithmic graph. Costa and Neff (1966) reported the following results : the specific activity of the heart norepinephrine at zero-time = about 7,000 dpm/μg; $T_{1/2}$ = 9 hr; rate constant (k) = 0.077; norepinephrine pool size = 0.64 μg/g; and the turnover rate of heart norepinephrine = 0.049 μg/g/hr.

V. 1. 2. Non-isotopic Method

A. *Principle*

α-Methyl-*p*-tyrosine, a synthetic amino acid which competitively inhibits tyrosine hydroxylase, can block the synthesis of catecholamines from tyrosine *in vivo* (Spector, Sjoerdsma and Udenfriend, 1965). Costa and Neff (1966), Neff and Costa (1966), and Brodie, Costa, Dlabac, Neff and Smookler (1966) reported that after administration of a sufficient amount of α-methyl-*p*-tyrosine the tissue catecholamine content declined as a single exponential and that the turnover rate of catecholamines could be estimated from the rate constant obtained by the semi-logarithmic decline of tissue catecholamines (μg/g). This method can be applied also to the turnover assay of norepinephrine or dopamine in the brain.

B. *Procedure*

Five groups of male Sprague-Dawley rats (180–210 g), each group consisting of 5 animals, were used for the experiment. At time zero 200 mg /kg of L-α-methyl-*p*-tyrosine was administered intravenously and at 3 hr, 75 mg/kg. At 0, 1, 2, 4, 8 hr, the animals were killed and decapitated. The brains and hearts were removed immediately and homogenized in 10 ml of 5 % trichloroacetic acid. The homogenate was centrifuged and catecholamines were isolated by adsorption and elution from alumina by the method of Crout (1961). The log [norepinephrine] against time was plotted on a semi-logarithmic graph. The results by Neff and Costa (1966) are shown in Table XIX. The turnover rates (μg/g/hr) obtained were : heart norepinephrine $= 0.049$; brain norepinephrine $= 0.036$; and brain dopamine $= 0.21$. The turnover rates obtained by this non-isotopic method agreed with those by the isotopic norepinephrine-H^3 method.

V. 2. Methods for the Estimation of the Synthesis Rate of Catecholamines

The turnover rate, though it is an indirect measurement of catecholamine synthesis in tissues, should be identical with the synthesis rate. However, it is possible to make direct measurement of the synthesis rate of catecholamines *in vivo* by assaying the formation of catecholamines in a given period of time from radio-labeled tyrosine.

TABLE XIX. The Turnover Rate of Catecholamines in Rat Heart and Brain (Neff and Costa, 1966).

Method	Tissue	Catecholamine	Pool size (μg/g)	$T_{\frac{1}{2}}$ (hr)	Rate constant (k) (hr^{-1})	Turnover rate (μg/g/hr)
Isotopic method (norepinephrine-H^3)	Heart	NE	0.64	9	0.077	0.049
Non-isotopic method	Heart	NE	0.64	9	0.077	0.048
	Brain	NE	0.31	5.9	0.12	0.036
		DM	0.75	2.5	0.28	0.21

NE = norepinephrine; DM = dopamine.

V. 2. 1. DIRECT ASSAY OF THE SYNTHESIS RATE OF CATECHOLAMINES BY
PERFUSION OF RADIOACTIVE TYROSINE THROUGH THE ISOLATED ORGAN

A. *Principle*

An isolated organ (for example, heart or vas deferens) is perfused with
radioactive tyrosine for a short period of time. The radioactive catecholamines formed during the perfusion are isolated, and their total radioactivity measured. The synthesis rate of catecholamine is calculated from
the specific activity of tyrosine.

B. *Procedure*

The estimation of the synthesis rate by the conversion of tyrosine-C^{14} to
norepinephrine in the perfused guinea pig heart was described by Spector,
Sjoerdsma, Zaltzman-Nirenberg, Levitt and Udenfriend (1963) and by
Levitt, Spector, Sjoerdsma and Udenfriend (1965).

Male Hartley guinea pigs weighing 180 to 225 g were used. The animals
were killed by a blow on the head. The hearts were removed and perfused
in a Langendorff heart apparatus with oxygenated Tyrode solution (pH
7.4) containing 0.1% glucose at 37°C and at a pressure of 65 cm water at
a perfusion rate of 5–7 cm/min. Any heart that failed to beat in a regular
manner during a 10-min preliminary perfusion was discarded. The hearts
were then perfused with 500 ml of the Tyrode solution containing 2 mg/l
of ascorbic acid and 10 μCi of L-tyrosine-U-C^{14} (1×10^{-4} M) for 1.5 hr.
The perfusate was not recycled. Following perfusion the hearts were
blotted, weighed, and homogenized in 10 ml of 5% trichloroacetic acid.
At this point 25 μg of non-radioactive norepinephrine was added as
a carrier. The homogenate was centrifuged, and the supernatant solutions
were treated with alumina to adsorb catecholamines (Crout, 1961). The
effluents were saved for the assay of specific activity of tyrosine. The
catecholamines were eluted from the alumina column with 0.2 N acetic acid.
The eluate was again chromatographed on Amberlite IRC-50 (Na$^+$) and
Dowex-50 (H$^+$) columns to isolate norepinephrine (Udenfriend and Zaltzman-Nirenberg, 1963), and the total radioactivity of norepinephrine
was measured. Tyrosine in the effluents from the alumina column was
in turn adosrbed on a Dowex-50 (H$^+$) column. It was then eluted with
a solution of 3 N ammonia. After removal of the ammonia, the tyrosine-
containing solutions were passed over an Amberlite IRC-50 column (buffered with ammonium acetate, pH 5) to remove basic metabolites such
as tyramine and normetanephrine. Aliquots of the perfusates and of
the effluents from the IRC-50 columns were taken for tyrosine assay

(Waalkes and Udenfriend, 1957) and for radioassay, and the specific radioactivity of tyrosine was calculated.

The norepinephrine synthesized during the period of perfusion was calculated using the following equation:

$$C = \frac{(B/A) \times 0.169}{T}$$

where C = the synthesis rate of norepinephrine (μg/g/hr),
B = total radioactivity of norepinephrine (cpm/g),
A = the specific activity of tyrosine (cpm/nmole),
T = perfusion time (hr), and
0.169 = norepinephrine μg/nmole.

When the perfusion rate was 5–7 ml/min, the norepinephrine concentration in the heart was usually maintained near control values. The reduction of the endogenous norepinephrine levels were 0– -30 %. Therefore, it was assumed that the depletion of norepinephrine during the perfusion is negligible. The half maximum rate of norepinephrine synthesis occurred at a tyrosine concentration of about 2×10^{-5} M. A maximum rate was obtained at a tyrosine concentration of 1×10^{-4} M as 0.2 μg (about 1 nmole)/g/hr.

This method for the assay of the synthesis rate of norepinephrine was also applied to the isolated guinea pig vas deferens and the hypogastric nerve (Roth, Stjärne and Euler, 1967). The synthesis rate of norepinephrine was : 0.15–0.20 μg/g/hr in the vas deferens; and about 3 μg/g/hr in the hypogastric nerve. In the vas deferens, nerve stimulation caused about a 3-fold increase in the synthesis of norepinephrine from tyrosine.

V. 2. 2. DIRECT ASSAY OF THE SYNTHESIS RATE OF CATECHOLAMINES BY INTRAVENOUS PERFUSION OF RADIOACTIVE TYROSINE IN THE WHOLE ANIMAL

The relative rate of norepinephrine synthesis was measured by the accumulation of norepinephrine-C^{14} after intravenous administration of tyrosine-C^{14} to the whole animal (Gordon, Reid, Sjoerdsma and Udenfriend, 1966; Gordon, Spector, Sjoerdsma and Udenfriend, 1966). This method requires only a single injection of tyrosine-C^{14} and can reflect rapid changes in the synthesis rate of norepinephrine. This method was modified to get estimates of norepinephrine synthesis rates (Sedvall, Weise and Kopin, 1968; DeQuattro, Nagatsu, Maronde and Alexander, 1969; Neff, Ngai, Wang and Costa, 1969).

A. *The method by Sedvall, Weise and Kopin* (1968)

1. *Principle.* For the direct assay of the synthesis rate of catechol-amines in the isolated organ, the organ was perfused with radioactive tyrosine at a constant rate, and the total radioactivities of catecholamines synthesized during the perfusion were measured. A similar method was described, in which the rates of formation of norepinephrine-C^{14} in the heart, brain and submaxillary glands were measured *in vivo* during intravenous infusion of tyrosine-C^{14} into unanesthetized rats. When tyrosine-C^{14} was injected intravenously by slow, constant infusion for up to 1 hr, the specific activity of tyrosine in the blood and organs increased curvilinearly (Fig. 35) (Sedvall, Weise and Kopin, 1968; Neff, Ngai and Costa, 1969). From a curve of increase in the specific activity of tyrosine in plasma or tissues as shown in Fig. 35, the mean specific activity of tyrosine was determined from the area under the curve. The total radioactivity of nor-

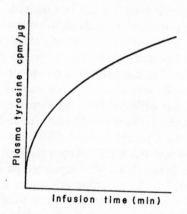

Fig. 35. Increase in the specific activity of tyrosine-C^{14} in plasma during the constant intravenous infusion of tyrosine-C^{14} (Sedvall, Weise and Kopin, 1968).

epinephrine was assayed after its chromatographic separation. Assuming that only a small fraction is lost during the relatively short intervals of perfusion, the total amount of norepinephrine-C^{14} formed is the product of the mean specific activity of the precursor tyrosine-C^{14} and the amount of tyrosine converted to norepinephrine during the interval (synthesis rate). Consequently, the rate of synthesis of norepinephrine was calculated from the following equation:

Synthesis rate of norepinephrine (μg/g/hr) =

$$\frac{\text{Total radioactivity of norepinephrine (cpm/}\mu\text{g)} \times 1.05}{\text{Mean specific activity of tyrosine (cpm/}\mu\text{g)} \times \text{Time of infusion (hr)}}$$

where 1.05 is a correction factor for the difference in molecular weight of tyrosine and norepinephrine and the loss of a carbon atom from uniformly labeled tyrosine-C^{14}.

Sedvall, Weise and Kopin (1968) reported that the specific activity of tyrosine in plasma was higher than that in an organ. The specific activity of the tyrosine at the site of catecholamine synthesis cannot exceed that in plasma. Thus, if the specific activity of plasma tyrosine is used to calculate the rate of norepinephrine synthesis, a minimum rate of synthesis may be obtained. On the other hand, it is not likely that the specific activity of tyrosine in sympathetic nerve endings is less than that of the whole tissue. Thus, if the mean specific activity of tissue tyrosine is used, a maximal estimate of norepinephrine synthesis can be obtained.

2. *Procedure.* The procedure by Sedvall, Weise and Kopin (1968) is as follows. Sixty μCi of L-tyrosine-U-C^{14} (350 mCi/mmole) were administered intravenously to male Sprague-Dawley rats (200–225 g) by slow, constant infusion for up to 1 hr. The animals (each group consisting of 6 animals) were sacrificed at 5, 10, 20, 40 and 60 min. Animals were killed by decapitation and the blood was collected from the carcasses in beakers. Tissues (brain, heart, salivary glands) were rapidly removed and tissues and plasma were homogenized in 0.4 N perchloric acid. Catecholamines were adsorbed on alumina and eluted with 0.2 N HCl (Anton and Sayre, 1962). Norepinephrine and dopamine in the eluate were separated on columns of Dowex-50-X4-W (K$^+$ form) (0.8 × 5 cm). After adjustment to pH 2, the alumina eluates were poured onto Dowex columns, which were then rinsed with 10 ml of water, 10 ml of 0.1 N phosphate buffer (pH 6.5), another 10 ml of water and 4 ml of 1 N HCl. Norepinephrine was eluted with 11 ml of 1 N HCl, and dopamine with 18 ml of 2 N HCl. Norepinephrine was determined fluorometrically with an aliquot of the eluate (Häggendal, 1963). The other aliquots of the remaining eluates were evaporated to dryness in a scintillation-counter vial in a stream of air at 75°C. The dry residues were taken up in water, and a scintillator solution was added. Radioactivity was counted in a liquid scintillation spectrometer.

The amount of tyrosine and its radioactivity was measured with the alumina effluent. Tyrosine was adsorbed on a Dowex-50 (H$^+$) column eluted with 3 N NH$_4$OH. After removal of the ammonia, the solution was passed through an Amberlite IRC-50 column (buffered with ammonium acetate, pH 5). An aliquot of the effluent was taken for tyrosine assay (Waalkes and Udenfriend, 1957). The rest of the solution was used for the radioassay of tyrosine.

Neff, Ngai, Wang and Costa (1969) used a Rexyn 102 column, 200–400 mesh (Fisher Scientific Company) buffered to pH 6.5 (50 mm × 78 mm²) for the separation of tyrosine. A 5-ml portion of the alumina effluent was added to a Rexyn column. The initial 2.5-ml effluent was discarded. The second 2.5-ml and a 5-ml water eluate were collected and analyzed for radioactivity and tyrosine (Waalkes and Udenfriend, 1957). The eluate was shown to contain a radioactive contaminant besides tyrosine by paper chromatography using n-butanol/acetic acid/water (120/30/50) as solvent (tyrosine : R_f = 0.45; and an unknown material : R_f = 0.21). The specific activities of tyrosine were corrected to account for the presence of this material.

The specific activity of tyrosine against time was plotted as shown in Fig. 35. The mean specific activity of tyrosine in plasma or tissues was determined from the areas under the curves. Synthesis rate of norepinephrine was calculated from the total radioactivity of norepinephrine and the mean specific activity of tyrosine either in plasma or in the tissue by the equation described above. If the mean specific activity of tyrosine in the plasma is used for the calculation, a minimum rate of synthesis can be obtained. If the mean specific activity of tissue tyrosine is used, a maximal estimate of synthesis can be obtained.

By using this method, Sedvall, Weise and Kopin (1968) showed that the synthesis rate of norepinephrine (μg/g/hr) in the brain (0.094–0.165), heart (0.060–0.106), and submaxillary gland (0.120–0.234) were 2- or 3-fold greater than the estimated turnover rates of norepinephrine. In order to explain the differences between the estimated synthesis rates and turnover rates, a hypothetical model of an open, two-compartment system for norepinephrine storage was proposed by Sedvall, Weise and Kopin (1968).

B. *The method by Neff, Ngai, Wang and Costa* (1969)

Neff, Ngai, Wang and Costa (1969) described a new method for the estimation of catecholamine synthesis rates in single, unanesthetized animals from the conversion of tyrosine-C^{14} to radioactive catecholamines. Their calculations accounted for the loss of newly formed norepinephrine with time. The catecholamine synthesis rates calculated by this method were shown to be comparable to those obtained from the decline of amine levels after blockade of catecholamine synthesis (Brodie, Costa, Dlabac, Neff and Smookler, 1966).

When tyrosine-C^{14} was infused at a constant rate into unanesthetized rats, the specific activity of plasma tyrosine increased curvilinearly with time, producing a concomitant increase in the specific activity of tissue catecholamines. By applying steady-state kinetics to this relationship, an open, single compartment model is developed. The fractional rate constant (k) of a catecholamine compartment was calculated, and the catecholamine synthesis rate was obtained by multiplying k by the steady-state amine level. The synthesis rate of catecholamines obtained by this method ($\mu g/g/$ hr) was: for brain norepinephrine, 0.12; and for heart norepinephrine, 0.095. These values were identical with those calculated from the decline of catecholamine levels after blockade of their synthesis with α-methyl-p-tyrosine.

APPENDIX*

I. Chemical Properties of Catecholamines

Catecholamines are a class of compounds possessing a catechol ring and a side chain of either ethylamine or ethanolamine, and the chemical properties of these compounds, together with related compounds, will be described in this section (references: Merck Index, 1968; Data for Biochem. Res., 1969). Dopamine, norepinephrine (noradrenaline) and epinephrine (adrenaline) are natural catecholamines (Fig. 1).

1. Dopamine

4-(2-Aminoethyl)pyrocatechol; 3-hydroxytyramine; 3,4-dihydroxyphenethylamine; α-(3,4-dihydroxyphenyl)-β-aminoethane. $C_8H_{11}NO_2$; mol wt 153.18. White stout prisms from H_2O, rapidly darkening on exposure to air. Highly sensitive to oxygen. Spontaneously oxidizes in aqueous solution at alkaline pHs. Stable at acidic pHs. pKa (25°C) 8.9 (OH), 10.6 (NH$_2$).

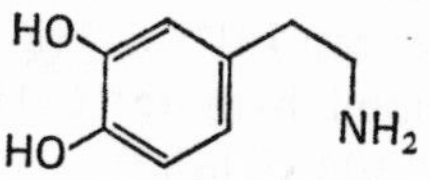

Dopamine

Hydrochloride: $C_8H_{11}NO_2 \cdot HCl$; mol wt 189.65, rosettes of needles from water, mp 237–41°C dec. Freely soluble in water, soluble in methanol, hot 95 % ethanol; practically insoluble in ether, petroleum ether, chloroform, benzene, toluene, soluble in aqueous solutions of alkali hydroxide.

Hydrobromide: $C_8H_{11}NO_2 \cdot HBr$; mol wt 234.10, plates, mp 210–214°C dec.

Picrate: $C_8H_{11}NO_2 \cdot C_6H_3N_3O_7$; mol wt 382.29, minute brownish yellow crystals from water, mp 189°C dec.

---

* I wish to thank Dr. Donald E. Wolf and Mrs. Idamarie Eggers (Merck Sharp and Dohme Research Laboratories, Rahway, New Jersey, U.S.A.) for their careful review of this appendix.

2. Norepinephrine

Noradrenaline; arterenol; α-(aminomethyl)-3,4-dihydroxybenzyl alcohol; 2-amino-1-(3,4-dihydroxyphenyl)ethanol; 1-(3,4-dihydroxyphenyl)-2-aminoethanol; 4-(α-hydroxy-β-aminoethyl)catechol. $C_8H_{11}NO_3$; mol wt 169.18. pKa (25°C) 8.82 (OH), 9.98 (NH₂). Natural (−)-form has D-configuration relative to mandelic acid. Aqueous solutions slowly racemize and oxidize under the influence of light and oxygen. Stable at acidic pHs. Stability maximal at pH 4. Solutions may be autoclaved at about pH 3.6.

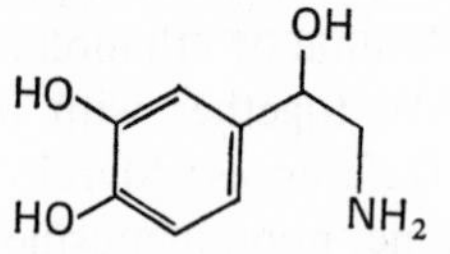

Norepinephrine

(±)-Form: crystals, mp 191°C dec. Sparingly soluble in water; very slightly soluble in alcohol, ether; rapidly soluble in dilute acids.

(+)-Form: mp 216–218°C, $[\alpha]_D^{25}$ +37.4° ($c=5$ in water with 1 equiv. HCl).

(−)-Form: occurs in animals and plants, microcrystals, mp 216.5–218°C dec. $[\alpha]_D^{25}$ −37.3° ($c=5$ in water with 1 equiv. HCl).

(−)-Form hydrochloride: $C_8H_{11}NO_3 \cdot HCl$; mol wt 205.65, crystals, mp 145.2–146.4°C, $[\alpha]_D^{25}$ −40° ($c=6$ in water). Freely soluble in water.

(±)-Form hydrochloride: mp 141°C.

(−)-Form D-bitartrate monohydrate: $C_8H_{11}NO_3$; $C_4H_6O_9 \cdot H_2O$; mol wt 337.29, crystals, mp 102–104°C, $[\alpha]_D^{25}$ −10.7° ($c=1.6$ in water). Freely soluble in water.

(−)-Form D-bitartrate anhydrate: mp 158–159°C (some decomposition).

3. Epinephrine

Adrenaline; 3,4-dihydroxy-α-[(methylamino)methyl]benzyl alcohol; 1-(3,4-dihydroxyphenyl)-2-(methylamino)ethanol; 3,4-dihydroxy-1-[1-hydroxy-

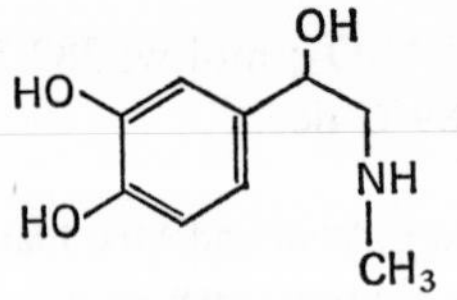

Epinephrine

2-(methylamino) ethyl] benzene; $C_9H_{13}NO_3$; mol wt 183.20. The (−)-form occurs in animals, and is the principal sympathomimetic hormone produced by the adrenal medulla in man. Configuration of natural (−)-form epinephrine is D- by relation to D-mandelic acid. Epinephrine has reducing properties owing to the catechol grouping. Redox potential + 0.81 V.

(±)-Form: Sparingly soluble in water, alcohol.

(±)-Form hydrochloride: $C_9H_{13}NO_3 \cdot HCl$; mol wt 219.68. Crystals from alchol, mp 157°C. Readily soluble in water, sparingly soluble in absolute alcohol.

(+)-Form: Crystals, mp 211–221°C dec, $[\alpha]_D{}^{20}$ +50.5°.

(−)-Form: Minute crystals gradually browning on exposure to light and air. mp 211–212°C, about 215°C dec when rapidly heated. $[\alpha]_D{}^{20}$ −50°– −53.5° (1 g in 20 ml of 0.5 N HCl, 200 mm tube). Sparingly soluble in water; insoluble in alcohol, chloroform, ether, acetone, oils. Readily solube in aqueous solutions of mineral acids and of sodium hydroxide or of potassium hydroxide, but not in aqueous solutions of ammonia and of the alkali carbonates. Aqueous solutions are slightly alkaline to litmus. Combines with acids, forming salts which are readily soluble in water. Solutions of epinephrine are likely to undergo oxidation in the presence of oxygen, especially in neutral or alkaline solutions; the red color formed by this oxidation is adrenochrome. Relatively stable below pH 5 in cold. LD50 orally in mice 50 mg/kg.

Adrenochrome

(−)-Form 3,4-cyclic borate: $C_9H_{12}BNO_4$.

(−)-Form D-bitartrate: $C_{19}H_{13}NO_3 \cdot C_4H_6O_6$; mol wt 333.29, crystals, darken slowly on exposure to air and light. mp 147–154°C some dec. One gram dissolves in about 3 ml water. Slightly soluble in alcohol.

4. DOPA

3-(3,4-Dihydroxyphenyl)-alanine; β-(3,4-dihydroxyphenyl)-alanine; 2-amino-3-(3,4-dihydroxyphenyl)propionic acid. $C_9H_{11}NO_4$; mol wt 197.19.

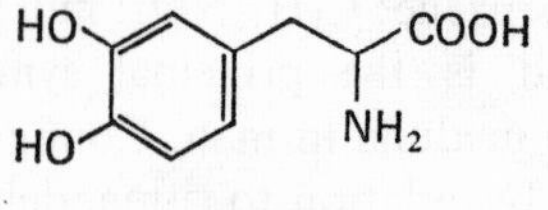

HO\
HO/ (structure) COOH, NH₂

DOPA

L-Form, the naturally occurring form. White needles or prisms from water, mp 276–278°C dec, $[\alpha]_D^{18}$ −13.1° ($c=5.12$ in 1 N HCl). pKa 1: 2.32 (COOH), 2: 8.72 (NH₂), 3: 9.96 (OH), 4: 11.79 (OH). λ_{max} (0.001 N HCl): 220.5 nm and 280 nm (log ε 3.79, 3.42). Solubility in water: 66 mg/40 ml. Rapidly oxidized in aqueous solutions, which become green. Relatively stable at acidic pHs. The solid should be stored away from light.

DL-Form: prisms from water or from aqueous NaHSO₃ solution, mp 270–272°C dec. Solubility in water: 144 mg/40 ml. Readily soluble in dilute acids and alkalies; slightly soluble in benzene, carbon disulfide, practically insoluble in absolute alcohol, ether, glacial acetic acid, petroleum ether, chloroform. Oxidizes readily.

D-Form: needles from water. mp 276–278°C dec. $[\alpha]_D^{11}$ +13.0° ($c=$ 5.27 in 1 N HCl). Solubility in water: 66 mg/40 ml.

5. *Normetanephrine*

α-(Aminomethyl)vanillyl alcohol; 4-hydroxy-3-methoxy-α-(aminomethyl) benzyl alcohol; 1-(4-hydroxy-3-methoxyphenyl)-2-aminoethanol; 3-O-methylarterenol; 3-O-methylnoradrenaline; 3-O-methylnorepinephrine. $C_9H_{13}NO_3$, mol wt 183.20.

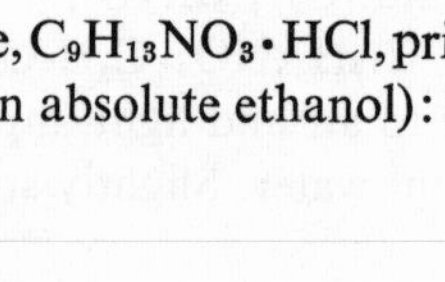

CH₃O\
HO/ (structure) OH, NH₂

Normetanephrine

($\pm$)-Form hydrochloride, $C_9H_{13}NO_3 \cdot$ HCl, prisms from absolute ethanol, mp 206–207°C dec. λ_{max} (in absolute ethanol): 232 nm ($\varepsilon=7,100$) and 282 nm ($\varepsilon=2,970$).

6. *Metanephrine*

α-(Methylaminomethyl)vanillyl alcohol; 4-hydroxy-3-methoxy-α-(methylaminomethyl) benzyl alcohol; 3-O-methylepinephrine; 3-O-methyladrenaline; 1-(4-hydroxy-3-methoxyphenyl)-2-methylaminoethanol. $C_{10}H_{15}NO_3$; mol wt 197.23.

($\pm$)-Form hydrochloride, $C_{10}H_{15}NO_3 \cdot HCl$, prisms from ethanol + ether. mp 175°C dec. λ_{max} (in ethanol): 231 nm ($\varepsilon = 7{,}600$) and 280 nm ($\varepsilon = 3{,}100$).

Metanephrine

7. Spectra of catecholamines

The absorption spectra of catecholamines have a maximum at 280 nm and a minimum at 250 nm (Fig. 36).

The fluorescence spectra of catecholamines has the activation maximum at 285 nm and the emission maximum at 325 nm (uncorrected) (Udenfriend, 1962).

294

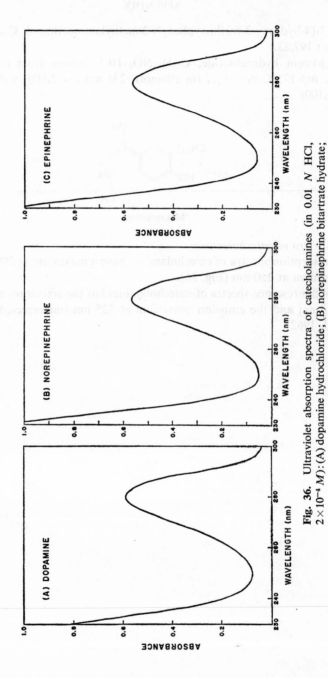

Fig. 36. Ultraviolet absorption spectra of catecholamines (in 0.01 N HCl, 2×10^{-4} M): (A) dopamine hydrochloride; (B) norepinephrine bitartrate hydrate; (C) epinephrine bitartrate.

IIa. Abbreviations of Catecholamines and the Related Compounds Frequently Used in Literatures

Compound	Abbreviation	Formula	Mol wt
Phenylalanine	Phe	$C_9H_{11}NO_2$	165.19
Tyrosine	Tyr	$C_9H_{11}NO_3$	181.19
3,4-Dihydroxy-phenylalanine	DOPA	$C_9H_{11}NO_4$	197.19
Dopamine	DM or DA	$C_8H_{11}NO_2$	153.18
hydrochloride		$C_8H_{11}NO_2 \cdot HCl$	189.65
hydrobromide		$C_8H_{11}NO_2 \cdot HBr$	234.10
picrate		$C_8H_{11}NO_2 \cdot C_6H_3N_3O_7$	382.29
Norepinephrine (Noradrenaline)	NE	$C_8H_{11}NO_3$	169.18
hydrochloride		$C_8H_{11}NO_3 \cdot HCl$	205.65
bitartrate monohydrate		$C_8H_{11}NI_3 \cdot C_4H_6O_6 \cdot H_2O$	337.29

Compound	Abbreviation	Formula	Mol wt
Epinephrine (Adrenaline)	EN		
		$C_9H_{13}NO_3$	183.20
hydrochloride		$C_9H_{13}NO_3 \cdot HCl$	219.68
bitartrate		$C_9H_{13}NO_3 \cdot C_4H_6O_6$	333.29
3-Methoxytyramine	MT		
		$C_9H_{13}NO_2$	167.21
Normetanephrine	NMN		
		$C_9H_{13}NO_3$	183.20
hydrochloride		$C_9H_{13}NO_3 \cdot HCl$	219.68
Metanephrine	MN		
		$C_{10}H_{15}NO_3$	197.23
hydrochloride		$C_{10}H_{15}NO_3 \cdot HCl$	233.70
3,4-Dihydroxyphenyl-acetic acid	DOPAC		
		$C_8H_8O_4$	168.15
3,4-Dihydroxymandelic acid	DOMA		
		$C_8H_8O_5$	184.15

Compound	Abbreviation	Formula	Mol wt
3-Methoxy-4-hydroxyphenylacetic acid (Homovanillic acid)	HVA	CH_3O—phenyl—CH_2COOH, HO— $C_9H_{10}O_4$	182.18
3-Methoxy-4-hydroxymandelic acid (Vanillylmandelic acid, Vanilmandelic acid)	VMA	CH_3O—phenyl—$CH(OH)COOH$, HO— $C_9H_{10}O_5$	198.18
3-4-Dihydroxyphenethanol	DHPE	HO—phenyl—CH_2CH_2OH, HO— $C_8H_{10}O_3$	154.17
3,4-Dihydroxyphenylglycol	DHPG	HO—phenyl—$CH(OH)CH_2OH$, HO— $C_8H_{10}O_4$	170.17
3-Methoxy-4-hydroxyphenethanol	MHPE	CH_3O—phenyl—CH_2CH_2OH, HO— $C_9H_{12}O_3$	168.20
3-Methoxy-4-hydroxyphenylglycol	MHPG	CH_3O—phenyl—$CH(OH)CH_2OH$, HO— $C_9H_{12}O_4$	184.20
3-Methoxy-4-hydroxybenzoic acid (Vanillic acid)		CH_3O—phenyl—$COOH$, HO— $C_8H_8O_4$	168.14

Compound	Abbreviation	Formula	Mol wt
Tyramine			
		$C_8H_{11}NO$	137.18
hydrochloride		$C_8H_{11}NO \cdot HCl$	173.74
Octopamine			
		$C_8H_{11}NO_2$	153.18
hydrochloride		$C_8H_{11}NO_2 \cdot HCl$	189.65
Tryptophan	Trp TP		
		$C_{11}H_{12}N_2O_2$	204.22
5-Hydroxytryptophan	5-HTP		
		$C_{11}H_{12}N_2O_3$	220.22
Tryptamine			
		$C_{10}H_{12}N_2$	160.21
hydrochloride		$C_{10}H_{12}N_2 \cdot HCl$	196.69
Serotonin (5-Hydroxytryptamine)	5-HT		
		$C_{10}H_{12}N_2O$	176.22
hydrochloride		$C_{10}H_{12}N_2O \cdot HCl$	212.69
picrate		$C_{10}H_{12}N_2O \cdot C_6H_3N_3O_7 \cdot H_2O$	423.35
creatinine sulfate complex		$C_{14}H_{23}N_5O_7S$	405.44

Compound	Abbreviation	Formula	Mol wt
Indoleacetic acid	IA	$C_{10}H_9NO_2$	175.19
5-Hydroxyindoleacetic acid	5-HIA	$C_{10}H_9NO_3$	191.19

IIb. Abbreviations of Enzymes Related to Catecholamine Metabolism Frequently Used in Literatures

TH   Tyrosine hydroxylase
DDC   DOPA decarboxylase
DBH   Dopamine-β-hydroxylase
PNMT   Phenylethanolamine-N-methyltransferase
COMT   Catechol-O-methyltransferase
MAO   Monoamine oxidase

SUPPLEMENT*

Fluorometric determination of primary amines with a new reagent, RO 20-7234, Fluorescamine

The structure of the fluorophor in the procedure for the fluorometric determination of primary amines using ninhydrin and phenylacetaldehyde (Samejima, Dairman and Udenfriend, 1971; Samejima, Dairman, Stone and Udenfriend, 1971) has been determined (Weigele M., Blount J.F., Tengi J.P., Czajkowski, R.C. and Leimgruber, W. 1972), and a novel reagent, 4-phenylspiro[furan-2(3H),1'-phthalan]-3,3'-dione (fluorescamine) synthesized. This reagent reacts with primary amines to yield a fluorophor identical to that produced by ninhydrin and phenylacetaldehyde (Udenfriend, personal communication, 1972).

RO 20-7234   Major fluorophor

Reaction of RO 20-7234 (fluorescamine) with primary amines

Conditions for reaction are as follows: The reaction is carried out at room temperature. Place 0.1 ml of the amine solution in a cuvette. Add 1.4 ml of 0.20 M sodium borate, pH 9.0 and mix. Add 0.5 ml of the reagent (fluorescamine) in acetone (60 mg/100 ml) and mix immediately and rapidly. Measure the fluorescence with the excitation at 390 nm and the emmission at 490 nm at a standard time after mixing. By using this new reagent in an automated flow system, a highly sensitive amino acid analyzer with a sensitivity in the picomole range has been constructed. Other column chromatographlc systems have also been developed for primary amines, peptides and proteins at the Roche Institute of Molecular Biology in Nutley, New Jersey (Udenfriend, S., personal communication, 1972).

---

* Supplement references on pages 352–353.

Catecholamines do not react with fluorescamine in borate buffer, but react in phosphate buffer. To 100 μl of a catecholamine sample, 1.4 ml of 0.05 M phosphate buffer, pH 8.0 and 0.5 ml of fluorescamine solution (30 mg/100 ml dioxane) are added in this order by mixing immediately at each addition. The fluorescence intesively is measured at 390 nm excitation and 475 nm emission.

Immunohistochemical localization of the enzymes of catecholamine biosynthesis.

Recent progress in purification of the enzymes of catecholamine biosynthesis made it possible to provide antibodies which are necessary for immunohistochemical localization. The first success in immunofluorescent localization was reported on dopamines-β-hydroxylase in adrenal medulla and brain (Hartman and Udenfriend, 1970; Livett, Geffen and Rush, 1969; Geffen, Livett and Rush, 1969). Immunohistochemical studies were also reported on other enzymes such as phenylethanolamine-N-methyltransferase (Fuxe, Goldstein, Hökfelt and Joh, 1971; Goldstein, Fuxe, Hökfelt and Joh, 1971). The immunohistochemical method for dopamine-β-hydroxylase (Hartman and Udenfriend, 1970) has been further improved so that it is now possible to observe noradrenergic cell bodies, non-terminal fibres and terminals in the rat brain (Hartman, Zide and Udenfriend, 1972). These immunohistochemical studies will certainly open an entirely new field in catecholamine research.

Assay of tyrosine hydroxylase activity by coupled decarboxylation of DOPA formed from L-tyrosine-1-C^{14}

A similar procedure as the $C^{14}O_2$ assay method for DOPA decarboxylase activity is applicable for the assay of tyrosine hydroxylase activity based on the coupled decarboxylation of DOPA formed from L-tyrosine-1-C^{14} (Waymire, Bjur and Weiner, 1971). Since aromatic L-amino acid decarboxylase has a higher affinity for L-DOPA compared to L-tyrosine (K_m for L-DOPA, $5.6 \times 10^{-4} M$; and K_m for L-tyrosine, $2.0 \times 10^{-2} M$), the L-DOPA-1-C^{14} which is formed enzymatically from L-tyrosine-1-C^{14} by tyrosine hydroxylase can preferentially decarboxylated to produce $C^{14}O_2$ by aromatic L-amino acid decarboxylase (Waymire, Bjur and Weiner, 1971). This method was reported to be highly sensitive and rapid. The incubation mixture (total volume, 0.5 ml) contained (in μmoles): sodium acetate buffer, pH 6.1, 100; ferrous sulfate, 0.5; 6,7-dimethyl-5,6,7,8-tetrahydropterin

(DMPH₄), 1.0; mercaptoethanol, 20; sodium phosphate, 1.0; L-tyrosine-1-C^{14}, 0.05 (10 $\mu Ci/\mu$mole, 1.1×10^6 dpm); a crude kidney aromatic L-amino acid decarboxylase preparation (ammonium sulfate stage), 7.5 units (nmole/30 min); and pyridoxal phosphate, 0.005. The incubation was carried out at 37°C for 20 min. The reactions were stopped by adding 0.5 ml of 10% trichloroacetic acid. The radioactive CO_2 preferentially liberated from the L-DOPA-1-C^{14} which is formed from tyrosine-1-C^{14} by tyrosine hydroxylase was adsorbed on a filter paper wetted with NCS solubilizer and measured as described in the assay of DOPA decarboxylase activity based on $C^{14}O_2$ evolution from (carboxy-C^{14}) DOPA.

Assay of DOPA decarboxylase activity based on $C^{14}O_2$ evolution from (carboxy-C^{14}) DOPA*

A highly sensitive and simple assay method of DOPA decarboxylase activity has been developed based on the enzymatic decarboxylation of (carboxy-C^{14}) DOPA using a reaction vessel with a side arm (Roads and Uden-

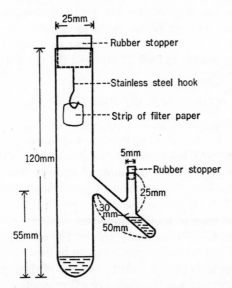

Reaction vessel for assay of DOPA decarboxylase activity
(Ellenbogen, Markley and Taylor, 1968)

---

* I wish to thank Drs. J. G. Christenson and W. Dairman for their personal information on this assay.

friend, 1968; Ellenbogen, Markley and Taylor, 1969; Christenson, Dairman and Udenfriend, 1970; Christenson, 1972). Assays were carried out in a glass test tube (25×120 mm) having a side arm, about 55 mm from the bottom, to which 0.3 ml of 35% trichloroacetic acid was added. The preincubation mixture (total volume 1.25 ml) contained (in μmole): phosphate buffer, pH 7.0, 120; pyridoxal phosphate, 0.105; mercaptoethanol, 15; and enzyme. This was preincubated at $37°C$ for 15 min, and then cooled in an ice bath. The blank, which contained water instead of enzyme, was also prepared and preincubated at the same time. Strips of Whatman 3 MM paper (about 15×23 mm) were suspended from rubber stoppers by a stainless steel hook, wetted with 0.05 ml of NCS solubilizer (Nuclear Chicago) to trap $C^{14}O_2$ formed, and allowed to dry for 10–20 min. Then 0.25 ml of 0.018 M DOPA containing 0.1 μCi of DL-(carboxy-C^{14}) DOPA in 0.02 N HCl was added to each tube. The tubes were stoppered with the paper strip centered in the tube and were incubated at $37°C$ for 15 min. After incubation, the tubes were placed in an ice bath and trichloroacetic acid in the side arm was immediately tipped in and mixed. The tubes were then incubated at $37°C$ for at least 30 min, and the paper strips were removed and counted in 10 ml of Omnifluor-dioxane scintillation mixture or Bray's scintillation mixture (Bray, 1960) to calculate the production of labeled CO_2. The CO_2 production was linear as a function of time and enzyme concentration for at least 20 min and the first 800 nmole of CO_2.

A rapid purification procedure of dopamine-β-hydroxylase

A rapid purification procedure for dopamine-β-hydroxylase from adrenal medulla of beef (Foldes, Jeffrey, Preston and Austin, 1972) and sheep (Rush and Geffen, 1972) has been reported. About 5 mg of the pure enzyme was obtained from 600 g of bovine adrenal medulla. The principle of the purification is based on the isolation of pure chromaffin granules from fresh adrenal medulla by the sucrose density gradient (Smith and Winkler, 1967a) and the subsequent solubilization and purification by DEAE-cellulose and Sephadex G-200 chromatographies. The entire purification takes only 1–2 weeks. Fresh adrenal medulla should be used as starting material. Frozen adrenal medulla cannot be used because of damage to chromaffin granules during freezing and thawing. The entire purification procedure is summarized in the following flow-chart:

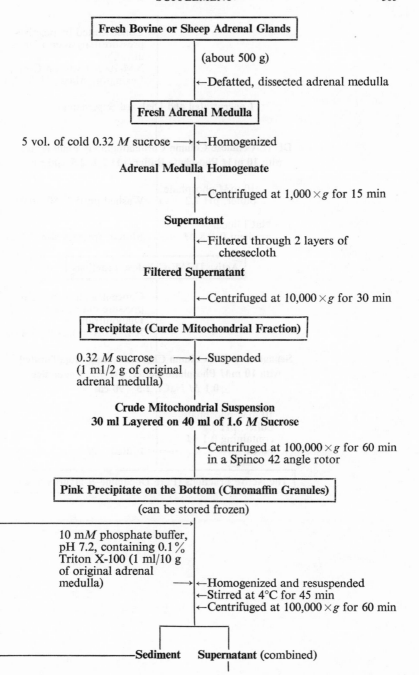

Fresh Bovine or Sheep Adrenal Glands

(about 500 g)

←Defatted, dissected adrenal medulla

Fresh Adrenal Medulla

5 vol. of cold 0.32 *M* sucrose ⟶ ←Homogenized

Adrenal Medulla Homogenate

←Centrifuged at 1,000 × *g* for 15 min

Supernatant

←Filtered through 2 layers of
   cheesecloth

Filtered Supernatant

←Centrifuged at 10,000 × *g* for 30 min

Precipitate (Curde Mitochondrial Fraction)

0.32 *M* sucrose ⟶ ←Suspended
(1 ml/2 g of original
adrenal medulla)

Crude Mitochondrial Suspension
30 ml Layered on 40 ml of 1.6 *M* Sucrose

←Centrifuged at 100,000 × *g* for 60 min
   in a Spinco 42 angle rotor

Pink Precipitate on the Bottom (Chromaffin Granules)

(can be stored frozen)

⟶

10 m*M* phosphate buffer,
pH 7.2, containing 0.1%
Triton X-100 (1 ml/10 g
of original adrenal
medulla)   ⟶ ←Homogenized and resuspended
                             ←Stirred at 4°C for 45 min
                             ←Centrifuged at 100,000 × *g* for 60 min

Sediment   Supernatant (combined)

←Concentrated by positive-
pressure dialysis on a Diafloultrafilter
XM-100A (Amicon Corp.,
Lexington, Mass., U. S. A.)

Concentrated and Dialyzed Supernatant

**DEAE-Cellulose Column Chromatography Equilibrated
with 10 mM Phosphate Buffer, pH 7.2, 2.5 × 40 cm**

10 mM phosphate
buffer, pH 7.2 ⟶ ←Washed until A280<0.05

NaCl linear
gradient 0–0.8 M ⟶ ←Eluted; fraction size, 10 ml

Active DEAE-Cellulose Fractions

←Concentrated by positive-
pressure dialysis on a
Diafloultrafilter
XM-100A to less than 4 ml

**Sephadex G-200 Column Chromatography Equilibrated
with 10 mM Phosphate Buffer, pH 7.2, Containing
0.1 M NaCl, 2.5 × 90 cm**

10 mM phosphate
buffer, pH 7.2
containing 0.1 M
NaCl   ⟶ ←Eluted

The Active Fractions (Pure Dopamine-β-Hydroxylase)

REVIEWS

Acheson, G. H., *ed*: Second symposium on catecholamines. Proceedings of the second symposium on catecholamines, Milan, July 1965. *Pharmacol. Rev.*, **18** (1966).

Bhagat, B. D.: "Recent Advances in Adrenergic Mechanisms." Charles C. Thomas Publ., Springfield, Illinois (1971).

Bulm, J. J., *ed*: "Biogenic Amines as Physiological Regulators." Prentice-Hall Inc., Englewood Cliffs, New Jersey (1970).

Cooper, J. R., Bloom, F. E. and Roth, R. H.: "The Biochemical Basis of Neuropharmacology." p. 80, Oxford University Press, London (1970).

Costa, E., Côte, L. and Yahr, M. D., *eds*: "Biochemistry and Pharmacology of the Basal Ganglia. Proceedings of the Second Symposium of Parkinson's Disease." Raven Press, New York (1966).

Costa, E. and Sandler, M., *eds*: "Monoamine Oxidase—New Vistas." Raven Press, New York (1972).

Creveling, C. R. and Daly, J. W.: Assay of enzymes of catecholamine biosynthesis and metabolism. In "Methods of Biochemical Analysis" (D. Glick, *ed*), p. 153, John Wiley & Sons, Inc., New York (1971).

Daly, J. W. and Witkop, B.: Neuere Untersuchungen über zentral wirkende endogene Amine. *Angew. Chem.*, **75**, 552 (1963).

De la Terre, J. C.: "Dynamics of Brain Monoamines." Plenum Press, New York (1972).

Euler, U. S. von: "Noradrenaline. Chemistry, Physiology, Pharmacology and Clinical Aspects." Charles C. Thomas Publ., Springfield, Illinois (1956).

Euler, U. S. von, *ed*: "Mechanism of Release of Biogenic Amines. Proceedings of the International Wenner-Gren Symposium, Stockholm, February 1965." Pergamon Press, Oxford (1966).

Finkle, B. J. and Runeckles, V. C., *eds*: "Phenolic Compounds and Metabolic Regulation." Appleton-Century-Crofts, New York (1967).

Franzen, F. and Eysell, K.: "Biologically Active Amines Found in Man." Pergamon Press, Oxford (1969).

Geffen, L. B. and Livett, B. G.: Synaptic vesicles in sympathetic neurons. *Physiol. Rev.*, **51**, 98 (1971).

Hermann, H. and Mornex, R. (translated by R. Crawford): "Human Tumours Secreting Catecholamines." Pergamon Press, Oxford (1964).

Himwich, H. E., *ed*: "Biochemistry, Schizophrenia, and Affective Illness." Williams & Wilkins Co., Baltimore (1970).

Himwich, H. E., Kety, S. S. and Symthies, J. R., *eds*: "Amines and Schizophrenia." Pergamon Press, Oxford (1967).

Hopper, G., *ed*: "Metabolism of Amines in the Brain. Proceedings of the Symposium of the British and Scandinavian Pharmacological Societies, Edinburg, 1968." Macmillan, London (1969).

Imaizumi, R., *ed*: "Catecholamine" (in Japanese), Igaku Shoin Ltd., Tokyo (1968).

Iversen, L. L.: "The Uptake and Storage of Noradrenaline in Sympathetic Nerves." Cambridge University Press, Cambridge (1967).

Kappeler-Adler, R.: "Amine Oxidase and Methods for Their Study." Wiley-Interscience, New York (1970).

Krayer, O., ed: Symposium on catecholamines. Proceedings of the first symposium on catecholamines, Bethesda, October 1958. Pharmacol. Rev., 11, (1959).

Malmfors, T. and Thoenen, H., eds: "6-Hydroxydopamine and Catecholamine Neurons." North-Holland Publ. Co., Amsterdam (1971).

Manger, W. M., ed: "Hormones and Hypertension." Charles C. Thomas Publ., Springfield, Illinois (1966).

Nagatsu, T.: Biosynthesis and metabolism of catecholamines. J. Jap. Biochem. Soc. (SEIKAGAKU) (in Japanese), 37, 697 (1965).

Pohorecky, L. A. and Wurtman, R. J.: Adrenocortical control of epinephrine synthesis. Pharmacol. Rev., 23, 1 (1971).

Reader, R., ed: Catecholamines in cardiovascular physiology and disease. Proceedings of a conference, Camberra, January 1967. Circ. Res., 21, 6, Suppl. III (1967).

Schümann, H. J. and Kronenberg, G., eds: "New Aspects of Storage and Release Mechanisms of Catecholamines. Bayer Symposium II, Grosse Ledder, Germany, October 1969." Springer-Verlag, Berlin (1970).

Udenfriends, S.: "Fluorescence Assay in Biology and Medicine, vol. 1." Academic Press, New York (1962).

Udenfriend, S.: "Fluorescence Assay in Biology and Medicine, vol. 2." Academic Press, New York (1969).

Udenfriend, S., Spector, S. (co-chairman) and Cotten, M. deV., eds: Regulation of catecholamine metabolism in the sympathetic nervous system. New York Heart Association Symposium, New York, February 1972. Pharmacol. Rev., 24, 2 (June 1972).

Umezawa, H.: "Enzyme Inhibitors of Microbial Origin." University of Tokyo Press, Tokyo (1972).

Vane, J. R., Wolstenholme, G. E. W. and O'Connor, M., eds: "Adrenergic Mechanisms (Ciba Foundation Symposium)." Churchill, London (1960).

Varley, H. and Gowenlock. A. H., eds: "The Clinical Chemistry of Monoamines. Proceedings of the Symposium on the Clinical Chemistry of Monoamines, Manchester, 1962." Elsevier Publ. Co., Amsterdam (1963).

Weil-Malherbe, H.: The estimation of total (free+conjugated) catecholamines and some catecholamine metabolites in human urine. In "Methods of Biochemical Analysis" (D. Glick, ed), vol. 16, p. 293, John Wiley & Sons, Inc., New York (1968).

Wolstenholme, G. E. W. and O'Connor, M., eds: "Adrenergic Neurotransmission (Ciba Foundation Study Groups No. 33)." Churchill, London (1968).

Wurtman, R. J.: Catecholamines. New Engl. J. Med., 273, 637, 693, 746 (1965).

REFERENCES

Abdel-Latif, A. A.: Reaction of catecholamines with hydroxylamine and its application to the assay of catechol O-methyl transferase. *Anal. Biochem.*, **29,** 468 (1969).

Abel, J. I. and Crawford, A. C.: On the blood-pressure-raising constituent of the suprarenal capsule. *Bull. Johns Hopkins Hosp.*, **8,** 151 (1897).

Ahtee, L., Sharman, D. F. and Vogt, M.: Acid metabolites of monoamines in avian brain; effects of probenecid and reserpine. *Brit. J. Pharmacol.*, **38,** 72 (1970).

Akopyan, Z. I., Stesina, L. N. and Gorkin, V. Z.: New properties of highly purified bovine liver mitochondrial monoamine oxidase. *J. Biol. Chem.*, **246,** 4610 (1971).

Aldrich, T. B.: A preliminary report on the active principle of the suprarenal gland. *Am. J. Physiol.*, **5,** 457 (1901).

Alousi, A. and Weiner, N.: The regulation of norepinephrine synthesis in sympathetic nerves: effect of nerve stimulation, cocaine, and catecholamine. *Proc. Natl. Acad. Sci. U. S. A.*, **56,** 1491 (1966).

Andén, N. E.: Serotonin and dopamine in the extrapyramidal system. Comments. *Adv. Pharmacol.*, **6,** 347 (1968).

Andén, N. E., Ross, B. E. and Werdinius, B.: On the occurrence of homovanillic acid in brain and cerebrospinal fluid and its determination by a fluorometric method. *Life Sci.*, **7,** 448 (1963).

Andén, N. E., Ross, B. E. and Werdinius, B.: Effects of chlorpromazine, haloperidol and reserpine on the levels of phenolic acids in rabbit corpus striatum. *Life Sci.*, **3,** 149 (1964).

Änggård, E. and Sedvall, G.: Gas chromatography of catecholamine metabolites using electron capture detection and mass spectrometry. *Anal. Chem.*, **41,** 1250 (1969).

Annino, J. S., Lipson, M. J. and Williams, L. A.: Quantitative determination of 3-methoxy-4-hydroxymandelic acid (VMA) in urine by thin layer chromatography. *Clin. Chem.*, **10,** 636 (1964).

Anton, A. H. and Sayre, D. F.: A study of the factors affecting the aluminum oxide. A trihydroxyindole procedure for the analysis of catecholamines. *J. Pharmacol. Exp. Therap.*, **138,** 360 (1962).

Anton, A. H. and Sayre, D. F.: The distribution of dopamine and dopa in various animals and a method for their determination in diverse biological material. *J. Pharmacol. Exp. Therap.*, **145,** 326 (1964).

Anton, A. H. and Sayre, D. F.: Distribution of metanephrine and normetanephrine in various animals and their analysis in diverse biological material. *J. Pharmacol. Exp. Therap.*, **153,** 15 (1966).

Armstrong, M. D., McMillan, A. and Shaw, K. N. F.: 3-Methoxy-4-hydroxy-D-mandelic acid, a urinary metabolite of norepinephrine. *Biochim. Biophys. Acta,* **25,** 422 (1957).

Armstrong, M. D., Shaw, K. N. F. and Wall P. E.: The phenolic acids in human

309

urine. Paper chromatography of phenolic acids. *J. Biol. Chem.*, **218**, 293 (1956).

Assicot, M. and Bohuon, C.: Purification and studies of catechol-*O*-methyltransferase of rat liver. *Eur. J. Biochem.*, **12**, 490 (1970).

Austin, L., Livett, B. G. and Chubb, I. W.: Biosynthesis of noradrenaline in sympathetic nervous tissue. *Circ. Res.*, **21**, Supple. 3, 111 (1967).

Awapara, J., Sandman, R. P. and Hanly C.: Activation of dopa decarboxylase by pyridoxal phosphate. *Arch. Biochem. Biophys.*, **98**, 520 (1962).

Axelrod, J.: *O*-Methylation of epinephrine and other catechols *in vitro* and *in vivo*. *Science*, **126**, 400 (1957).

Axelrod, J.: Presence, formation, and metabolism of normetanephrine in the brain. *Science*, **127**, 754 (1958).

Axelrod, J.: Metabolism of epinephrine and other sympathomimetic amines. *Physiol. Rev.*, **39**, 751 (1959).

Axelrod, J.: *N*-Methyladrenaline, a new catecholamine in the adrenal gland. *Biochim. Biophys. Acta*, **45**, 614 (1960 a).

Axelrod, J.: Enzymatic conversion of metanephrine to normetanephrine. *Experientia*, **16**, 502 (1960 b).

Axelrod, J.: Catechol-*O*-methyltransferase from rat liver. In "Methods in Enzymology" (S. P. Colowick and N. O. Kaplan, *eds*), Vol. 5, p. 748. Academic Press, New York (1962 a).

Axelrod, J.: Purification and properties of phenylethanolamine *N*-methyl transferase. *J. Biol. Chem.*, **237**, 1657 (1962 b).

Axelrod, J.: The enzymatic *N*-methylation of serotonin and other amines. *J. Pharmacol. Exp. Therap.*, **138**, 28 (1962 c).

Axelrod, J.: Enzymatic formation of adrenaline and other catechols from monophenols. *Science*, **140**, 499 (1963 a).

Axelrod, J.: The formation, metabolism, uptake and release of noradrenaline and adrenaline. In "The Clinical Chemistry of Monoamines" (H. Varley and A. H. Gowenlock, *eds*), p. 5. Elsevier Publ. Co., Amsterdam (1963 b).

Axelrod, J.: The uptake and release of catecholamines and the effect of drugs. In "Progress in Brain Research, Biogenic Amines" (H. E. Himwich and W. A. Himwich, eds), Vol. 8, p. 81. Elsevier Publ. Co., Amsterdam (1964 a).

Axelrod, J.: Enzymic oxidation of epinephrine to adrenochrome by the salivary gland. *Biochim. Biophys. Acta*, **85**, 247 (1964 b).

Axelrod, J.: The metabolism, storage and release of catecholamines. *Recent. Prog. Horm. Res.*, **21**, 597 (1965).

Axelrod, J.: Methylation reactions in the formation and metabolism of catecholamines and other biogenic amines. *Pharmacol. Rev.*, **18**, 95 (1966).

Axelrod, J.: Noradrenaline: fate and control of its biosynthesis. *Science*, **173**, 598 (1971a).

Axelrod, J.: Phenylethanolamine-*N*-methyltransferase (mammalian adrenal glands). In "Methods in Enzymology" (H. Tabor and C. W. Tabor, *eds*), vol. 17B, p. 761. Academic Press, New York (1971b).

Axelrod, J., Albers, W. and Clemente, C. D.: Distribution of catechol-*O*-methyl transferase in the nervous system and other tissues. *J. Neurochem.*, **5**, 68 (1959).

Axelrod, J., Hertting, G. and Patrick, R. W.: Inhibition of H^3-norepinephrine release by monoamine oxidase inhibitors. *J. Pharmacol. Exp. Therap.*, **134**, 325 (1961).

Axelrod, J., Inscoe, J K., Senoh, S. and Witkop, B.: O-Methylation, the principal pathway for the metabolism of epinephrine and norepinephrine in the rat. *Biochim. Biophys. Acta,* **27,** 210 (1958).

Axelrod, J., Kopin, I. J. and Mann, J. D.: 3-Methoxy-4-hydroxyphenylglycol sulfate, a new metabolite of epinephrine and norepinephrine. *Biochim. Biophys. Acta,* **36,** 576 (1959).

Axelrod, J. and Laroche, M. J.: Inhibition of O-methylation of epinephrine and norepinephrine *in vitro* and *in vivo. Science,* **130,** 800 (1959).

Axelrod, J. and Lerner, A. B.: O-Methylation in the conversion of tyrosine to melanin. *Biochim. Biophys. Acta,* **71,** 650 (1963).

Axelrod, J., Mueller, R. A., Henry, J. P. and Stephens, P. M.: Changes in enzymes involved in the biosynthesis and metabolism of noradrenaline and adrenaline after psychosocial stimulation. *Nature,* **225,** 1059 (1970).

Axelrod, J., Senoh, S. and Witkop, B.: O-Methylation of catecholamines *in vivo. J. Biol. Chem.,* **233,** 697 (1958).

Axelrod, J. and Tomchick, R.: Enzymatic O-methylation of catecholamines. *J. Biol. Chem.,* **233,** 702 (1958).

Axelrod, J., Weil-Malherbe, H. and Tomchick, R.: The physiological disposition of ^{3}H-epinephrine and its metabolite metanephrine. *J. Pharmacol. Exp. Therap.,* **127,** 251 (1959).

Ayukawa, S., Hamada, M., Kojiri, K., Takeuchi, T., Hara, T., Nagatsu, T. and Umezawa, H.: Studies on a new pigment antibiotic chrothiomycin. *J. Antibiotics,* **22,** 303 (1969).

Ayukawa, S., Takeuchi, T., Sezaki, M., Hara, T., Umezawa, H. and Nagatsu, T.: Inhibition of tyrosine hydroxylase by aquayamycin. *J. Antibiotics,* **21,** 350 (1968).

Bacq, Z. M., Gosselin, L., Dresse, A. and Renson, J.: Inhibition of O-methyltransferase by catechol and sensitization to epinephrine. *Science,* **130,** 453 (1959).

Bagchi, S. P. and Zarycki, E. P.: *In vivo* formation of tyrosine from phenylalanine in brain. *Life Sci.,* **9,** 111 (1970).

Banks, P. and Helle, K.: The release of protein from the stimulated adrenal medulla. *Biochem. J.,* **97,** 40 C (1965).

Barbato, L. M. and Abood, L. G.: Purification and properties of monoamine oxidase. *Biochim. Biophys. Acta,* **67,** 531 (1963).

Baudhuin, P., Beaufay, H., Rahman-Li, Y., Sellinger, O. Z. and Wattiaux, R., Jacques, P. and de Duve, C.: Tissue fractionation studies 17. Intracellular distribution of monoamine oxidase, aspartate aminotransferase, alanine aminotransferase, D-amino acid oxidase and catalase in rat liver tissue. *Biochem. J.,* **92,** 179 (1964).

Beaven, M. A. and Maickel, R. P.: Stereoselectivity of norepinephrine storage sites in the heart. *Biochem. Biophys. Res. Commun.,* **14,** 509 (1964).

Bell, C. E. and Somercille, A. R.: Identity of the "pink spot." *Nature,* **211,** 1405 (1966).

Belleau, B. and Burba, J.: Occupancy of adrenergic receptors and inhibition of pyrocatechol O-methyltransferase by tropolones. *J. Med. Chem.,* **6,** 755 (1963).

Belleau, B. and Burba, J.: Tropolones: a unique class of potent non-competitive inhibitors of S-adenosylmethionine-catechol methyltransferase. *Biochim. Bio-*

phys. Acta, **54,** 195 (1961).

Bertler, A., Carlsson, A. and Rosengren, E.: A method for the fluorimetric determination of adrenaline and noradrenaline in tissues. *Acta Physiol. Scand.,* **44,** 273 (1958).

Bertler, A., Carlsson, A. and Rosengren, E.: Fluorimetric method for differential estimation of the 3-*O*-methylated derivatives of adrenaline and noradrenaline (metanephrine and normetanephrine). *Clin. Chim. Acta,* **4,** 456 (1959).

Bertler, A., Hillarp, N.-Å. and Rosengren, E.: "Bound" and "free" catecholamines in the brain. *Acta Physiol. Scand.,* **50,** 113 (1960).

Bhagat, B. and Shideman, F. E.: Repletion of cardiac catecholamines in the rat: importance of adrenal medulla and synthesis from precursors. *J. Pharmacol. Exp. Therap.,* **143,** 77 (1964).

Birkmayer, W. and Mentasti, M.: Weitere experimentelle Untersuchungen über Catecholaminestoffwechsel bei extra-pyramidalen Erkrankungen (Parkinson und Chorea Syndrom). *Arch. Psychiat. Nervenks.,* **210,** 29 (1967).

Blaschko, H.: Amine oxidase. In: "The Enzymes" (P. D. Boyer, H. Lardy and K. Myrbäck, *eds*) vol. 8, p. 337. Academic Press, New York (1963).

Blaschko, H.: "Hypotensive drugs" (M. Harington, *ed*). p. 23. Pergamon Press, London (1956).

Blaschko, H.: The specific action of *l*-dopa decarboxylase. *J. Physiol.,* **96,** 50P (1939).

Blaschko, H. and Bonney, R.: Spermine oxidase and benzylamine oxidase. Distribution, development and substrate specificity. *Proc. Roy. Soc. B.,* **156,** 268 (1962).

Blaschko, H., Comline, R. S., Schneider, F. H., Silver, M. and Smith, A. D.: Secretion of a chromaffin granule protein, chromogranin, from the adrenal gland after splanchnic stimulation. *Nature,* **215,** 59 (1967).

Blaschko, H., Hagen, P. and Welch, A. D.: Observations on the intracellular particles of the adrenal medulla. *J. Physiol.,* **129,** 27 (1955).

Blaschko, H. and Helle, K.: Interaction of soluble protein fractions from bovine adrenal medullary granules with adrenaline and adenosine triphosphate. *J. Physiol.,* **169,** 120P (1963).

Blaschko, H., Richter, D. and Schlossmann, H.: The inactivation of adrenaline. *J. Physiol.,* **90,** 1 (1937 a).

Blaschko, H., Richter, D. and Schlossmann H.: The oxidation of adrenaline and other amines. *Biochem. J.,* **31,** 2187 (1937 b).

Blaschko, H. and Schlossmann, H.: Decomposition of adrenaline in tissue. *Nature,* **137,** 110 (1936).

Blaschko, H. and Welch, A. D.: Localization of adrenaline in cytoplasmic particles of the bovine adrenal medulla. *Arch. Exp. Path. Pharmakol.,* **219,** 17 (1953).

Bohuon, C. and Guerinot, F.: Dopamine-β-hydroxylase humaine et bovine. Activité vis à vis de la dopamine et de la méthoxytryptamine. *Clin. Chim. Acta,* **19,** 125 (1968).

Bornstein, P., Kang, A. H. and Piez, K. A.: The nature and location of intramolecular cross-links in collagen. *Proc. Natl. Acad. Sci. U. S. A.,* **55,** 417 (1966).

Boulton, A. A. and Felton, C. A.: The "pink spot" and schizophrenia. *Nature,* **211,** 1404 (1966).

Bray, G. A.: A simple efficient liquid scintillator for counting aqueous solutions in a liquid scintillation counter. *Anal. Biochem.,* **1,** 279 (1960).

Breese, G. R., Chase, T. N. and Kopin, I. J.: Metabolism of some phenylethylamines and their β-hydroxylated analogs in brain. *J. Pharmacol. Exp. Therap.,* **165,** 136 (1968).

Brenneman, A. R. and Kaufman, S.: The role of tetrahydropteridine in the enzymatic conversion of tyrosine to 3,4-dihydroxyphenylalanine. *Biochem. Biophys. Res. Commun.,* **17,** 177 (1964).

Brenneman, A. R. and Kaufman, S.: Characteristics of the hepatic phenylalanine-hydroxylating system in newborn rats. *J. Biol. Chem.,* **240,** 3617 (1965).

Bridgers, W. F. and Kaufman, S.: The enzymatic conversion of epinine to epinephrine. *J. Biol. Chem.,* **237,** 526 (1962).

Brodie, B. B., Costa, E., Dlabac, A., Neff, N. H. and Smookler, N. H.: Application of steady state kinetics to the estimation of synthesis rate and turnover time of tissue catecholamines. *J. Pharmacol. Exp. Therap.,* **154,** 493 (1966).

Brodie, B. B., Davies, J. I., Hynie, S., Krishna, G. and Weiss, B.: Interrelationships of catecholamines with other endocrine systems. *Pharmacol. Rev.,* **18,** 273 (1966).

Brodie, B. B., Spector, S. and Shore, P. A.: Interaction of drugs with norepinephrine in the brain. *Pharmacol. Rev.,* **11,** 548 (1959).

Brunjes, S., Wybenga, D. and Johns, V. J., Jr.: Fluorometric determination of urinary metanephrine and normetanephrine. *Clin. Chem.,* **10,** 1 (1964).

Bublitz, C.: A direct assay for liver phenylalanine hydroxylase. *Biochim. Biophys. Acta,* **191,** 249 (1969).

Bülbring, E.: Methylation of noradrenaline by minced suprarenal tissue. *Brit. J. Pharmacol.,* **4,** 234 (1949).

Bu'Lock, J. and Harley-Mason, J.: The chemistry of adrenochrome. Part II. Some analogues and derivatives. *J. Chem. Soc.,* 712 (1951).

Burack, W. R. and Draskóczy, P. R.: The turnover of endogenously labelled catecholamines in several regions of the sympathetic nervous system. *J. Pharmacol. Exp. Therap.,* **144,** 66 (1964).

Burkard, W. P., Pavlin, R., Pletscher, A. and Gey, K. F.: Effect of psychotropic drugs on decarboxylase of aromatic amino acids in rat brain. *Int. J. Neuropharmacol.,* **1,** 233 (1962).

Carlsson, A.: Detection and assay of dopamine. *Pharmacol. Rev.,* **11,** 300 (1959 a).

Carlsson, A.: The occurrence, distribution and physiological role of catecholamines in the nervous system. *Pharmacol. Rev.,* **11,** 490 (1959 b).

Carlsson, A., Hillarp, N.-Å. and Waldeck, B.: Analysis of the Mg^{++} - ATP dependent storage mechanism in the amine granules of the adrenal medulla. *Acta Physiol. Scand.,* **59,** supple. 215 (1963).

Carlsson, A. and Lindqvist, M.: A method for the determination of normetanephrine in brain. *Acta Physiol. Scand.,* **54,** 83 (1962).

Carlsson, A. and Lindqvist, M., Magnusson, T. and Waldeck, B.: On the presence of 3-hydroxytyramine in brain. *Science,* **127,** 471 (1958).

Carlsson, A. and Waldeck, B.: A fluorimetric method for the determination of dopamine (3-hydroxytyramine). *Acta Physiol. Scand.,* **44,** 293 (1958).

Carlsson, A. and Waldeck, B.: A method for the fluorimetric determination of 3-

methoxytyramine in tissues and the occurrence of this amine in brain. *Scand. J. Clin. Lab. Invest.,* **16,** 133 (1964).

Carver, M. L.: Influence of phenylalanine administration on the free amino acids of brain and liver in the rat. *J. Neurochem.,* **12,** 45 (1965).

Ceasar, P. M., Ruthven, C. R. J. and Sandler, M.: Catecholamine and 5-hydroxy-indole metabolism in immunosympathectomized rats. *Brit. J. Pharmacol.,* **36,** 70 (1969).

Chang, C. C., Costa, E. and Brodie, B. B.: Interaction of guanethidine with ad-renergic neurons. *J. Pharmacol. Exp. Therap.,* **147,** 303 (1965).

Chirigos, M. A., Greengard, P. and Udenfriend, S.: Uptake of tyrosine by rat brain *in vivo. J. Biol. Chem.,* **235,** 2075 (1960).

Christenson, J. G., Dairman, W. and Udenfriend, S.: Preparation and properties of a homogeneous aromatic L-amino acid decarboxylase. *Archs. Biochem. Biophys.,* **141,** 356 (1970).

Chruściel, T. L.: Observations on the localization of noradrenaline in homo-genates of dog's hypothalamus. In " Adrenergic Mechanisms" (J. R. Vane, G. E. W. Wolstenholme and M. O'Connor, *eds*), p.539. J. & A. Churchill Ltd., London (1960).

Ciaranello, R. D., Barchas, R. E., Byers, G. S., Stemmle, D. W. and Barchas, J. P.: Enzymatic synthesis of adrenaline in mammalian brain. *Nature,* **221** 368 (1969).

Clark, C. T., Weissbach, H. and Udenfriend, S.: 5-Hydroxytryptophan decar-boxylase: preparation and properties. *J. Biol. Chem.,* **210,** 139 (1954).

Clarke, D. D., Wilk, S., Gitlow, S. E. and Franklin, M. J.: Gas-chromatographic determination of dopamine at the nanogram level. *J. Gas Chromatog.,* **5,** 307 (1967).

Clark, W. G.: Studies on inhibition of L-DOPA-decarboxylase *in vitro* and *in vivo. Pharmacol. Rev.,* **11,** 330 (1959).

Clark, W. G., Akawie, R. I., Pogrund, R. S. and Geissman, T. A.: Conjugation of epinephrine *in vivo. J. Pharmacol. Exp. Therap.,* **101,** 6 (1951).

Clineschmidt, B. V. and Horita, A.: The monoamine oxidase catalyzed degrada-tion of phenelzine-1-^{14}C, an irreversible inhibitor of monoamine oxidase-I. Studies *in vitro. Biochem. Pharmacol.,* **18,** 1011 (1969 a).

Clineschmidt, B. V. and Horita, A.: The monoamine oxidase catalyzed degrada-tion of phenelzine-1-^{14}C, an irreversible inhibitor of monoamine oxidase-II. Studies *in vivo. Biochem. Pharmacol.,* **18,** 1021 (1969 b).

Cohen, G. and Goldenberg, M.: The simultaneous fluorimetric determination of adrenaline and noradrenaline in plasma. *J. Neurochem.,* **2,** 58 (1957).

Collins, G. G. S., Sandler, M., Williams, E. D. and Youdim, M. B. H.: Multiple forms of human brain mitochondrial monoamine oxidase. *Nature,* **225,** 817 (1970).

Collins, G. G. S. and Youdim, M. B. H.: Further properties of multiple forms of mitochondrial monoamine oxidase. *Biochem. J.,* **114,** 80p (1969).

Collins, G. G. S. and Youdim, M. B. H. and Sandler, M.: Isoenzymes of human and rat liver monoamine oxidase. *FEBS Letters,* **1,** 215 (1968).

Conner, J. D.: Caudate nucleus neurons: correlation of the effects of substantia nigra stimulation with iontophoretic dopamine. *J. Physiol.,* **208,** 691 (1970).

Connett, R. J. and Kirshner, N.: Purification and properties of bovine phenyl-ethanolamine *N*-methyltransferase. *J. Biol. Chem.,* **245,** 329 (1970).

Corrodi, H. and Hillarp, N.-Å.: Fluoreszenzmethoden zur histochemischen Sichtbarmachung von Monoaminen. 1. Identifizierung der fluoreszierenden Produkte aus Modellversuchen mit 6,7-dimethoxy-isochinolinderivaten und Formaldehyd. *Helv. Chim. Acta,* **46,** 2425 (1963).

Corrodi, H. and Hillarp, N.-Å.: Fluoreszenzmethoden zur histochemischen Sichtbarmachung von Monoaminen. 2. Identifizierung des fluoreszierenden Produktes aus Dopamine und Formaldehyd. *Helv. Chim. Acta,* **47,** 911 (1964).

Corrodi, H., Hillarp, N.-Å. and Jonsson, G.: Fluorescence methods for the histochemical demonstration of monoamines. Sodium borohydride reduction of the fluorescent compounds as a specificity test. *J. Histochem. Cytochem.,* **12,** 582 (1964).

Corrodi, H. and Jonsson, G.: Fluorescence methods for the histochemical demonstration of monoamines. 4. Histochemical differentiation between dopamine and noradrenaline in models. *J. Histochem. Cytochem.,* **13,** 484 (1965).

Costa, E., Boullin, D. J., Hammer, W., Vogel, W. and Brodie, B. B.: Interactions of drugs with adrenergic neurons. *Pharmacol. Rev.,* **18,** 577 (1966).

Costa, E. and Neff, N. E.: Isotopic and non-isotopic measurements of the rate of catecholamine biosynthesis. In: "Biochemistry and Pharmacology of Basal Ganglia. Proceedings of the second symposium of Parkinson's disease" (E. Costa, L. Côté and M. D. Yahr, *eds*), p. 141, Raven Press, New York (1966).

Cotton, R. G. H.: Phenylalanine hydroxylase of *Macaca Irus.* Purification of two components of the enzyme. *Biochim. Biophys. Acta,* **235,** 61 (1971).

Cotzias, G. C. and Dole, V. P.: Metabolism of amines; mitochondrial localization of monoamine oxidase. *Proc. Soc. Exp. Biol. Med.,* **78,** 157 (1951).

Cotzias, G. C., Papavasiliou, P. S. and Gellene, R.: Modification of parkinsonism —chronic treatment with L-DOPA. *New Engl. J. Med.,* **280,** 337 (1969).

Cotzias, G. C., Serlin, I. and Greenough, J. J.: Preparation of soluble monoamine oxidase. *Science,* **120,** 144 (1954).

Coward, R. F. and Smith, P.: A new screening test for pheochromocytoma. *Clin. Chim. Acta,* **13,** 538 (1966).

Craig, C. R., Azzaro, A. J., Frame, B. K. and Hunt, W. A.: Automated fluorometric method for the determination of dopamine (3-hydroxytyramine). *Advan. Automat. Anals.,* **2,** 189 (1970).

Crawford, T. B. B.: Derivatives of adrenaline and noradrenaline in an extract of an adrenal medullary tumour. *Biochem. J.,* **48,** 203 (1951).

Crawford, T. B. B. and Yates, C. M.: A method for the estimation of the catecholamines and their metabolites in brain tissue. *Brit. J. Pharmacol.,* **38,** 56 (1970).

Creasey, N. H.: Factors which interfere in the manometric assay of monoamine oxidase. *Biochem. J.,* **64,** 178 (1956).

Creveling, C. R.: Studies on dopamine-β-oxidase. Doctoral Thesis, George Washington University, Washington, D. C. (1962).

Creveling, C. R., Barchas, J., Nagatsu, T., Levitt, M. and Udenfriend, S.: The anatomical distribution of tyrosine hydroxylase and DOPA decarboxylase in canine brain. Unpublished results (1972).

Creveling, C. R. and Daly, J. W.: Identification of 3,4-dimethoxyphenethylamine from schizophrenic urine by mass spectrometry. *Nature,* **216,** 190 (1967).

Creveling, C. R. and Daly, J. W.: The use of dancyl derivatives for the identification and quantitation of amines. In "Methods in Enzymology" (H. Tabor and

C. W. Tabor, *eds*), vol. 17B, p. 846. Adademic Press, New York (1971).

Creveling, C. R., Daly, J. W., Witkop, B. and Udenfriend, S.: Substrates and inhibitors of dopamine-β-oxidase. *Biochim. Biophys. Acta,* **64,** 125 (1962).

Creveling, C. R., Levitt, M. and Udenfriend, S.: An alternative route for biosynthesis of norepinephrine. *Life. Sci.,* No. 10, 523 (1962).

Creveling, C. R., van der Schoot, J. B. and Udenfriend, S.: Phenethylamine isosters as inhibitors of dopamine-β-oxidase. *Biochem. Biophys. Res. Commun.,* **8,** 215 (1962).

Crout, J. R.: Catecholamines in urine. In "Standard Methods of Clinical Chemistry" (Seligson D., *ed*), vol. 3, p. 62. Academic Press, New York (1961).

Crout, J. R.: Sampling and analysis of catecholamines and metabolites. *Anesthesiology,* **29,** 661 (1968).

Crout, J. R., Creveling, C. R. and Udenfriend, S.: Norepinephrine metabolism in rat brain and heart. *J. Pharmacol. Exp. Therap.,* **132,** 269 (1961).

Dahlström, A. and Fuxe, K.: Evidence for the existence of monoamine-containing neurons in the central nervous system. *Acta Physiol. Scand.,* **62,** Suppl. 232 (1964).

Dairman, W. and Udenfriend, S.: Decrease in adrenal tyrosine hydroxylase and increase in norepinephrine synthesis in rats given L-DOPA. *Science,* **171,** 1022 (1971).

Dairman, W. and Udenfriend, S.: Increased conversion of tyrosine to catecholamines in the intact rat following elevation of tissue tyrosine hydroxylase levels by administered phenoxybenzamine. *Mol. Pharmacol.,* **6,** 350 (1970).

Daly, J. W., Axelrod, J. and Witkop, B.: Dynamic aspects of enzymatic O-methylation and O-demethylation of catechols *in vitro* and *in vivo. J. Biol. Chem.,* **235,** 1155 (1960).

Daly, J. W., Benigni, J., Minnis, R., Kanaoka, Y. and Witkop, B.: Synthesis and metabolism of 6-hydroxycatecholamines. *Biochemistry,* **4,** 2513 (1965).

Daly, J. W. and Guroff, G.: Production of *m*-methyltyrosine and *p*-hydroxymethylphenylalanine from *p*-methylphenylalanine by phenylalanine hydroxylase. *Arch. Biochem. Biophys.,* **125,** 136 (1968).

Daly, J. W., Horner, L. and Witkop, B.: Chemical and enzymatic routes to methoxydopamines. *J. Am. Chem. Soc.,* **83,** 4787 (1961).

Daly, J. W., Levitt, M., Guroff, G. and Udenfriend, S.: Isotope studies on the mechanism of action of adrenal tyrosine hydroxylase. *Arch. Biochem. Biophys.,* **126,** 593 (1968).

Daly, J. W. and Witkop, B.: Neuere Untersuchungen über zentral wirkende endogene Amine. *Angew. Chem.,* **75,** 552 (1963).

Davis, V. E. and Awapara, J.: A method for the determination of some amino acid decarboxylase. *J. Biol. Chem.,* **235,** 124 (1960).

Davison, A. N.: Physiological role of monoamine oxidase. *Physiol. Rev.,* **38,** 729 (1958).

Dawson, R. M. C., Elliott, D. C., Elliott, W. H. and Jones, K. M., (eds): "Data for Biochemical Research," 2nd Ed. Clarendon Press, Oxford (1969)

De Champlain, J., Mueller, R. A. and Axelrod, J.: Subcellular localization of monoamine oxidase in rat tissues. *J. Pharmacol. Exp. Therap.,* **166,** 339 (1969).

DeEds, F., Booth, A. N. and Jones, F. F.: Methylation and dehydroxylation of phenolic compounds by rats and rabbits. *J. Biol. Chem.,* **225,** 615 (1957).

Deitrich, R. A. and Erwin, V. G.: A convenient spectrophotometric assay for monoamine oxidase. *Anal. Biochem., 30,* 395 (1969).

Demis, D. J., Blaschko, H. and Welch, A. D.: The conversion of dihydroxyphenylalanine-2-^{14}C (dopa) to norepinephrine by bovine adrenal medullary homogenates. *J. Pharmacol. Exp. Therap., 113,* 14 (1955).

Demis, D. J., Blaschko, H. and Welch, A. D.: The conversion of dihydroxyphenylalanine-2-^{14}C (dopa) to norepinephrine by bovine adrenal medullary homogenates. *J. Pharmacol. Exp. Therap., 117,* 208 (1956).

Denber, H. C. B.: Some current biochemical theories concerning schizophrenia. In "Biochemistry of Brain and Behavior" (R. E. Bowman and S. P. Datta, *eds*) p. 171. Plenum Press, New York-London (1970).

De Potter, W. P., Vochten, R. F. and de Schaepdryver, A. F.: Thin-layer chromatography of catecholamines and their metabolites. *Experientia, 21,* 482 (1965).

DeQuattro, V., Nagatsu, T., Maronde, R. and Alexander, N.: Catecholamine synthesis in rabbits with neurogenic hypertension. *Circ. Res., 24,* 545 (1969).

DeQuattro, V., Wybenga, D., Studnitz, W. von. and Brunjes, S.: Determination of urinary 3,4-dihydroxymandelic acid. *J. Lab. Clin. Med., 63,* 864 (1964).

De Robertis, E.: Adrenergic endings and vesicles isolated from brain. *Pharmacol. Rev., 18,* 413 (1966).

De Robertis, E., Pellegrino de Iraldi, A., Rodríguez de Lores Arnaiz, G. and Zieher, L. M.: Synaptic vesicles from the rat hypothalamus. *Life Sci., 4,* 193 (1965).

Diliberto, E. J. and DiStefano, V.: Unidimensional chromatographic separation of dansyl catecholamines. *Anal. Biochem., 32,* 281 (1969).

Dodgson, K. S., Garton, G. A. and Williams, R. T.: The conjugation of *d*-adrenaline and certain catechol derivatives in the rabbit. *Biochem. J., 41,* 1 (1947).

Dominic, J. A. and Moore, K. E.: Behavioral and catechol amine depleting effects of α-methyl-5-hydroxytryptophan. *Europ. J. Pharmacol., 8,* 292 (1969).

Douglas, W. W.: Stimulus-secretion coupling: the concept and clues from chromaffin and other cells. *Brit. J. Pharmacol., 34,* 451 (1968).

Douglas, W. W. and Rubin, R. P.: The role of calcium in the secretory response of the adrenal medulla to acetylcholine. *J. Physiol., 159,* 40 (1961).

Drain, D. J., Horlington, M., Lazare, R. and Poulter, G. A.: The effect of α-methyl dopa and some decarboxylase inhibitors on brain 5-hydroxytryptamine. *Life Sci., 1,* 93 (1962).

Drujan, B. D., Alvarez, N. and Díaz Borges, J. M.: A method for determination of 3,4-dihydroxyphenylacetic acid and 3,4-dihydroxymandelic acid in urine. *Anal. Biochem., 15,* 8 (1966).

Drujan, B. D., Sourkes, T. L., Layne, D. S. and Murphy, G. F.: The differential determination of catecholamines in urine. *Can. J. Biochem. Biophys., 37,* 1153 (1959).

Duch, D. S. and Kirshner, N.: Isolation and partial characterization of an endogenous inhibitor of dopamine-β-hydroxyrase. *Biochim. Biophys. Acta, 236,* 628 (1971).

Duch, D. S., Vireros, O. H. and Kirshner, N.: Endogenous inhibitor(s) in adrenal medulla of dopamine-β-hydroxylase. *Biochem. Pharmacol., 17,* 255 (1968).

Dutton, G. J. and Storey, I. D. E.: Uridine compounds in glucuronic acid metabolism; formation of glucuronides in liver suspensions. *Biochem. J.,* **57,** 275 (1954).

Ehrlén, I.: Fluorimetric determination of adrenaline II. *Farm. Revy.,* **47,** 242 (1948).

Ellenbogen, L., Taylor, R. J., Jr. and Brundage, G. B.: On the role of pteridines as cofactors for tyrosine hydroxylase. *Biochem. Biophys. Res. Commun.,* **19,** 708 (1965).

Elmadjian, F., Lamson, E. T. and Neri, R.: The nature of adrenaline and noradrenaline in normal human urine. *J. Clin. Endocrinol, Metab.,* **16,** 216 (1956).

Engelman, K. and Portnoy, B.: A sensitive double-isotope derivative assay for norepinephrine and epinephrine. *Circ. Res.,* **26,** 53 (1970).

Engelman, K., Portnoy, B. and Lovenberg, W.: A sensitive and specific double-isotope derivative method for the determination of catecholamines in biological specimens. *Am. J. Med. Sci.,* **255,** 259 (1968).

Eränko, O.: The histochemical demonstration of noradrenaline in the adrenal medulla of rats and mice. *J. Histochem. Cytochem.,* **4,** 11 (1955).

Erspamer, V. and Boretti, G.: Identification and characterization, by paper chromatography, of enteramine, octopamine, tyramine, histamine and allied substances in extracts of posterior salivary glands of octopoda and in other tissue extracts of vertebrates and invertebrates. *Arch. Int. Pharmacodyn. Thér.,* **88,** 296 (1951).

Erwin, V. G. and Hellerman, L.: Mitochondrial monoamine oxidase I. Purification and characterization of the bovine kidney enzyme. *J. Biol. Chem.,* **242,** 4230 (1967).

Euler, U. S. von: Presence of a substance with sympathin E properties in spleen extracts. *Acta Physiol. Scand.,* **11,** 168 (1946 a).

Euler, U. S. von: Presence of a sympathomimetic substance in extracts of mammalian heart. *J. Physiol.,* **105,** 38 (1946 b).

Euler, U. S. von: A specific sympathomimetic ergone in adrenergic nerve fibres (sympathin) and its relation to adrenaline and nor-adrenaline. *Acta Physiol. Scand.,* **12,** 73 (1946 c).

Euler, U. S. von.: "Noradrenaline," p. 166. Charles C. Thomas Publ., Springfield, Illinois (1956).

Euler, U. S. von: The presence of the adrenergic neurotransmitter in intraaxonal structures. *Acta Physiol. Scand.,* **43,** 155 (1958).

Euler, U. S. von: Twenty years of noradrenaline. *Pharmacol. Rev.,* **18,** 29 (1966 a).

Euler, U. S. von: Release and uptake of noradrenaline in adrenergic nerve granules. *Acta Physiol. Scand.,* **67,** 430 (1966 b).

Euler, U. S. von: Adrenergic neurotransmitter functions. *Science,* **173,** 202 (1971).

Euler, U. S. von. and Floding, I.: A fluorimetric method for differential estimation of adrenaline and noradrenaline. *Acta Physiol. Scand.,* **33,** Suppl. 118, 45 (1955 a).

Euler, U. S. von and Floding, I.: Fluorimetric estimation of noradrenaline and adrenaline in urine. *Acta Physiol. Scand.,* **33,** Suppl. 118, 57 (1955 b).

Euler, U. S. von and Hamberg, U.: *l*-Noradrenaline in the suprarenal medulla. *Nature,* **163,** 642 (1949 a).

Euler, U. S. von and Hamberg, U.: Colorimetric determination of noradrenaline and adrenaline. *Acta Physiol. Scand.*, **19**, 74 (1949 b).

Euler, U. S. von and Hillarp, N.-Å.: Evidence for the presence of noradrenaline in submicroscopic structures of adrenergic axons. *Nature*, **177**, 44 (1956).

Euler, U. S. von and Lishajko, F.: The estimation of catechol amines in urine. *Acta physiol. Scand.*, **45**, 122 (1959).

Euler, U. S. von and Lishajko, F.: Release of noradrenaline from adrenergic transmitter granules by tyramine. *Experientia*, **16**, 376 (1960).

Euler, U. S. von and Lishajko, F.: Noradrenaline release from isolated nerve granules. *Acta Physiol. Scand.*, **51**, 193 (1961 a).

Euler, U. S. von and Lishajko, F.: Improved technique for the fluorimetric estimation of catecholamines. *Acta Physiol. Scand.*, **51**, 348 (1961 b).

Euler, U. S. von and Lishajko, F.: Effect of adenine nucleotides on catecholamine release and uptake in isolated adrenergic nerve granules. *Acta Physiol. Scand.*, **59**, 454 (1963 a).

Euler, U. S. von and Lishajko, F.: Effect of reserpine on the uptake of catecholamines in isolated nerve storage granules. *Int. J. Neuropharmacol.*, **2**, 127 (1963 b).

Euler, U. S. von, Lishajko, F. and Stjärne, L.: Catecholamines and adenosine triphosphate in isolated adrenergic nerve granules. *Acta Physiol. Scand.*, **59**, 495 (1963).

Euler, U. S. von and Orwén, I.: Preparation of extracts of urine and organs for estimation of free and conjugated noradrenaline. *Acta Physiol. Scand.*, **33**, Suppl. 118, 1 (1955).

Euler, U. S. von, Stjärne, L. and Lishajko, F.: Uptake of radioactively labeled DL-catecholamines in isolated adrenergic nerve granules with and without reserpine. *Life Sci.*, No. **11**, 878 (1963).

Fahn, S., Rodman, J. S. and Côté, L. J.: Association of tyrosine hydroxylase with synaptic vesicles in bovine caudate nucleus. *J. Neurochem.*, **16**, 1293 (1969).

Falck, B.: Observations on the possibilities of the cellular localization of monoamines by a fluorescence method. *Acta Physiol. Scand.*, **56**, Suppl. 197 (1962).

Falck, B., Hillarp, N.-Å., Thieme, G. and Torp, A.: Fluorescence of catecholamines and related compounds condensed with formaldehyde. *J. Histochem. Cytochem.*, **10**, 348 (1962).

Falck, B. and Owman, C.: A detailed methodological description of the fluorescence method for the cellular demonstration of biogenic monoamines. *Acta Univ. Lund.* Sectio II, No. 7 (1965).

Fellman, J. H.: Purification and properties of adrenal L-DOPA decarboxylase. *Enzymologia*, **20**, 366 (1959).

Finkle, B. J. and Nelson, R. F.: Enzyme reaction with phenolic compounds by a meta O-methyl transferase in plants. *Biochim. Biophys. Acta*, **78**, 747 (1963).

Fischer, A. G., Schulz, A. R. and Oliner, L.: The possible role of thyroid monoamine oxidase in iodothyronine synthesis. *Life Sci.*, **5**, 995 (1966).

Fisher, D. B. and Kaufman, S.: The effect of enzyme concentration, ionic strength, and temperature on the stoichiometry of the phenylalanine hydroxylase reaction. *Biochem. Biophys. Res. Communs.*, **38**, 663 (1970).

Fisher, D. B., Kirkwood, R. and Kaufman, S.: Rat liver phenylalanine hydroxylase, an iron enzyme. *J. Biol. Chem.*, **247**, 5161 (1972).

Fischer, J. E., Kopin, I. J. and Axelrod, J.: Evidence for extraneuronal binding of norepinephrine. *J. Pharmacol. Exp. Therap.,* **147,** 181 (1965).

Fischer, P.: Sur la substance responsable de la fluorescence de l'adrenaline. *Bull. Soc. Chim. Belges.,* **58,** 205 (1949).

Fleming, R. M., Clark, W. G., Fenster, E. D. and Towne, J. C.: Single extraction method for the simultaneous fluorometric determination of serotonin, dopamine and norepinephrine in brain. *Anal. Chem.,* **37,** 692 (1965).

Forn, J., Maling, H. M. and Gessa, G. L.: Homovanillic and 5-hydroxyindoleacetic acids in cerebrospinal fluid after probenecid: measurement of brain monoamine oxidase inhibition *in vivo. Proc. Soc. Exp. Biol. Med.,* **133,** 1310 (1970).

Franklin, M. J. and Mayer, J.: Advantages of the double isotope approach to catecholamine analysis. *Atomlight,* No. **67,** p. 1, New England Nuclear Corp., Boston, Mass. (1968).

Friedhoff, A. J. and Van Winkle, E.: Isolation and characterization of a compound from the urine of schizophrenics. *Nature,* **194,** 897 (1962).

Friedhoff, A. J. and Van Winkle, E.: Conversion of dopamine to 3,4-dimethoxyphenylacetic acid in schizophrenic patients. *Nature,* **199,** 1271 (1963).

Friedman, S. and Kaufman, S.: 3,4-Dihydroxyphenylethylamine β-hydroxylase: a copper protein *J. Biol. Chem.,* **240,** PC552 (1965 a).

Friedman, S. and Kaufman, S.: 3,4-Dihydroxyphenylethylamine β-hydroxylase. Physical properties, copper content, and role of copper in the catalytic activity. *J. Biol. Chem.,* **240,** 4763 (1965 b).

Friedman, S. and Kaufman, S.: An electron paramagnetic resonance study of 3,4-dihydroxyphenylethylamine β-hydroxylase. *J. Biol. Chem.,* **241,** 2256(1966).

Fuller, R. W. and Hunt, J. M.: Substrate specificity of phenylethanolamine *N*-methyl transferase. *Biochem. Pharmacol.,* **14,** 1896 (1965).

Fuller, R. W. and Hunt, J. M.: Activity of phenylethanolamine *N*-methyl transferase in the adrenal glands of foetal and neonatal rats. *Nature,* **214,** 190 (1967).

Gál, E. M. and Millard, S. A.: The mechanism of inhibition of hydroxylases *in vivo* by *p*-chlorophenylalanine: the effect of cycloheximide. *Biochim. Biophys. Acta,* **227,** 32 (1971).

Gewirtz, G. D. and Kopin, I. J.: Release of dopamine-β-hydroxylase with norepinephrine during cat splenic nerve stimulation. *Nature,* **227,** 406 (1970).

Ghisla, S. and Hemmerich, P.: Synthesis of the flavocoenzyme of monoamine oxidase. *FEBS Letters,* **16,** 229 (1971).

Giarman, N. J.: Symposium and conference reports (monoamine oxidase inhibitors). *Biochem. Pharmacol.,* **2,** 73 (1959).

Gibb, J. W., Spector, S. and Udenfriend, S.: Production of antibodies to dopamine-β-hydroxylase of bovine adrenal medulla. *Mol. Pharmacol.,* **3,** 473 (1967).

Gitlow, S. E., Bertani, L. M., Rausen, A., Gribetz, D. and Dziedzic, S. W.: Diagnosis of neuroblastoma by qualitative and quantitative determination of catecholamine metabolites in urine. *Cancer,* **25,** 1377 (1970).

Gitlow, S. E., Mendlowitz, M., Franklin, M. J., Carr, H. E. and Clarke, D. D.: A quantitative assay for vanillylmandelic acid (VMA) by gas-liquid chromatography. *Anal. Biochem.,* **13,** 544 (1965).

Gitlow, S. E., Mendlowitz, M., Khassis, S., Cohen, G. and Sha, J.: The diagnosis of pheochromocytoma by determination of urinary 3-methoxy-4-hydroxyman-delic acid. *J. Clin. Invest.*, **36**, 221 (1960).

Gjessing, L. R.: Studies of functional neural tumors. I. Urinary 3-methoxy-4-hydroxy-phenyl-metabolites. *Scand. J. Clin. Lab. Invest.*, **15**, 463 (1963 a).

Gjessing, L. R.: Studies of functional neural tumors V. Urinary excretion of 3-methoxy-4-hydroxy-phenyl-lactic acid. *Scand. J. Clin. Lab. Invest.*, **15**, 649 (1963 b).

Gjessing, J. R.: Biochemistry of functional neural crest tumors. *Advan. Clin. Chem.*, **11**, 82 (1968).

Glenner, G. G., Burtner, H. J. and Brown, G. W.: The histochemical demonstration of monoamine oxidase activity by tetrazolium salts. *J. Histochem. Cytochem.*, **5**, 591 (1957).

Glowinski, J. and Axelrod, J.: Effect of drugs on the uptake, release, and metabolism of H^3-norepinephrine in the rat brain. *J. Pharmacol. Exp. Therap.*, **149**, 43 (1965).

Glowinski, J. and Axelrod, J.: Effects of drugs on the disposition of H^3-norepinephrine in the rat brain. *Pharmacol. Rev.*, **18**, 775 (1966).

Glowinski, J., Kopin, I. and Axelrod, J.: Metabolism of H^3-norepinephrine in the rat brain. *J. Neurochem.*, **12**, 25 (1965).

Gödicke, W. and Brosowski, K. H.: Die Isolierung der 3-Methoxy-4-hydroxymandelsäure aus dem Urin unter Verwendung der Keilstreifenmethode. *J. Chromatog.*, **15**, 88 (1964).

Goldberg, I. H. and Delbrück, A.: Transfer of sulfate from 3'-phosphoadenosine-5'-phosphosulfate to lipids, mucopolysaccharides and aminoalkylphenols. *Fed. Proc.*, **18**, 235 (1959).

Goldstein, M.: Inhibition of norepinephrine biosynthesis at the dopamine-β-hydroxylation stage. *Pharmacol. Rev.*, **18**, 77 (1966).

Goldstein, M., Anagnoste, B., Lauber, E. and McKereghan, M. R.: Inhibition of dopamine-β-hydroxylase by disulfiram. *Life Sci.*, **3**, 763 (1964).

Goldstein, M., Freedman, L. S. and Bonnay, M.: An assay for dopamine-β-hydroxylase activity in tissues and serum. *Experientia*, **27**, 632 (1971).

Goldstein, M., Friedhoff, A. J., Pomerantz, S. and Simmons, C.: The characterization of a new metabolite of dopamine. *Biochim. Biophys. Acta*, **39**, 189 (1960).

Goldstein, M., Friedhoff, A. J. and Simmons, C.: Metabolic pathways of 3-hydroxytyramine. *Biochim. Biophys. Acta*, **33**, 572 (1959).

Goldstein, M., Gang, H. and Anagnoste, B.: The inhibition of tyrosine hydroxylase by isopropyltropolone *in vivo* and *in vitro*. *Bulletin de Chimie thérapeutique*, **6**, 442 (1968).

Goldstein, M., Joh, T. H., Garvey, T. Q., III: Kinetic studies of the enzymatic dopamine-β-hydroxylase reaction. *Biochemistry*, **7**, 2724 (1968).

Goldstein, M., Lauber, E. and McKereghan, M. R.: The inhibition of dopamine-β-hydroxylase by tropolone and other chelating agents. *Biochem. Pharmacol.*, **13**, 1103 (1964).

Goldstein, M., Lauber, E. and McKereghan, M. R.: Studies on the purification and characterization of 3,4-dihydroxyphenylethylamine β-hydroxylase. *J. Biol. Chem.*, **240**, 2066 (1965).

Goldstein, M. and Nakajima, K.: The effect of disulfiram on catecholamine levels in the brain. *J. Pharmacol. Exp. Therap.*, **157**, 96 (1967).

Gomes, B., Igaue, I., Kloepfer, H. G. and Yasunobu, K. T.: Amine oxidase XIV. Isolation and characterization of the multiple beef liver amine oxidase components. *Arch. Biochem. Biophys.*, **132**, 16 (1969).

Gomes, B., Naguwa, G., Kloepfer, H. G. and Yasunobu, K. T.: Amine oxidase XV. The sulfhydryl groups of beef liver mitochondrial amine oxidase. *Arch. Biochem. Biophys.*, **132**, 28 (1969).

Goodall, McC.: Dihydroxyphenylalanine and hydroxytyramine in mammalian suprarenals. *Acta. Chem. Scand.*, **4**, 550 (1950 a).

Goodall, McC.: Hydroxytyramine in mammalian heart. *Nature,* **166**, 738 (1950 b).

Goodall, McC.: Studies of adrenaline and noradrenaline in mammalian heart and suprarenals. *Acta Physiol. Scand.*, **24**, Supple. 85 (1951).

Goodall, McC. and Kirshner, N.: Biosynthesis of adrenaline and noradrenaline by sympathetic nerves and ganglia. *Fed. Proc.*, **16**, 49 (1957).

Goodall, McC. and Kirshner, N.: Biosynthesis of epinephrine and norepinephrine by sympathetic nerves and ganglia. *Circulation* **17**, 366 (1958).

Goodall, McC., Kirshner, N. and Rosen, M.: Metabolism of noradrenaline in human. *J. Clin. Invest.*, **38**, 707 (1959).

Gordon, R., Reid, J. V. O., Sjoerdsma, A. and Udenfriend, S.: Increased synthesis of norepinephrine in the rat heart on electrical stimulation of the stellate ganglia. *Mol. Pharmacol.*, **2**, 606 (1966).

Gordon, R., Spector, S., Sjoerdsma, A. and Udenfriend, S.: Increased synthesis of norepinephrine and epinephrine in the intact rat during exercise and exposure to cold. *J. Pharmacol. Exp. Therap.*, **153**, 440 (1966).

Gorkin, V. Z.: Partial separation of rat liver mitochondrial amine oxidase. *Nature,* **200**, 77 (1963).

Gorkin, V. Z.: Separation of rat liver mitochondrial amine oxidase. *Experientia,* **25**, 1142 (1969).

Gorkin, V. Z. and Orekhovitch, W. N.: Monoamine oxidases: New data on their nature, possible biological role and specific inhibition by pharmaceutical preparations. *Biochimica Applicata*, **14**, 343 (1967).

Gorkin, V. Z. and Tatyanenko, L. V.: "Transformation" of mitochondrial monoamine oxidase into a diamine oxidase-like enzyme *in vitro*. *Biochem. Biophys. Res. Commun.*, **27**, 613 (1967).

Grabartis, F., Chessick, R. and Lal, H.: Changes in brain norepinephrine after decapitation. *Biochem. Pharmacol.*, **15**, 127 (1966).

Green, A. L.: The inhibition of dopamine-β-oxidase by chelating agent. *Biochim. Biophys. Acta*, **81**, 391 (1964).

Green, M. and Walker, G.: Dietary vanillin does not affect the VMA [vanillylmandelic acid] method of Pisano, *et al. Clin. Chim. Acta,* **29**, 189 (1970).

Guha, S. R. and Krishna Murti, C. R.: Purification and solubilization of monoamine oxidase of rat liver mitochondria. *Biochem. Biophys. Commun.,* **18**, 350 (1965).

Guilbault, G. G., Brignac, P. J., Jr. and Juneau, M.: New substrates for the fluorometic determination of oxidative enzymes. *Anal. Chem.*, **40**, 1256 (1968).

Gunne, L. M. and Jonsson, J.: On the occurrence of tyramine in the rabbit brain. *Acta. Physiol. Scand.*, **64**, 434 (1965).

Gurin, S. and Delluva, A. M.: The biological synthesis of radioactive adrenaline from phenylalanine. *J. Biol. Chem.*, **170**, 545 (1947).

Guroff, G.: Irreversible *in vivo* inhibition of rat liver phenylalanine hydroxylase by *p*-chlorophenylalanine. *Arch. Biochem. Biophys.,* **134,** 610 (1969 a).

Guroff, G.: The hydroxylation-induced migration of tritium: Practical aspects. *Atomlight,* No. **69,** p. 1, New England Nuclear, Boston, Mass. (1969 b).

Guroff, G.: Phenylalanine hydroxylase (Pseudomonas). In "Methods in Enzymology" (H. Tabor and C. W. Tabor, *eds*), vol. 17A, p. 597. Academic Press, New York (1970).

Guroff, G. and Abramowitz, A.: A simple radioisotope assay for phenylalanine hydroxylase. *Anal. Biochem.,* **19,** 548 (1967).

Guroff, G., Daly, J. W., Jerina, D., Renson, J., Witkop, B. and Udenfriend, S.: Hydroxylation-induced migration: The NIH Shift. *Science,* **157,** 1524 (1967).

Guroff, G. and Ito, T.: Induced, soluble phenylalanine hydroxylase from Pseudomonas sp. grown on phenylalanine or tyrosine. *Biochim. Biophys. Acta,* **77,** 159 (1963).

Guroff, G. and Ito, T.: Phenylalanine hydroxylation by Pseudomonas species (ATCC 11299 a). *J. Biol. Chem.,* **240,** 1175 (1965).

Guroff, G., Kondo, K. and Daly, J. W.: The production of *meta*-chlorotyrosine from *para*-chlorophenylalanine by phenylalanine hydroxylase. *Biochem. Biophys. Res. Commun.,* **25,** 622 (1966).

Guroff, G., Levitt, M., Daly, J. W. and Udenfriend, S.: The production of *meta*-tritiotyrosine from *p*-tritiophenylalanine by phenylalanine hydroxylase. *Biochem. Biophys. Res. Commun.,* **25,** 253 (1966).

Guroff, G., Reifsnyder, C. A. and Daly, J. W.: Retention of deuterium in *p*-tyrosine formed enzymatically from *p*-deuterophenylalanine. *Biochem. Biophys. Res. Commun.,* **24,** 720 (1966).

Guroff, G. and Rhoads, C. A.: Phenylalanine hydroxylase from Pseudomonas species (ATCC 11299 a). Purification of the enzyme and activation by various metal ions. *J. Biol. Chem.,* **242,** 3641 (1967).

Guroff, G., Rhoads, C. A. and Abramowitz, A.: A simple radioisotope assay of phenylalanine hydroxylase cofactor. *Anal. Biochem.,* **21,** 273 (1967).

Guroff, G. and Udenfriend, S.: Studies on aromatic amino acid uptake by rat brain *in vivo. J. Biol. Chem.,* **237,** 803 (1962).

Haeusler, G., Haefely, W. and Thoenen, H.: Chemical sympathectomy of the cat with 6-hydroxydopamine. *J. Pharmacol. Exp. Therap.,* **170,** 50 (1969).

Hagen, P.: The storage and release of catecholamines. *Pharmacol. Rev.,* **11,** 361 (1959).

Hagen, P.: Observations on the substrate specificity of dopa decarboxylase from ox adrenal medulla, human phaeochromocytoma and human argentaffinoma. *Brit. J. Pharmacol.,* **18,** 175 (1962).

Häggendal, J.: Fluorimetric determination of 3-*O*-methylated derivatives of adrenaline and noradrenaline in tissues and body fluids. *Acta Physiol. Scand.,* **56,** 258 (1962).

Häggendal, J.: An improved method for fluorimetric determination of small amounts of adrenaline and noradrenaline in plasma and tissues. *Acta Physiol. Scand.,* **59,** 242 (1963).

Hamberger, B., Malmfors, T., Norberg, K. A. and Sachs, C.: Uptake and accumulation of catecholamines in peripheral adrenergic neurons of reserpinized animals, studied with a histochemical method. *Biochem. Pharmacol.,* **13,** 841

(1964).

Hansson, E., Fleming, R. M. and Clark, W. G.: Effect of some benzylhydrazines and benzyloxyamines on dopa and 5-hydroxytryptophan decarboxylase *in vivo*. *Int. J. Neuropharmacol.*, **3**, 177 (1964).

Harada, M., Mizutani, K. and Nagatsu, T.: Purfication and properties of mitochondrial monoamine oxidase in beef brain. *J. Neurochem.*, **18**, 559 (1971).

Harada, M. and Nagatsu, T.: Identification of flavin in the purified beef brain mitochondrial monoamine oxidase. *Experientia*, **25**, 583 (1969).

Harada, M., Ôya, H., Nakano, G., Kuzuya, H. and Nagatsu, T.: Intracellular localization of monoamine oxidase in mammalian salivary glands. *J. Dent. Res.*, **50**, 1290 (1970).

Hare, M. L. C.: Tyramine oxidase: New enzyme system in liver. *Biochem.J.*, **22**, 968 (1928).

Harley-Mason, J.: The structure of adrenochrome and its reduction products. *Experientia*, **4**, 307 (1949).

Harley-Mason, J.: The chemistry of adrenochrome and its derivatives. *J. Chem. Soc.*, p. 1276 (1950).

Harley-Mason, J. and Laird, A. H.: Isolation and structure of the fluorescent substances formed in the oxidative reaction of adrenaline and noradrenaline with ethylenediamine. *Tetrahedron*, **7**, 70 (1959).

Harrison, W. H., Levitt, M. and Udenfriend, S.: Norepinephrine synthesis and release *in vivo* mediated by 3,4-dihydroxyphenethylamine. *J. Pharmacol. Exp. Therap.*, **142**, 157 (1963).

Hartman, W. J., Akawie, R. I. and Clark, W. G.: Competitive inhibition of 3,4-dihydroxyphenylalanine (dopa) decarboxylase *in vitro*. *J. Biol. Chem.*, **216**, 507 (1955).

Hartman, B. K. and Udenfriend, S.: Immunofluorescent localization of dopamine β-hydroxylase in tissues. *Mol. Pharmacol.*, **6**, 85 (1970).

Hashimoto, Y. and Okuyama, T.: Chromatographycal purification of monoamine oxidase from chicken brain and its properties. *J. Jap. Biochem. Soc.* (in Japanese), **42**, 350 (1970).

Hawkins, J.: Localization of amine oxidase in liver cell. *Biochem. J.*, **50**, 577 (1952 a).

Hawkins, J.: Amine oxidase activity of rat liver in riboflavin deficiency. *Biochem. J.*, **51**, 399 (1952 b).

Hayaishi, O.: Oxygenases. In *Proceeding of the Plenary Sessions. Sixth International Congress of Biochemistry*. I.U.B. vol. 33, p. 31 (1964).

Hayaishi, O., Okuno, S., Fujisawa, H. and Umezawa, H.: Inhibition of brain tryptophan 5-monooxygenase by aquayamycin. *Biochem., Biophys. Res. Commun.*, **39**, 643 (1970).

Helle, K. B.: Antibody formation against soluble protein from bovine adrenal chromaffin granules. *Biochim. Biophys. Acta*, **117**, 107 (1966 a).

Helle, K. B.: Comparative studies on the soluble protein fractions of bovine, equine, porcine and ovine adrenal chromaffin granules. *Biochem. J.*, **100**, 6C (1966 b).

Hertting, G.: The fate of H^3-isoproterenol in the rat. *Biochem. Pharmacol.*, **13**, 1119 (1964).

Hertting, G.: Effect of drugs and sympathetic denervation on noradrenaline uptake and binding in animal tissues. In "Pharmacology of Cholinergic and Adrenergic Transmission" (Koelle, Dougla sand Carlsson, eds), Pergamon Press, Oxford (1965).

Hertting, G., Axelrod, J., Kopin, I. J. and Whitby, L. G.: Lack of uptake of catecholamines after chronic denervation of sympathetic nerves. Nature, 189, 66 (1961).

Hertting, G. and LaBrosse, E. H.: Biliary and urinary excretion of metabolites of 7-H³-epinephrine in the rat. J. Biol. Chem., 237, 2291 (1962).

Hertting, G. and Schiefthaler, T.: The effect of stellate ganglion excision on the catecholamine content and the uptake of H³-norepinephrine in the heart of the cat. Int. J. Neuropharmacol., 3, 65 (1964).

Hidaka, H., Nagatsu, T., Nagasaka, A. and Ishizuki, Y.: Monoamine oxidase activity of the thyroid glands in thyroid disease. Clin. Chim. Acta, 23, 383 (1969).

Hidaka, H., Nagatsu, T., Takeya, K., Takeuchi, T., Suda, H., Kojiri, K., Matsuzaki, M. and Umezawa, H.,: Fusaric acid a hypotensive agent produced by fungi. J. Antibiotics, 22, 228 (1969).

Hidaka, H., Nagatsu, T. and Yagi, K.: Microdetermination of monoamine oxidase using serotonin as substrate. J. Biochem. (Tokyo) 62, 621 (1967).

Hillarp, N.-Å.: Adenosinephosphates and inorganic phosphate in the adrenaline and noradrenaline containing granules of the adrenal medulla. Acta Physiol. Scand., 42, 321 (1958 a).

Hillarp, N.-Å.: Isolation and some biochemical properties of the catecholamine granules in the cow adrenal medulla. Acta Physiol. Scand., 43, 82 (1958 b).

Hillarp, N.-Å., Högberg, B. and Nilson, B.: Adenosine triphosphate in the adrenal medulla of the cow. Nature, 176, 1032 (1955).

Hillarp, N.-Å. and Hökfelt, B.: Evidence of adrenaline and noradrenaline in separate adrenal medullary cells. Acta Physiol. Scand., 30, 55 (1953).

Hillarp, N.-Å., Lagerstedt, S. and Nilson, B.: The isolation of a granular fraction from the suprarenal medulla, containing the sympathomimetic catechol amines. Acta Physiol. Scand. 29, 251 (1953).

Hoeldtke, R. D. and Sloan, J. W.: Acid hydrolysis of urinary catecholamines. J. Lab. Clin. Med., 75, 159 (1970).

Hoffer, A.: Adrenochrome in blood plasma. Am. J. Psychiat., 114, 752 (1958 a).

Hoffer, A.: Relationship of epinephrine metabolites to schizophrenia. In "Chemical Concepts of Psychosis" (M. Rinkel and H. C. B. Denber, eds), p. 127. McDowell, Obolensky, New York (1958 b).

Hogans, A. F.: A sensitive method for the simultaneous estimation of norepinephrine and dopamine in tissue. Personal communication (1968).

Hollister, L. E. and Friedhoff, A. J.: Effects of 3,4-dimethoxyphenylethylamine in man. Nature, 210, 1377 (1966).

Hollunger, G. and Oreland, L.: Preparation of soluble monoamine oxidase from pig liver mitochondria. Arch. Biochem. Biophys., 139, 320 (1970).

Holtz, P.: Dopadecarboxylase. Naturwissenschaften, 27, 724 (1939).

Holtz, P.: Role of L-DOPA decarboxylase in the biosynthesis of catecholamines in nervous tissue and the adrenal medulla. Pharmacol. Rev., 11, 317 (1959).

Holtz, P. and Bachmann, F.: Activierung der Dopadecarboxylase des Nebennierenmarks durch Nebennieren-Rindenextrakt. Naturwissenschaften, 39, 116

(1952).

Holtz, P., Credner, K. and Koepp, W.: Die enzymatische Entstehung von Oxytyramine in Organismus und die physiologische Bedeutung der Decarboxylase. *Arch. exp. Path. Pharmakol.,* **200,** 356 (1942).

Holtz, P., Credner, K. and Kroneberg, G.: Über das sympathicomimetische pressorische Prinzip des Harns ("Urosympathin"). *Arch Exp. Path. Pharmakol.,* **204,** 228 (1947).

Holtz, P., Credner, K. and Strübing, C.: Über das Vorkommen der Dopadecarboxylase im Pankreas. *Arch. exp. Path. Pharmakol.,* **199,** 145 (1942).

Holtz, P., Heise, R. and Lüdtke, K.: Fermentativer Abbau von *l*-Dioxyphenylalanin (Dopa) durch Niere. *Arch. exp. Path. Pharmakol.,* **191,** 87 (1938).

Holtz, P., Stock, K. and Westermann, E.: Pharmakologie des Tetrahydropapaverolins und seine Entstehung aus Dopamin. *Naunyn-Schmiedebergs Arch. exp. Path. Pharmakol.,* **248,** 387 (1964).

Holtz, P. and Westermann, E.: Über die Dopadecarboxylase und Histidindecarboxylase des Nervengewebes. *Arch. Exp. Path. Pharmakol.,* **227,** 538 (1956).

Horita, A. and Chinn, C.: An analysis of the interaction of reversible and irreversible monoamine oxidase inhibitors. *Biochem. Pharmacol.,* **13,** 371 (1964).

Horita, A. and McGrath, W. R.: The interaction between reversible and irreversible monoamine oxidase inhibitors. *Biochem. Pharmacol.,* **3,** 206 (1960).

Igaue, I., Gomes, B. and Yasunobu, K.: Beef mitochondrial monoamine oxidase, a flavin dinucleotide enzyme. *Biochem. Biophys. Res. Commun.,* **29,** 562 (1967).

Ikeda, M., Fahien, L. and Udenfriend, S.: Kinetic study of bovine adrenal tyrosine hydroxylase. *J. Biol. Chem.,* **241,** 4452 (1966).

Ikeda, M., Levitt, M. and Udenfriend, S.: Hydroxylation of phenylalanine by purified preparations of adrenal and brain tyrosine hydroxylase. *Biochem. Biophys. Res. Commun.,* **18,** 482 (1965).

Ikeda, M., Levitt, M. and Udenfriend, S.: Phenylalanine as substrate and inhibitor of tyrosine hydroxylase. *Arch. Biochem. Biophys.,* **120,** 420 (1967).

Imai, K. and Tamura, Z.: Selective and sensitive method for determination of vanillylmandelic acid in urine. *Chem. Pharm. Bull.,* **18,** 1055 (1970).

Imaizumi, R.: On the precursor of adrenaline (1) (in Japanese). *J. Osaka Med. Soc.,* **37,** 1631 (1938).

Inouye, A., Kataoka, K. and Shinagawa, Y.: Intracellular distribution of brain noradrenaline and de Robertis' non-cholinergic nerve endings. *Biochim. Biophys. Acta,* **71,** 491 (1963).

Inscoe, J. E., Daly, J. and Axelrod, J.: Factors affecting the enzymatic formation of *O*-methylated dihydroxy derivatives. *Biochem. Pharmacol.,* **14,** 1257 (1965).

Isselbacher, K. and Axelrod, J.: Enzymic formation of corticosteroid glucuronides. *J. Am. Chem. Soc.,* **77,** 1070 (1955).

Itoh, C., Yoshinaga, K., Sato, T., Ishida, N. and Wada, Y.: Presence of *N*-methylmetadrenaline in human urine and tumour tissue of phaeochromocytoma. *Nature,* **193,** 477 (1962).

Itoh, T., Matsuoka, M., Nakazima, K., Tagawa, K. and Imaizumi, R.: An isolation method of catecholamine and effect of reserpine on the enzyme systems related to the formation and inactivation of catecholamines in brain. *Jap. J. Pharmacol.,* **12,** 130 (1962).

Iversen, L. L.: The uptake of norepinephrine by the isolated perfused rat heart.

Brit. J. Pharmacol. Chemother., **21**, 523 (1963).

Iversen, L. L.: The uptake of catecholamines at high perfusion concentrations in the rat isolated heart: A novel catecholamine uptake process. *Brit. J. Pharmacol. Chemotherap.*, **25**, 18 (1965 a).

Iversen, L. L.: The inhibition of noradrenaline uptake by drugs. In "Advances in Drug Research" (N. J. Harper and A. B. Simmonds, *eds*), p. 1. Academic Press, London (1965 b).

Iversen, L. L.: "The Uptake and Storage of Norepinephrine in Sympathetic Nerves." Cambridge University Press, Cambridge (1967).

Iversen, L. L.: Biosynthesis and inactivation of the adrenergic transmitter substance. *J. Physiol.*, **201**, 1 (1969).

Iversen, L. L., Glowinski, J. and Axelrod, J.: The uptake and storage of ^{3}H-norepinephrine in the reserpine-pretreated rat heart. *J. Pharmacol. Exp. Therap.*, **150**, 173 (1965 a).

Iversen, L. L., Glowinski, J. and Axelrod, J.: Reduced uptake of tritiated noradrenaline in tissues of immunosympathectomized animals. *Nature*, **206**, 1222 (1965 b).

Izumi, F., Oka, M., Yoshida, H. and Imaizumi, R.: Effect of reserpine on monoamine oxidase activity in guinea pig heart. *Life Sci.*, **6**, 2333 (1967).

Izumi, F., Oka, M., Yoshida, H. and Imaizumi, R.: Stimulatory effect of reserpine on monoamine oxidase in guinea pig heart. *Biochem. Pharmacol.*, **18**, 1739 (1969).

Jacobs, S. L., Sobel, C. and Henry, R. J.: Excretion of 3-methoxy-4-hydroxymandelic acid and catecholamines in patients with pheochromocytoma. *J. Clin. Endocrinol.*, **21**, 315 (1961).

James, W. O.: Demonstration and separation of noradrenaline, adrenaline and methyladrenaline. *Nature*, **161**, 851 (1948).

Janakidevi, K., Dewey, V. C. and Kidder, G. W.: The biosynthesis of catecholamines in two genera of protozoa. *J. Biol. Chem.*, **241**, 2576 (1966).

Jequier, E., Robinson, D. S., Lovenberg, W. and Sjoerdsma, A.: Further studies on tryptophan hydroxylase in rat brain stem and beef pineal. *Biochem. Pharmacol.*, **18**, 1071 (1969).

Jervis, G. A.: Phenylpyruvic oligophrenia deficiency of phenylalanine-oxidizing system. *Proc. Soc. Exp. Biol. Med.*, **82**, 514 (1953).

Johnson, G. A. and Boukma, S. J.: A rapid method for separation of dopa, dopamine and norepinephrine. *Anal. Biochem.*, **18**, 143 (1967).

Johnson, G. A., Boukma, S.J. and Kim, E.G.: Inhibition of dopamine β-hydroxylase by aromatic and alkyl thioureas. *J. Pharmacol. Exp. Therap*, **168**, 229 (1969).

Johnson, G. A., Boukma, S. J. and Kim, E. G.: *In vivo* inhibition of dopamine β-hydroxylase by 1-phenyl-3-(2-thiazolyl)-2-thiourea (U-14,624). *J. Pharmacol. Exp. Therap.*, **171**, 80 (1970).

Jonsson, J., Grobecker, H. and Gunne, L.-M.: Phenylethyldithiocarbamate: A new dopamine β-hydroxylase inhibitor. *J. Pharm. Pharmacol.*, **19**, 201 (1967).

Justice, P., O'Flynn, M. E. and Hsia, D. Y. Y.: Phenylalanine-hydroxylase activity in hyperphenylalaninaemia. *Lancet*, **1**, 928 (1967).

Kakimoto, Y. and Armstrong, M. D.: The phenolic amines of human urine. *J. Biol. Chem.*, **237**, 208 (1962 a).

Kakimoto, Y. and Armstrong, M. D.: On the identification of octopamine in mammals. *J. Biol. Chem.*, **237**, 422 (1962 b).

Kariya, T. and Aprison, M. H.: Microdetermination of norepinephrine, 3,4-dihydroxyphenylethylamine, and 5-hydroxytryptamine from single extracts of specific rat brain areas. *Anal. Biochem.*, **31**, 102 (1969).

Karlson, P. and Ammon, H.: Zum Tyrosinstoffwechsel der Insekten. XI. Biogenese und Schicksal der Acetylgruppe des N-Acetyl-dopamins. *Hoppe-Seyl. Z. Physiol. Chem.*, **330**, 161 (1963).

Karlson, P. and Liebau, H.: Zum Tyrosinstoffwechsel der Insekten. V. Reindarstellung, Kristallisation und Substrat Spezifität der O-Diphenoloxydase aus Calliphora erythrocephala. *Hoppe-Seyler's Z. Physiol. Chem.*, **326**, 135 (1961).

Karlson, P., Mergenhagen, D. and Sekeris, C. E.: Zum Tyrosinstoffwechsel der Insekten. XV. Weitere Untersuchungen über das O-Diphenoloxydase System von Calliphora erythrocephala. *Hoppe-Seyler's Z. Physiol. Chem.*, **338**, 42 (1964).

Karlson, P. and Schweiger, A.: Zum Tyrosinstoffwechsel der Insekten. IV. Das Phenoloxydase System von Calliphora erythrocephala und seine Beeinflussung durch das Hormon Ecdyson. *Hoppe-Seyler's Z. Physiol. Chem.*, **323**, 199 (1961).

Karlson, P. and Sekeris, C. E.: Zum Tyrosinstoffwechsel der Insekten. IX. Kontrolle des Tyrosinstoffwechsels durch Ecdyson. *Biochim, Biophys. Acta*, **63**, 489 (1962).

Karlson, P., Sekeris, C. E. and Sekeri, K.: Zum Tyrosinstoffwechsel der Insekten. VI. Identifizierung von N-Acetyl-3,4-dihydroxy-β-phenäthylamin (N-Acethydopamin) als Tyrosinmetabolit. *Hoppe-Seyler's Z. Physiol. Chem.*, **327**, 86 (1962).

Karoum, F., Anah, C. O., Ruthven, C. R. J. and Sandler, M.: Further observations on the gas chromatographic measurement of urinary, phenolic and indolic metabolites. *Clin. Chim. Acta*, **24**, 341 (1969).

Käser, H.: 3-Methoxytyramine, a catecholamine catabolite regularly present in human urine. *Experientia*, **26**, 138 (1970).

Kaufman, S.: The enzymatic conversion of phenylalanine to tyrosine. *J. Biol. Chem.*, **226**, 511 (1957).

Kaufman, S.: The participation of tetrahydrofolic acid in the enzymic conversion of phenylalanine to tyrosine. *Biochim, Biophys. Acta*, **27**, 428 (1958 a).

Kaufman, S.: A new cofactor required for the enzymatic conversion of phenylalanine to tyrosine. *J. Biol. Chem.*, **230**, 931 (1958 b).

Kaufman, S.: Phenylalanine hydroxylation cofactor in phenylketonuria. *Science*, **128**, 1506 (1958 c).

Kaufman, S.: Studies on the mechanism of the enzymatic conversion of phenylalanine to tyrosine. *J. Biol. Chem.*, **234**, 2677 (1959).

Kaufman, S.: The nature of the primary oxidation product formed from tetrahydropteridines during phenylalanine hydroxylation. *J. Biol. Chem.*, **236**, 804 (1961).

Kaufman, S.: On the structure of the phenylalanine hydroxylation cofactor. *J. Biol. Chem.*, **237**, PC 2712 (1962 a).

Kaufman, S.: Aromatic hydroxylations. In "Oxygenases" (O. Hayaishi, *ed*), p. 129. Academic Press, New York (1962 b).

Kaufman, S.: Phenylalanine hydroxylase. In "Methods in Enzymology" (S. P.

Colowick and N. O. Kaplan, *eds*), p. 809. Academic Press, New York (1962 c).

Kaufman, S.: The structure of the phenylalanine-hydroxylation cofactor. *Proc. Natl. Acad. Sci. U. S. A., 50,* 1085 (1963 a).

Kaufman, S.: Phenylalanine hydroxylation. In "The Enzymes" (P. D. Boyer, H. Lardy and K. Myrbäck, *eds*), p. 373. Academic Press, New York (1963 b).

Kaufman, S.: Pteridine transformations during the enzymatic conversion of phenylalanine to tyrosine. In "Pteridine Chemistry" (W. Pfleiderer and E. C. Taylor, *eds*), p. 307. Pergamon Press, Oxford (1964).

Kaufman, S.: Coenzymes and hydroxylases: ascorbate and dopamine-β-hydroxylase; tetrahydropteridines and phenylalanine and tyrosine hydroxylases. *Pharmacol. Rev., 18,* 61 (1966 a).

Kaufman, S.: The phenylalanine hydroxylase system of mammalian liver and the dopamine-β-hydroxylase of adrenal medulla. In "Biological and Chemical Aspects of Oxygenases" (K. Bloch and O. Hayaishi, *eds*), p. 261. Maruzen Co., Ltd., Tokyo (1966 b).

Kaufman, S.: Metabolism of the phenylalanine hydroxylation cofactor. *J. Biol. Chem., 242,* 3934 (1967 a).

Kaufman, S.: Pteridine cofactors. In "Ann. Rev. Biochem.," vol.36, Part I, p. 171. Annual Reviews, Inc., Palo Alto (1967 b).

Kaufman, S.: Phenylalanine hydroxylase of human liver: assay and some properties. *Arch. Biochem. Biophys., 134,* 249 (1969).

Kaufman, S.: A protein that stimulates rat liver phenylalanine hydroxylase. *J. Biol. Chem., 245,* 4751 (1970).

Kaufman, S.: Phenylalanine hydroxylase (rat liver). In "Methods in Enzymology" (H. Tabor and C. W. Tabor, *eds*), vol. 17A, p. 603. Academic Press, New York (1970).

Kaufman, S.: Dopamine β-hydroxylase (beef adrenal). In "Methods in Enzymology" (H. Tabor and C. W. Tabor, *eds*), vol. 17B, p. 754. Academic Press, New York (1971).

Kaufman, S., Bridgers, W. F., Eisenberg, F. and Friedman, S.: The source of oxygen in the phenylalanine hydroxylase and the dopamine-β-hydroxylase catalyzed reactions. *Biochem. Biophys. Res. Commun., 9,* 497 (1962).

Kaufman, S. and Fisher, D. B.: Purification and some physical properties of phenylalanine hydroxylase from rat liver. *J. Biol. Chem., 245,* 4745 (1970).

Kaufman, S. and Levenberg, B.: Further studies on the phenylalanine-hydroxylation cofactor. *J. Biol. Chem., 234,* 2683 (1959).

Kaufman, S., Storm, C. B. and Fisher, D. B.: Studies on the mechanism of the enzymatic conversion of phenylalanine to tyrosine. In "Chemistry and Biology of Pteridines" (K. Iwai, M. Akino, M. Goto and Y. Iwanami, *eds*), p. 209. International Academic Printing Co., Tokyo (1970).

Kawai, S., Nagatsu, T., Imanari, T. and Tamura, Z.: Gas chromatography of catecholamines and related compounds. *Chem. Pharm. Bull., 14,* 618 (1966).

Kawai, S. and Tamura, Z.: Dimethylsulfoxide as a suitable solvent for trimethylsilylation of catecholamines. *J. Chromatog., 25,* 471 (1966).

Kawai, S. and Tamura, Z.: Gas chromatography of catecholamines using dimethyl sulfoxide as an effective solvent for trimethylsilylation. *Chem. Pharm. Bull., 15,* 1493 (1967).

Kawai, S. and Tamura, Z.: Gas chromatography of catecholamines as their trifluoroacetates. *Chem. Pharm. Bull.,* **16,** 699 (1968 a).

Kawai, S. and Tamura, Z.: Gas chromatography of the catecholamines as their trifluoroacetates in urine and tumor. *Chem. Pharm. Bull.,* **16,** 1091 (1968 b).

Kearney, E. B., Salach, J. I., Walker, W. H., Seng, R. and Singer, T. P.: Structure of the covalently bound flavin of monoamine oxidase. *Biochem. Biophys. Res. Commun.,* **42,** 490 (1971).

Keller, E. B., Boissonnas, R. A. and du Vigneaud, V.: The origin of the methyl group of epinephrine. *J. Biol. Chem.,* **183,** 627 (1950).

Kirshner, A. G. and Kirshner, N.: A specific soluble protein from the catechola-mine storage vesicles of bovine adrenal medulla. II. Physical characterization. *Biochim. Biophys. Acta,* **181,** 219 (1969).

Kirshner, N.: Pathway of noradrenaline formation from dopa. *J. Biol. Chem.,* **226,** 821 (1957).

Kirshner, N.: Uptake of catecholamines by a particulate fraction of the adrenal medulla, *J. Biol. Chem.,* **237,** 2311 (1962).

Kirshner, N. and Goodall, McC.: Separation of adrenaline, noradrenaline, and hydroxytyramine by ion exchange chromatography. *J. Biol. Chem.,* **226,** 207 (1957 a).

Kirshner, N. and Goodall, McC.: The formation of adrenaline from noradrena-line. *Biochim. Biophys. Acta,* **24,** 658 (1957 b).

Kirshner, N., Goodall, McC. and Rosen, L.: Metabolism of *dl*-adrenaline-2-C^{14} in the human. *Proc. Soc. Exp. Biol. Med.,* **98,** 627 (1958).

Kirshner, N., Goodall, McC. and Rosen, L.: The effect of iproniazid on the metabolism of *dl*-epinephrine-2-C^{14} in the human. *J. Pharmacol. Exp. Therap.,* **127,** 1 Proc. (1959).

Kirshner, N., Kirshner, A. G. and Kamin, D. L.: Adenosine triphosphatase ac-tivity of adrenal medulla catecholamine granules. *Biochim. Biophys. Acta,* **113,** 332 (1966).

Kirshner, N., Rorie, M. and Kimin, D. L.: Inhibition of dopamine uptake *in vitro* by reserpine administration *in vivo. J. Pharmacol. Exp. Therap.,* **141,** 285 (1963).

Kirshner, N., Sage, H. J., Smith, W. J. and Kirshner, A. G.: Release of catechol-amines and specific protein from adrenal glands. *Science,* **154,** 529 (1966).

Kitabchi, A. E. and Williams, R. H.: Phenylethanolamine-*N*-methyltransferase in human adrenal gland. *Biochim. Biophys. Acta,* **171,** 181 (1969).

Kitani, K., Imai, K. and Tamura, Z.: Detection of catecholamines after *N*-dansy-lation on the surface of alumina. *Chem. Pharm. Bull.,* **18,** 1495 (1970).

Knox, W. E. and Hsia, D. Y.-Y.: Pathogenic problems in phenylketonuria. *Am. J. Med.,* **22,** 687 (1957).

Kopin, I. J.: Technique for the study of alternate metabolic pathways; epine-phrine metabolism in man. *Science,* **131,** 1372 (1960).

Kopin, I. J.: Biochemical aspects of release of norepinephrine and other amines from sympathetic nerve endings. *Pharmacol. Rev.,* **18,** 513 (1966).

Kopin, I. J. and Axelrod, J.: 3,4-Dihydroxyphenylglycol, a metabolite of epine-phrine. *Arch. Biochem. Biophys.,* **89,** 148 (1960 a).

Kopin, I. J. and Axelrod, J.: Presence of 3-methoxy-4-hydroxyphenylglycol and metanephrine in phaeochromacytoma tissue. *Nature,* **185,** 788 (1960 b).

Kopin, I. J., Axelrod, J. and Gordon, E.: The metabolic fate of H^3-epinephrine and C¹⁴-metanephrine in the rat. *J. Biol. Chem.*, **236,** 2109 (1961).

Kopin, I. J. and Gordon, E. K.: Origin of norepinephrine in the heart. *Nature,* **199,** 1289 (1963).

Kopin, I. J., Gorden, E. K. and Horst, W. D.: Studies of uptake of L-norepinephrine-C¹⁴. *Biochem. Pharmacol.,* **14,** 753 (1965).

Krakoff, L. R. and Axelrod, J.: Inhibition of phenylethanolamine-*N*-methyl transferase. *Biochem. Pharmacol.,* **16,** 1384 (1967).

Kraml, M.: A rapid microfluorimetric determination of monoamine oxidase. *Biochem. Pharmacol.,* **14,** 1683 (1965).

Kuehl, F. A., Ormond, R. E. and Vandenheuvel, W. J. A.: Occurrence of 3,4-dimethoxyphenylacetic acid in urines of normal and schizophrenic individuals. *Nature,* **211,** 606 (1966).

Kumagai, H., Matsui, H., Ogata, K., Yamada, H. and Fukami, H.: Oxidation of dopamine by crystalline tyramine oxidase from Sarcina lutea. *Memoirs of the Research Institute for Food Science, Kyoto University,* No. 29, p. 69 (1968).

Kuzuya, H. and Nagatsu, T.: Flavins and monoamine oxidase activity in the brain, liver and kidney of the developing rat. *J. Neurochem.,* **16,** 123 (1969 a).

Kuzuya, H. and Nagatsu, T.: A simple assay of dopamine-β-hydroxylase activity in the homogenate of the adrenal medulla. *Enzymologia,* **36,** 31 (1969 b).

Laasberg, L. H. and Shimosato, S.: Paper chromatographic identification of catecholamines. *J. Appl. Physiol.* 21, 1929 (1966).

LaBrosse, E. H., Axelrod, J. and Kety, S. S.: *O*-Methylation, the principal route of metabolism of epinephrine in man. *Science,* **128,** 593 (1958).

LaBrosse, E. H., Axelrod, J., Kopin, I. J. and Kety, S. S.: Metabolism of 7-H³-epinephrine-*d*-bitartrate in normal young men. *J. Clin. Invest.,* **40,** 253 (1961).

Laduron, P. and Belpaire, F.: Transport of noradrenaline and dopamine-β-hydroxylase in sympathetic nerves. *Life Sci.* **7,** 1 (1968 a).

Laduron. P. and Belpaire, F.: A rapid assay and partial purification of Dopa decarboxylase. *Anal. Biochem.,* **26,** 210 (1968 b).

Laduron, P. and Belpaire, F.: Tissue fractionation and catecholamines-II. Intracellular distribution patterns of tyrosine hydroxylase, dopa decarboxylase, dopamine-β-hydroxylase, phenylethanolamine *N*-methyltransferase and monoamine oxidase in adrenal medulla. *Biochem. Pharmacol.,* **17,** 1127 (1968 c).

Langeman, H.: Enzymes and their substrates in the adrenal gland of the ox. *Brit. J. Pharmacol.* **6,** 318 (1951).

Laverty, R., Michaelson, I. A., Sharman, D. F. and Whittaler, V. P.: The subcellular localization of dopamine and acetylcholine in the dog caudate nucleus. *Brit. J. Pharmacol.,* **21,** 482 (1963).

Laverty, R. and Robertson, A.: Effects of α-methyl tyrosine in normotensive and hypertensive rats. *Circ. Res.,* **21,** Suppl. III, 127 (1967).

Laverty, R. and Sharman, D. F.: The estimation of small quantities of 3,4-dihydroxyphenylethylamine in tissues. *Brit. J. Pharmacol.,* **24,** 538 (1965).

Laverty, R., Sharman, D. F. and Vogt, M.: Action of 2,4,5-trihydroxyphenylethylamine on the storage and release of noradrenaline. *Brit. J. Pharmacol.,* **24,** 549 (1965).

Laverty, R. and Taylor, K. M.: The fluorometric assay of catecholamines and related compounds: Improvements and extensions to the hydroxyindole technique. *Anal. Biochem.,* **22,** 269 (1968).

Leeper L. C. and Udenfriend, S.: Dihydroxyphenylethylamine as a precursor of adrenal epinephrine in the intact rat. *Fed, Proc.,* **15,** 298 (1956).

Leeper, L. C., Weissbach, H. and Udenfriend, S.: Studies on the metabolism of norepinephrine, epinephrine and their O-methyl analogs by partially purified enzyme preparations. *Arch. Biochem. Biophys.,* **77,** 417 (1958).

Levi, R. and Maynert, E. W.: The subcellular localization of brain-stem norepinephrine and 5-hydroxytryptamine in stressed rats. *Biochem. Pharmacol.,* **13,** 615 (1964).

Levi-Montalcini, R. and Angeletti, P. U.: Noradrenaline and monoamine oxidase content in immunosympathectomized animals. *Int. J. Neuropharmacol.,* **1,** 161 (1962).

Levi-Montalcini, R. and Angeletti, P. U.: Immunosympathectomy. *Pharmacol. Rev.,* **18,** 619 (1966).

Levin, E. Y. and Kaufman, S.: Studies on the enzyme catalyzing the conversion of 3,4-dihydroxyphenylethylamine to norepinephrine. *J. Biol. Chem.,* **236,** 2043 (1961).

Levin, E. Y., Levenberg, B. and Kaufman, S.: The enzymatic conversion of 3,4-dihydroxyphenylethylamine to norepinephrine. *J. Biol. Chem.,* **235,** 2080 (1960).

Levitt, M., Gibb, J. W., Daly J. W., Lipton M. and Udenfriend, S.: A new class of tyrosine hydroxylase inhibitors and a simple assay of inhibition *in vivo. Biochem. Pharmacol.,* **16,** 1313 (1967).

Levitt, M., Spector, S., Sjoerdsma, A. and Udenfriend, S.: Elucidation of the rate-limiting step in norepinephrine biosynthesis in the perfused guinea-pig heart. *J. Pharmacol. Exp. Therap.,* **148,** 1 (1965).

Livett, B. G., Geffen, L. B. and Rush, R. A.: Immunohistochemical evidence for the transport of dopamine-β-hydroxylase and a catecholamine-binding protein in sympathetic nerves. *Biochem. Pharmacol.,* **18,** 923 (1969).

Lovenberg, W.: Aromatic L-amino acid decarboxylase (guinea pig kidney). In "Methods in Enzymology" (H. Tabor and C. W. Tabor, *eds*), vol. 17B, p. 652. Academic Press, New York (1971).

Lovenberg, W., Barchas, J., Weissbach, M. and Udenfriend, S.: Characteristics of the inhibition of aromatic L-amino acid decarboxylase by α-methylamino acids. *Arch. Biochem. Biophys.,* **103,** 9 (1963).

Lovenberg, W., Dixon, E., Keiser, H. R. and Sjoerdsma, A.: A comparison of amine oxidase activity in human skin, rat skin and rat liver: relevant to collagen cross-linking. *Biochem. Pharmacol.,* **17,** 1117 (1968).

Lovenberg, W., Levine, R. J. and Sjoerdsma, A.: A sensitive assay of monoamine oxidase activity *in vitro*: application to heart and sympathetic ganglia. *J. Pharmacol. Exp. Therap.,* **135,** 7 (1962).

Lovenberg, W., Weissbach, H. and Udenfriend, S.: Aromatic L-amino acid decarboxylase. *J. Biol. Chem.,* **237,** 89 (1962).

Lowry, O. H., Rosebrough, N. J., Farr, A. L. and Randall, R. J.: Protein measurement with the Folin phenol reagent. *J. Biol. Chem.,* **193,** 265 (1951).

Lund, A.: Fluorimetric determination of adrenaline in blood. I. Isolation of the fluorescent oxidation product of adrenaline. *Acta Pharmacol. Toxicol.,* **5,** 75 (1949 a).

Lund, A.: Fluorimetric determination of adrenaline in blood. II. The chemical constitution of adrenolutine (the fluorescent oxidation product of adrenaline). *Acta Pharmacol. Toxicol.*, **5**, 121 (1949 b).

Maickel, R. P., Beaven, M. A. and Brodie, B. B.: Implications of uptake and storage of norepinephrine by sympathetic nerve endings. *Life Sci.*, **2**, 953 (1963).

Mann, J. D., Fales, H. M. and Mudd, H. S.: Alkaloids and plant metabolism: O-methylation *in vitro* of norbelladine, a precursor of amarylliaceae alkaloids. *J. Biol. Chem.*, **238**, 3820 (1963).

Mannarino, E., Kirshner, N. and Nashold, B. S., Jr.: The metabolism of C^{14}-noradrenaline by cat brain *in vivo*. *J. Neurochem.*, **10**, 373 (1963).

Margolis, F. L., Roffi, J. and Jost, A.: Norepinephrine methylation in fetal rat adrenals. *Science*, **154**, 275 (1966).

Märki, F., Axelrod, J. and Witkop, B.: Catecholamines and methyltransferases in the South American toad (Bufo marinus). *Biochim. Biophys. Acta*, **58**, 367 (1962).

Marshall, C. S.: The use of Sephadex G-25 for the separation of catecholamines from plasma. *Biochim. Biophys. Acta*, **74**, 158 (1963).

Martin, L. E. and Harrison, C.: An automated method for determination of noradrenaline and adrenaline in tissues and biological fluid. *Anal. Biochem.*, **23**, 529 (1968).

Mason, W. D. and Olson, C. L.: Differential amperometric measurement of monoamine oxidase activity at tubular carbon electrodes. *Anal. Chem.*, **42**, 488 (1970).

Masuoka, D.: Monoamines in isolated nerve ending particles. *Biochem. Pharmacol.*, **14**, 1688 (1965).

Masuoka, D. T., Schott, H. F., Akawie, R. I. and Clark, W. G.: Conversion of ^{14}C-arterenol to epinephrine *in vivo*. *Proc. Soc. exp. Biol. Med.*, **93**, 5 (1956).

Matsubara, M., Katoh, S., Akino, M. and Kaufman, S.: Sepiapterin reductase. *Biochim. Biophys. Acta*, **122**, 202 (1966).

Matsuoka, M., Ishii, S., Shimizu, N. and Imaizumi, R.: Effect of win 18501-2 on the content of catecholamines and the number of catechol-containing granules in the rabbit hypothalamus. *Experientia*, **21**, 121 (1965)..

Mattok, G. L., Wilson, D. L. and Heacock, R. A.: Differential estimation of adrenaline, noradrenaline, dopamine, metanephrine and normetanephrine in urine. *Clin. Chim. Acta*, **14**, 99 (1966).

Maynert, E. W., Levi, R. and de Lorenzo, A. J. D.: The presence of norepinephrine and 5-hydroxytryptamine in vesicles from disrupted nerve ending particles. *J. Pharmacol. Exp. Therap.*, **144**, 385 (1964).

McEwen, C. M., Jr.: Human plasma monoamine oxidase I. Purification and identification. *J. Biol. Chem.*, **240**, 2003 (1965).

McEwen, C. M. and Cohen, J. D.: An amine oxidase in normal human serum. *J. Lab. Clin. Med.*, **62**, 766 (1963).

McGeer, E. G. and McGeer, P. L.: *In vitro* screen of inhibitors of rat brain tyrosine hydroxylase. *Can. J. Biochem.*, **45**, 115 (1967).

McGeer, E. G., McGeer, P. L. and Peters, D. A.: Inhibition of brain tyrosine hydroxylase by 5-halotryptophans. *Life Sci.*, **6**, 2221 (1967).

McGeer, P. L. and McGeer, E. G.: Formation of adrenaline by brain tissue. *Biochem. Biophys. Res. Commun.*, **17**, 502 (1964).

McGeer, P. L., Bagchi, S. P. and McGeer, E. G.: Subcellular fractionation of tyrosine hydroxylase in beef caudate nucleus. *Life Sci., 4,* 1859 (1965).

Meisch, J. J., Carlsson, A. and Waldeck, B.: Effect of desipramine and reserpine on the *in vivo* β-hydroxylation of α-methyl-*m*-tyramine and α-methyldopamine. *J. Pharm. Pharmacol., 19,* 63 (1967).

Mendell, J. R., Chase, T. N. and Engel, W. K.: Modification by L-DOPA of a case of progressive supranuclear palsy. *Lancet, 1,* 593 (1970).

Merrills, R. J.: An autoanalytical method for the estimation of adrenaline and noradrenaline. *Nature, 193,* 988 (1962).

Merrills, R. J.: A semiautomatic method for determination of catecholamines. *Anal. Biochem., 6,* 272 (1963).

Milhaud, G. and Glowinski, J.: Metabolisme de la dopamine ^{14}C dans le cerveau du rat. Etude du mode d'administration. *C. R. Acad. Sci., Paris, 255,* 203 (1962).

Milhaud, G. and Glowinski, J.: Metabolism de la noradrenaline ^{14}C dans le cerveau du rat. *C. R. Acad, Sci., Paris, 256,* 1033 (1963).

Missala, K., Lloyd, K., Gregoriads, G. and Sourkes, T. L.: Conversion of ^{14}C-dopamine to cardiac ^{14}C-noradrenaline in the copper-deficient rat. *Europ. J. Pharmacol., 1,* 6 (1967).

Mitoma, C.: Studies on partially purified phenylalanine hydroxylase. *Arch. Biochem. Biophys., 60,* 476 (1956).

Miyake, H., Yoshida, H. and Imaizumi, R.: Determination methods for urinary 3-methoxy-4-hydroxymandelic acid and 3,4-dihydroxymandelic acid. *Jap. J. Pharmacol., 12,* 79 (1962).

Mizutani, K., Nagatsu, T., Asajima, M. and Kinoshita, S.: Inhibition of tyrosine hydroxylase by naphthoquinone pigments in Echinodermata. *J. Jap. Biochem. Soc., 43,* 747 (1971).

Molinoff, P. B. and Axelrod, J.: Octopamine: normal occurrence in sympathetic nerves of rats. *Science, 164,* 428 (1969).

Molinoff, P B., Landsberg, L. and Axelrod, J.: An enzymatic assay for ocopamine and other β-hydroxylated phenylethylamines. *J. Pharmacol. Exp. Therap., 170,* 253 (1969).

Molinoff, P. B., Weinshilboum, R. and Axelrod, J.: A sensitive enzymatic assay for dopamine-β-hydroxylase. *J. Pharmacol. Exp. Therap., 178,* 425 (1971).

Montanari, R., Beaven, M. A., Costa, E. and Brodie, B. B.: Turnover rates of norepinephrine in hearts of intact mice, rats and guinea pigs using tritiated norepinephrine. *Life Sci., 2,* 232 (1963).

Mueller, R. A., deChamplain, J. and Axelrod, J.: Increased monoamine oxidase activity in isoproterenol-stimulated submaxillary glands. *Biochem. Pharmacol., 17,* 2455 (1968).

Mueller, R. A., Thoenen, H. and Axelrod, J.: Adrenal tyrosine hydroxylase: compensating increase in activity after chemical sympathectomy. *Science, 163,* 468 (1969 a).

Mueller, R. A., Thoenen, H. and Axelrod, J.: Increase in tyrosine hydroxylase activity after reserpine administration. *J. Pharmacol. Exp. Therap., 169,* 74 (1969 b).

Murphy, G. F., Robinson, D. and Sharman, D. F.: The effect of tropolone on the formation of 3,4-dihydroxyphenylacetic acid and 4-hydroxy-3-methoxyphenyl-acetic acid in the brain of the mouse. *Brit. J. Pharmacol.*, **36**, 107 (1969).

Murphy, G. F. and Sourkes, T. L.: The action of antidecarboxylases on the conversion of 3,4-dihydroxyphenylalanine to dopamine *in vivo. Arch. Biochem. Biophys.*, **93**, 338 (1961).

Musacchio, J. M.: Subcellular distribution of adrenal tyrosine hydroxylase. *Biochem. Pharmacol.*, **17**, 1470 (1968).

Musacchio, J. M., Julou, L., Kety, S. S. and Glowinski, J.: Increase in rat brain tyrosine hydroxylase activity produced by electroconvulsive shock. *Proc. Natl. Acad. Sci. U. S. A.*, **63**, 117 (1969).

Musacchio, J. M., Kopin, I. J. and Weise, V. K.: Subcellular distribution of some sympathomimetic amines and their β-hydroxylated derivatives in the rat heart. *J. Pharmacol. Exp. Therap.*, **148**, 22 (1965).

Musacchio, J. M., Wurzburger, R. J. and D'Angelo, G. L.: Different molecular forms of bovine adrenal tyrosine hydroxylase. *Mol. Pharmacol.*, **7**, 136 (1971).

Nagai (Matsubara), M.: Studies on sepiapterin reductase: Further characterization of the reaction product. *Arch. Biochem. Biophys.*, **126**, 426 (1968).

Nagatsu, I., Nagatsu, T., Mizutani, K., Umezawa, H., Matsuzaki, M. and Takeuchi, T.: Adrenal tyrosine hydroxylase and dopamine β-hydroxylase in spontaneously hypertensive rats. *Nature,* **230**, 381 (1971).

Nagatsu, I., Nagatsu, T., Mizutani, K., Umezawa, H., Matsuzaki, M. and Takeuchi, T.: Adrenal enzymes of catecholamine biosynthesis and metabolism in spontaneously hypertensive rats. *Experientia,* **27**, 10103 (1971).

Nagatsu, T.: Partial separation and properties of mitochondrial monoamine oxidase in brain. *J. Biochem. (Tokyo),* **59**, 606 (1966).

Nagatsu, T., Ayukawa, S. and Umezawa, H.: Inhibition of dopamine β-hydroxylase by aquayamycin. *J. Antibiotics,* **21**, 354 (1968).

Nagatsu, T., Hidaka, H., Kuzuya, H., Takeya, K., Umezawa, H., Takeuchi, T. and Suda, H.: Inhibition of dopamine β-hydroxylase by fusaric acid (5-butylpicolinic acid) *in vitro* and *in vivo. Biochem. Pharmacol.*, **19**, 35 (1970).

Nagatsu, T., Kuzuya, H. and Hidaka, H.: Inhibition of dopamine β-hydroxylase by sulfhydryl compounds and the nature of the natural inhibitors. *Biochim. Biophys. Acta,* **139**, 319 (1967).

Nagatsu, T., Levitt, M. and Udenfriend, S.: Conversion of L-tyrosine to 3,4-dihydroxy phenylalanine by cell-free preparations of brain and sympathetically innervated tissues. *Biochem. Biophys. Res. Commun.*, **14**, 543 (1964 a).

Nagatsu, T., Levitt, M. and Udenfriend, S.: Tyrosine hydroxylase: The initial step in norepinephrine biosynthesis. *J. Biol. Chem.*, **239**, 2910 (1964 b).

Nagatsu, T., Levitt, M. and Udenfriend, S.: A rapid and simple radio assay for tyrosine hydroxylase activity. *Anal. Biochem.*, **9**, 122 (1964 c).

Nagatsu, T., Levitt, M. and Udenfriend, S.: Properties of the mammalian tyrosine hydroxylase associated with norepinephrine biosynthesis. *Fed. Proc.*, **23**, 480 (1964 d).

Nagatsu, T., Mizutani, K. and Nagatsu, I.: Enzyme of catecholamine biosynthesis and metabolism in human adrenal gland and pheochromocytoma. *Clin. Chim. Acta,* **39**, 417 (1972).

Nagatsu, T., Mizutani, K., Nagatsu, I., Matsuura, S. and Sugimoto, T.: Pteridines as cofactor or inhibitor of tyrosine hydroxylase. *Biochem. Pharmacol.*, **21**, 1945 (1972).

Nagatsu, T. and Nagatsu, I.: Subcellular distribution of tyrosine hydroxylase and monoamine oxidase in the bovine caudate nucleus. *Experientia*, **26**, 722 (1970).

Nagatsu, T., Nagatsu, I., Umezawa, H. and Takeuchi, T.: Effect of oudenone on adrenal tyrosine hydroxylase activity *in vivo* and on tissue catecholamine concentrations. *Biochem. Pharmacol.*, **20**, 2505 (1971).

Nagatsu, T., Nakano, G., Mizutani, K. and Harada, M.: Purification and properties of amine oxidases in brain and connective tissue (dental pulp). In "Advances in Biochemical Pharmacology" (E. Costa and M. Sandler, *eds*), p. 25. Raven Press, New York (1966).

Nagatsu, T., Rust, L. A. and DeQuattro, V.: The activity of tyrosine hydroxylase and related enzymes of catecholamine biosynthesis and metabolism in dog kidney. Effect of denervation. *Biochem. Pharmacol.*, **18**, 1441 (1969).

Nagatsu, T., Sudo, Y. and Nagatsu, I.: Studies on catecholamine biosynthesis. Tyrosine hydroxylase in caudate nucleus. *Bull. Jap. Neurochem. Soc.*, **9**, Suppl., 36 (1970).

Nagatsu, T., Sudo, Y. and Nagatsu, I.: Tyrosine hydroxylase in bovine caudate nucleus. *J. Neurochem.*, **18**, 2179 (1971).

Nagatsu, T. and Takeuchi, T.: The effect of high phenylalanine concentration on the formation of DOPA from phenylalanine and tyrosine by tyrosine hydroxylase. *Experientia*, **23**, 532 (1967).

Nagatsu, T. and Udenfriend, S.: Photometric assay of dopamine-β-hydroxylase in human blood. *Clin. Chem.*, **18**, 980 (1972).

Nagatsu, T., van der Schoot, J. B., Levitt, M. and Udenfriend, S.: Factors influencing dopamine β-hydroxylase activity and epinephrine levels in guinea pig adrenal gland. *J. Biochem. (Tokyo)*, **64**, 39 (1968).

Nagatsu, T. and Yagi, K.: Identification of the main ethylenediamine condensate of noradrenaline with that of catechol. *Nature*, **193**, 484 (1962 a).

Nagatsu, T. and Yagi, K.: Crystalline picrate of the condensation product of ethylenediamine with noradrenaline or with catechol. *J. Biochem. (Tokyo)*, **52**, 452 (1962 b).

Nagatsu, T. and Yagi, K.: A simple assay of monoamine oxidase and D-amino acid oxidase by measuring ammonia. *J. Biochem.*, **60**, 219 (1966).

Nagatsu, T. and Yamamoto, T.: Fluorescence assay of tyrosine hydroxylase activity in tissue homogenate. *Experientia*, **24**, 1183 (1968).

Nagatsu, T., Yamamoto, T. and Harada, M.: Purification and properties of human brain mitochondrial monoamine oxidase. *Enzymologia* **39**, 15 (1970).

Nagatsu, T., Yamamoto, T. and Nagatsu, I.: Partial separation and properties of tyrosine hydroxylase from the human pheochromocytoma. *Biochim. Biophys. Acta*, **198**, 210 (1970).

Nagatsu, T., Yamamoto, T. and Nagatsu, I.: Tyrosine hydroxylase in human pheochromocytoma: effect of tetrahydropteridine and norepinephrine. In "Chemistry and Biology of Pteridines" (K. Iwai, M. Akino, M. Goto and Y. Iwanami, *eds*), p. 235. International Academic Printing, Tokyo (1970).

Nair, P. M. and Vining, L. C.: Phenylalanine hydroxylase from spinach leaves. *Phytochemistry*, **4**, 401 (1965).

Nakano, G., Kuzuya, H. and Nagatsu, T.: Catecholamines in the dental pulp. *J. Dent. Res.*, **49**, 1549 (1970).

Nakano, G. and Nagatsu, T.: Purification and properties of an amine oxidase in boving dental pulp. *Experientia*, **27**, 1399 (1971).

Nara, S., Gomes, B. and Yasunobu, K. T.: Amine oxidase VII. Beef liver mito-chondrial monoamine oxidase, a copper-containing protein. *J. Biol. Chem.*, **241**, 2774 (1966).

Nara, S., Igaue, I., Gomes, B. and Yasunobu, K. L.: The prosthetic groups of animal amine oxidases. *Biochem. Biophys. Res. Commun.*, **23**, 324 (1966).

Natelson, S., Lugovoy, J. K. and Pincus, J. B.: A new fluorimetric method for the determination of epinephrine. *Arch. Biochem.*, **23**, 157 (1949).

Neff, N.H. and Costa, E.: The influence of monoamine oxidase inhibition on catecholamine synthesis. *Life Sci.*, **5**, 951 (1966).

Neff, N. H., Ngai, S. H., Wang, C. T. and Costa, E.: Calculation of the rate of catecholamine synthesis from the rate of conversion of tyrosine-^{14}C to catechol-amines. Effect of adrenal demedullation on synthesis rates. *Mol. Pharmacol.*, **5**, 90 (1969).

Nielsen, K. H., Simonsen, V. and Lind, K. E.: Dihydropteridine reductase. A method for the measurement of activity, and investigations of the specificity for NADH and NADPH. *Europ. J. Biochem.*, **9**, 497 (1969).

Nikodijevic, B., Creveling, C. R. and Udenfriend, S.: Inhibition of dopamine β-hydroxylase *in vivo* by benzyloxyamine and benzylhydrazine analogs. *J. Phar-macol. Exp. Therap.*, **140**, 224 (1963).

Nikodijevic, B., Daly, J. and Creveling, C. R.: Catechol-*O*-methyltransferase. I. An enzymatic assay for cardiac norepinephrine. *Biochem. Pharmacol.*, **18**, 1577 (1969).

Nikodijevic, B., Senoh, S., Daly, J. W. and Creveling, C. R.: Catechol-*O*-methyl-transferase. II. New class of inhibitors of catechol-*O*-methyltransferase; 3,5-dihydro-4-methoxy-benzoic acid and related compounds. *J. Pharmacol. Exp. Therap.*, **174**, 83 (1970).

Norberg, K. A. and Hamberger, B.: The sympathetic adrenergic neurone. *Acta Physiol. Scand.*, **63**, Supple. 238 (1964).

Obata, F., Ushiwata, A. and Nakamura, Y.: Spectrophotometric assay of mono-amine oxidase using 2,4,6-trinitrobenzene-1-sulfonic acid. *J. Biochem.*, **69**, 349 (1971).

O'Dell, B. L., Elsden, D. F., Thomas, J., Partridge, S. M., Smith, R. H. and Palmer, R.: Inhibition of the biosynthesis of the cross-links in elastin by a lathyrogen. *Nature*, **209**, 401 (1966).

Oestlund, E.: The distribution of catecholamine in lower animals and their effect on the heart. *Acta Physiol. Scand.*, **112**, Supple. 31 (1954).

Oh, Y. H., Leitch, W. H., Axelrod, S., Small, S. M., Winzler, R. J. and Sanders, B. E.: Binding of biologically active amines to plasma protein fractions. *Biochem. Pharmacol.*, **16**, 849 (1967).

Ohno, M., Okamoto, M., Kawabe, N., Umezawa, H., Takeuchi, T., Iinuma, H. and Takahashi, S.: Oudenone, a nobel tyrosine hydroxylase inhibitor from microbial origin. *J. Am. Chem. Soc.*, **93**, 1285 (1971).

Okamoto, H., Yamamoto, S., Nozaki, M. and Hayaishi, O.: On the submito-chondrial localization of L-kynurenine-3-hydroxylase. *Biochem. Biophys. Res. Commun.*, **26**, 309 (1967).

Olivecrona, T. and Oreland, L.: Reassociation of soluble monoamine oxidase with lipid-depleted mitochondria in the presence of phospholipids. *Biochemis-*

try, **10,** 332 (1971).

Oreland, L. and Olivecrona, T.: The role of acidic phospholipids in the binding of monoamine oxidase to the mitochondrial structure. *Arch. Biochem. Biophys.,* **142,** 710 (1971).

Otsuka, S. and Kobayashi, Y.: A radioisotopic assay for monoamine oxidase determinations in human plasma. *Biochem. Pharmacol.,* **13,** 995 (1964).

Ozaki, M., Weissbach, H., Ozaki, A., Witkop, B. and Udenfriend, S.: Monoamine oxidase inhibitors and procedures for their evaluation *in vivo* and *in vitro. J. Medicinal and Pharmaceutical Chem.,* **2,** 591 (1960).

Perry, T. L., Hensen, S. and MacDougall, L.: Identity and significance of some pink spots in schizophrenia and other conditions. *Nature,* **214,** 484 (1967).

Perry, T. L., Hensen, S., MacDougall, L. and Schwarz, C. J.: Urinary amines in chronic schizophrenia. *Nature,* **212,** 146 (1966).

Persson, T. and Waldeck, B.: Some problems encountered in attempting to estimate catecholamine turnover using labeled tyrosine. *J. Pharm. Pharmac.,* **22,** 473 (1970).

Petrack, B., Sheppy, F. and Fetzer, V.: Studies on tyrosine hydroxylase from bovine adrenal medulla. *J. Biol. Chem.,* **243,** 743 (1968).

Philippu, A. and Schümann, H. J.: Der Einfluss von Calcium auf die Brenzcatechinamin-Freisetzung. *Experientia,* **18,** 138 (1962).

Philippu, A. and Schümann, H. J.: Effect of ribonuclease on the ribonuleic acid, adenosine triphosphate and catecholamine content of medullary granules. *Nature,* **198,** 795 (1963).

Philippu, A. and Schümann, H. J.: Die Bedeutung divalenter Kationen für die Speicherung der Nebennierenmark-Hormone in den chromaffinen Granula. *Arch. exp. Path. Pharmakol.,* **247,** 295 (1964 a).

Philippu, A. and Schümann, H. J.: Ribonucleaseaktivität isolierter Nebennierenmarkgranula. *Experientia,* **20,** 547 (1964 b).

Philippu, A. and Schümann, H. J.: Significance of calcium and magnesium ions for the storage of adrenomedullar hormones. *Arch. exp. Path. Pharmakol.,* **252,** 339 (1966).

Philpott, J. E., Zarrow, M. X., Denenberg, V. H., Lu, K-H., Fuller, R. W. and Hunt, J. M.: Phenethanolamine *N*-methyl transferase and adrenocortical activity in the neonatal rat. *Life Sci.,* **8,** 367 (1969).

Pisano, J. J.: A simple analysis of normetanephrine and metanephrine in urine. *Clin. Chim. Acta,* **5,** 406 (1960).

Pisano, J. J., Creveling, C. R. and Udenfriend, S.: Enzymic conversion of *p*-tyramine to *p*-hydroxyphenylethanolamine (norsynephrine). *Biochim. Biophys. Acta,* **43,** 566 (1960).

Pisano, J. J., Crout, J. R. and Abraham, D.: Determination of 3-methoxy-4-hydroxymandelic acid in urine. *Clin. Chim. Acta,* **7,** 285 (1962).

Pisano, J. J., Oates, J. A., Jr., Karmen, A., Sjoerdsma, A. and Udenfriend, S.: Identification of *p*-hydroxy-*α*-(methylaminomethyl)benzyl alcohol (synephrine) in human urine. *J. Biol. Chem.,* **236,** 898 (1961).

Pletscher, A.: Monoamine oxidase inhibitors. *Pharmacol. Rev.,* **18,** 121 (1966).

Pletscher, A., Burkard, W. P. and Gey, K. F.: The effect of monoamine releasers and decarboxylase inhibitors on endogenous 5-hydroxyindole derivatives in the brain. *Biochem. Pharmacol.,* **13,** 385 (1964).

Pletscher, A. and Gey, K. F.: The effect of a new decarboxylase inhibitor on endogenous and exogenous amines. *Biochem. Pharmacol.*, **12**, 223 (1963).

Pletscher, A., Gey, K. F. and Burkard, W. P.: Inhibitors of monoamine oxidase and decarboxylase of aromatic amino acids. In "Handbuch der experimentellen Pharmakologie" vol. 19, p. 593. Springer-Verlag, Heidelberg (1965).

Pletscher, A., Gey, K. F. and Zeller, P.: Monoaminoxydase-Hemmer. In "Progress in Drug Research" (E. Jucker, *ed*). vol. 2, p. 417. Birkhäuser-Verlag, Basel (1960).

Pomerantz, S. H.: Separation, purification, and properties of two tyrosinases from hamster melanoma. *J. Biol. Chem.*, **238**, 2351 (1963).

Pomerantz, S. H. and Warner, M. C.: Identification of 3,4-dihydroxyphenylalanine as tyrosinase cofactor in melanoma. *Biochem. Biophys. Res. Commun.*, **24**, 25 (1966).

Pool, P. E., Covell, J. W., Levitt, M., Gibb, J. and Braunwald, E.: Reduction of cardiac tyrosine hydroxylase activity in experimental congestive heart failure. *Circ. Res.*, **20**, 349 (1967).

Porter, C. C., Watson, L. S., Titus, D. C., Totaro, J. A. and Byer, S. S.: Inhibition of dopa decarboxylase by the hydrazine analog of α-methyldopa. *Biochem. Pharmacol.*, **11**, 1067 (1962).

Potter, L. T. and Axelrod, J.: Storage of norepinephrine and the effect of drugs. *J. Pharmacol. Exp. Therap.*, **140**, 199 (1963 a).

Potter, L. T. and Axelrod, J.: Subcellular localization of catecholamines in tissues of the rat. *J. Pharmacol. Exp. Therap.*, **142**, 291 (1963 b).

Potter, L. T., Cooper, T., Willman, V. L. and Wolfe, D. E.: Synthesis, binding, release and metabolism of norepinephrine in normal and transplanted dog hearts. *Circ. Res.*, **16**, 468 (1965).

Pryor, M. G. M.: Sclerotization. In "Comparative Biochemistry" (M. Florkin and H. S. Mason, *eds*) vol. 4, p.371, Academic Press, New York (1964).

Pütter, J. and Kroneberg, G.: Untersuchungen über die Stereospezifität der decarboxylasehemmenden Wirkung von α-Methyldopa. *Arch. exp. Path. Pharmakol.*, **249**, 470 (1964).

Racker, E.: Liver aldehyde dehydrogenase. In "Methods in Enzymology" (S. P. Colowick and N. O. Kaplan, *eds*) vol. 1, p. 514. Academic Press, New York (1955).

Renson, J., Weissbach, H. and Udenfriend, S.: Hydroxylation of tryptophan by phenylalanine hydroxylase. *J. Biol. Chem.*, **237**, 2261 (1962).

Renson, J., Weissbach, H. and Udenfriend, S.: Studies on the biological activities of the aldehyde derived from norepinephrine, serotonin, tryptamine and histamine. *J. Pharmacol. Exp. Therap.*, **143**, 326 (1964).

Richter, D.: Inactivation of adrenaline *in vivo* in man. *J. Physiol.*, **98**, 361 (1940).

Richter, D. and MacIntosh, F. C.: Adrenaline ester. *Am. J. Physiol.*, **135**, 1 (1941).

Robinson, R., Ratcliffe, J. and Smith, P.: A screening test for phaeochromocytoma. *J. Clin. Path.*, **12**, 541 (1959).

Robinson, R. J. and Watts, D. T.: An automated trihydroxyindole procedure for the differential analysis of catecholamines. *Clin. Chem.*, **11**, 986 (1965).

Rodrígues DeLores Arnaiz, G. and de Robertis, E.: 5-Hydroxytryptophan decarboxylase activity in nerve endings of the rat brain. *J. Neurochem.*, **11**, 213

(1964).

Rosano, C. L.: Enzymatic method for determination of vanillylmandelic acid. *Clin. Chem.,* **10,** 673 (1964).

Rosenfeld, G., Leeper, L. C. and Udenfriend, S.: Biosynthesis of norepinephrine and epinephrine by the isolated perfused calf adrenal. *Arch. Biochem. Biophys.,* **74,** 252 (1958).

Rosengren, E.: On the role of monoamine oxidase for the inactivation of dopamine in brain. *Acta Physiol. Scand.,* **49,** 370 (1960).

Roth, R. H. and Stjärne, L.: Monoamine oxidase activity in the bovine splenic nerve granule preparation. *Acta. Physiol. Scand.,* **68,** 342 (1966).

Roth, R. H., Stjärne, L. and Euler, U. S. von: Acceleration of noradrenaline biosynthesis by nerve stimulation. *Life Sci.,* **5,** 1071 (1966).

Roth, R. H., Stjärne, L. and Euler, U. S. von: Factors influencing the rate of norepinephrine biosynthesis in nerve tissue. *J. Pharmacol. Exp. Therap.,* **158,** 373 (1967).

Roth, R. H., Stjärne, L., Levine, R. J. and Giarman, N. J.: Abnormal regulation of catecholamine synthesis in pheochromocytoma. *J. Lab. Clin. Med.,* **72,** 397 (1968).

Rubin, R. P.: The role of energy metabolism in calcium-evoked secretion from the adrenal medulla. *J. Physiol.,* **206,** 181 (1970).

Rucker, R. B., Rogler, J. C. and Parker, H. E.: The partial characterization of an amine oxidase in bone tissue. *Proc. Soc. Exp. Biol. Med.,* **130,** 1150 (1969).

Ruthven, C. R. J. and Sandler, M.: The estimation of homovanillic acid in urine. *Biochem. J.,* **83,** 30 P (1962).

Ruthven, C. R. J. and Sandler, M.: Estimation of homovanillic acid in urine. *Anal. Biochem.,* **8,** 282 (1964).

Ruthven, C. R. J. and Sandler, M.: The estimation of 4-hydroxy-3-methoxyphenyl glycol and total metadrenalines in human urines. *Clin. Chim. Acta,* **12,** 318 (1965).

Rutledge, C. O. and Weiner, N.: The effect of reserpine upon the synthesis of norepinephrine in the isolated rabbit heart. *J. Pharmacol. Exp. Therap.,* **157,** 290 (1967).

Saari, W. S., Williams, J., Britcher, S. F., Wolf, D. E. and Kuehl, F. A., Jr.: Tyrosine hydroxylase inhibitors. Synthesis and activity of substituted aromatic amino acids. *J. Med. Chem.,* **10,** 1008 (1967).

Saelens, J. K., Schoen, M. S. and Kovacsics, G. B.: An enzyme assay for norepinephrine in brain tissue. *Biochem. Pharmacol.,* **16,** 1043 (1967).

Sakamoto, Y., Ogawa, Y. and Hayashi, K.: Studies on monoamine oxidase. *J. Biochem. (Tokyo),* **54,** 292 (1963).

Samejima, K., Dairman, W. and Udenfriend, S.: Condensation of ninhydrin, aldehydes and primary amines to yield highly fluorescent ternary products. I. Mechanism of the reaction and partial characterization of the condensation product. *Anal. Biochem.,* **42,** 222 (1971).

Samejima, K., Dairman, W., Stone, J. and Udenfriend, S.: Condensation of ninhydrin with aldehydes and primary amines to yield highly fluorescent ternary products. II. Application to the detection and assay of peptides, amino acids, amines and amino sugars. *Anal. Biochem.,* **42,** 237 (1971).

Sandler, M.: Biosynthesis and metabolism of the catecholamines. *Schweiz. med.*

Wschr., **100**, 526 (1970).

Sandler, M. and Ruthven, C. R. J.: The estimation of 4-hydroxy-3-methoxyman-delic acid in urine. *Biochem. J.*, **80**, 78 (1961).

Sandler, M. and Ruthven, C. R. J.: The measurement of 4-hydroxy-3-methoxy-mandelic acid and homovanillic acid. *Pharmacol. Rev.*, **18**, 343 (1966).

Sankoff, I. and Sourkes, T. L.: Determination by thin-layer chromatography of urinary homovanillic acid in normal and disease states. *Can. J. Biochem. Phys-iol.*, **41**, 1381 (1963).

Sano, I., Gamo, T., Kakimoto, Y., Taniguchi, K., Takesada, M. and Nishinuma, K.: Distribution of catechol compounds in human brain. *Biochim. Biophys. Acta*, **32**, 586 (1959).

Sato, T. L.: The quantitative determination of 3-methoxy-4-hydroxyphenylacetic acid (homovanillic acid) in urine. *J. Lab. Clin. Med.*, **66**, 517 (1965).

Sato, T. and DeQuattro, V.: Enzymatic assay for 3,4-dihydroxymandelic acid (DOMA) in human urine, plasma, and tissues. *J. Lab. Clin. Med.*, **74**, 672 (1969).

Sato, T. L., Jequier, E., Lovenberg, W. and Sjoerdsma, A.: Characterization of a tryptophan hydroxylating enzyme from malignant mouse mast cell. *Eur. J. Pharmacol.*, **1**, 18 (1967).

Sato, T., Ono, I., Miura, Y. and Yoshinaga, K.: Increased catecholamine excre-tion during normotensive phase in paroxysmal type of pheochromocytoma. *Jap. Heart J.*, **12**, 214 (1971).

Sato, T., Yoshinaga, K., Ishida, N., Itoh, C. and Wada, Y.: A new simple screening test for pheochromocytoma. *Tohoku J. Exp. Med.*, **74**, 37 (1961).

Sato, T., Yoshinaga, K., Ishida, N., Itoh, C. and Wada, Y.: Advanced screening test for pheochromocytoma and argentaffinoma. *Tohoku J. Exp. Med.*, **77**, 78 (1962).

Schales, O.: Amino acid decarboxylases of animals. In "Methods in Enzymology" (S. P. Colowick and N. O. Kaplan, *eds*), vol. 2, p. 195. Academic Press Inc., New York. (1955).

Schales, O. and Schales, S. S.: Dihydroxyphenylalanine decarboxylase: Prepara-tion and properties of a stable dry powder. *Arch. Biochem. Biophys.*, **24**, 83 (1949).

Schmid, E. and Henning, N.: Über den Nachweis der 3-Methoxy-4-hydroxy-mandelsäure im Harn. *Klin. Wschr.*, **41**, 566 (1963).

Schmid, E., Zicha, L., Krautheim, J. and Blumberg, J.: Dünnschicht-Chromato-graphische Trennung von Substanzen des Katecholamin—und Serotonin—stoffwechsels. *Med. exp.*, **7**, 8 (1962).

Schnaitman, C., Erwin, V. G. and Greenwalt, J. W.: The submitochondrial loca-lization of monoamine oxidase. An enzymatic marker for the outer membrane of rat liver mitochondria. *J. Cell. Biol.*, **32**, 719 (1967).

Schneider, F. H. and Gillis, C. N.: Catecholamine biosynthesis *in vivo*: An ap-plication of thin-layer chromatography. *Biochem, Pharmacol.*, **14**, 623 (1965).

Schott, H. F. and Clark, W. G.: Dopa decarboxylase inhibition through the interaction of coenzyme and substrate. *J. Biol. Chem.*, **196**, 449 (1952).

Schümann, H. J.: Nachweis von Oxytyramin (Dopamin) in sympathischen Nerven und Ganglien. *Arch. exp. Path. Pharmakol.*, **227**, 566 (1956).

Schümann, H. J.: Über den Noradrenalin- und ATP- Gehalt sympathischer

Nerven. *Arch. exp. Path. Pharmakol.*, **233**, 296 (1958 a).

Schümann, H. J.: Über die Verteilung von Noradrenalin und Hydroxytyramin in Sympathischen Nerven (Milznerven). *Arch. exp. Path. Pharmakol.*, **234**, 17 (1958b).

Schümann, H. J.: Hormon- und ATP-Gehalt des menschlichen Nebennierenmarks und des Phäochromocytomgewebes. *Klin. Wschr.*, **38**, 11 (1960).

Schümann, H. J.: Medullary particles. *Pharmacol. Rev.*, **18**, 433 (1966).

Schümann, H. J. and Philippu, A.: Untersuchungen zum Mechanismus der Freisetzung von Brenzcatechinaminen durch Tyramin. *Arch. exp. Path. Pharmakol.*, **241**, 273 (1961).

Schümann, H. J. and Philippu, A.: Zum Mechanismus der durch Calcium und Magnesium verursachten Freisetzung der Nebennierenmark-Hormone. *Arch. exp. Path. Pharmakol.*, **244**, 466 (1963).

Schümann, H. J., Schnell, K. and Philippu, A.: Subcelluläre Verteilung von Noradrenalin und Adrenalin im Meerschweinchenherzen. *Arch. exp. Path. Pharmakol.*, **249**, 251 (1964).

Schweitzer, J. W. and Friedhoff, A. J.: A new method for the determination of labeled dopamine, norepinephrine and their metabolites in rat brain homogenate. *Life Sci.*, **8**, 173 (1969).

Sedvall, G. C. and Kopin, I. J.: Influence of sympathetic denervation and nerve impulse activity of tyrosine hydroxylase in the rat submaxillary gland. *Biochem. Pharmacol.*, **16**, 39 (1967).

Sedvall, G. C., Weise, V. K. and Kopin, I. J.: The rate of norepinephrine synthesis measured *in vivo* during short intervals; influence of adrenergic nerve impulse activity. *J. Pharmacol. Exp. Therap.*, **159**, 274 (1968).

Segura-Cardona, R. and Soehring, K.: Dünnschichtchromatographischer Nachweis kleinster Mengen von Katecholaminen und deren Derivaten. *Med. exp.*, **10**, 251 (1964).

Sekeris, C. E.: Zum Tyrosinstoffwechsel der Insekten. XII. Reinigung, Eigenschaften und Substratspezifität der Dopa-Decarboxylase. *Hoppe-Seyler Z. Physiol. Chem.*, **332**, 70 (1963).

Sekeris, C. E.: Action of ecdysone on the RNA and protein metabolism of the Calliphora erythrocephala. In "Mechanisms of Hormone Action" (Karlson ed), p.149. Academic Press, New York, and Springer-Verlag, Berlin (1965).

Sekeris, C. E. and Herrlich, P.: Vorkommen von Arylamin-Transacetylase im Säugetierorganismus. *Hoppe-Seyler Z. Physiol. Chem.*, **336**, 130 (1964).

Sekeris, C. E. and Karlson, P.: On the mechanisms of hormone action. II. Ecdysone and protein biosynthesis. *Arch. Biochem. Biophys.*, **105**, 483 (1964).

Sekeris, C. E. and Karlson, P.: Biosynthesis of catecholamines in insects. *Pharmacol. Rev.*, **18**, 89 (1966).

Sekeris, C. E. and Mergenhagen, D.: Phenol oxidase system of the blowfly, *Calliphora erythrocephala. Science*, **145**, 68 (1964).

Senoh, S., Creveling, C. R., Udenfriend, S. and Witkop, B.: Chemical, enzymatic and metabolic studies on the mechanism of oxidation of dopamine. *J. Am. Chem. Soc.*, **81**, 6236 (1959).

Senoh, S., Daly, J., Axelrod, J. and Witkop, B.: Enzymatic p-O-methylation by catechol O-methyl transferase. *J. Am. Chem. Soc.*, **81**, 6240 (1959).

Senoh, S. and Witkop, B.: Non-enzymatic conversions of dopamine to norepinephrine and trihydroxyphenethylamines. *J. Am. Chem. Soc.,* **81,** 6222 (1959).

Senoh, S., Witkop, B., Creveling, C. R. and Udenfriend, S.: 2,4,5-Trihydroxyphenethylamine, a new metabolite of 3,4-dihydroxyphenethylamine. *J. Am. Chem. Soc.,* **81,** 1768 (1959).

Sezaki, M., Hara, T., Ayukawa, S., Takeuchi, T., Okami, Y., Hamada, M., Nagatsu, T. and Umezawa, H.: Studies on a new antibiotic pigment, aquayamycin. *J. Antibiotics,* **21,** 91 (1968).

Sezaki, M., Kondo, S., Maeda, K., Umezawa, H. and Ohno, M.: The structure of aquayamycin. *Tetrahedron,* **26,** 5171 (1970).

Sharman, D. F.: A fluorometric method for the estimation of homovanillic acid and its identification in brain tissue. *Brit. J. Pharmacol.,* **20,** 204 (1963).

Sharman, D. F.: Glycol metabolites of noradrenaline in brain tissue. *Brit. J. Pharmacol.,* **36,** 523 (1969).

Shaw, F. H.: The estimation of adrenaline. *Biochem. J.,* **32,** 19 (1938).

Shaw, K. N. F., McMillan, A. and Armstrong, M. D.: The metabolism of 3,4-dihydroxyphenylalanine. *J. Biol. Chem.,* **226,** 255 (1957).

Shepherd, D. M. and West, G. B.: Hydroxytyramine and the adrenal medulla. *J. Physiol.,* **120,** 15 (1953).

Shiman, R., Akino, M. and Kaufman, S.: Solubilization and partial purification of tyrosine hydroxylase from bovine adrenal medulla. *J. Biol. Chem.,* **246,** 1330 (1971).

Shiman, R. and Kaufman, S.: Tyrosine hydroxylase (bovine adrenal glands). In "Methods in Enzymology" (H. Tabor and C. W. Tabor, *eds*), vol. 17A, p. 609. Academic Press, New York (1970).

Shimizu, H. and LaBrosse, E. H.: Metabolism of catecholamines-identification and quantification of 3-methoxy-4-hydroxyphenylglycol glucuronide in human urine. *Biochem. Pharmacol.,* **18,** 1643 (1969).

Shore, P. A.: A simple technique involving solvent extraction for the estimation of norepinephrine and epinephrine in tissues. *Pharmacol. Rev.,* **11,** 276 (1959).

Shore, P. A. and Olin, J. S.: Identification and chemical assay of norepinephrine in brain and other tissues. *J. Pharmacol. Exp. Therap.,* **122,** 295 (1958).

Siegel, R. C. and Martin, G. R.: Collagen cross-linking. Enzymatic synthesis of lysine-derived aldehydes and the production of cross-linked components. *J. Biol. Chem.,* **245,** 1653 (1970).

Sjoerdsma, A.: Catecholamines and the drug therapy of hypertension. *Circ. Res.,* **21,** Suppl. III. 119 (1967).

Sjoerdsma, A., Oates, J. A., Zaltzman, P. and Udenfriend, S.: Serotonin synthesis in carcinoid patients. Its inhibition by α-methyl-dopa with measurement of associated increases in urinary 5-hydroxytryptophan. *New Engl. J. Med.,* **263,** 585 (1960).

Sjökvist, F., Titus, I., Michelson, A., Taylor, F., Jr. and Richardson, K. C.: Uptake and metabolism of *d, l*-norepinephrine-7-H³ in tissues of immunosympathectomized mice and rats. *Life Sci.,* **4,** 1125 (1965).

Smith, A. D. and Winkler, H.: A simple method for the isolation of adrenal chromaffin granules on a large scale. *Biochem. J.,* **103,** 480 (1967 a).

Smith, A. D. and Winkler, H.: Purification and properties of an acidic protein from chromaffin granules of bovine adrenal medulla. *Biochem. J.,* **103,** 483 (1967 b).

Smith, E. R. B. and Weil-Malherbe, H.: Metanephrine and normetanephrine in human urine: method and results. *J. Lab. Clin. Med.,* **60,** 212 (1962).

Smith, T. E., Weissbach, H. and Udenfriend, S.: Studies on the mechanism of action of monoamine oxidase: Metabolism of *N,N*-dimethyltryptamine and *N,N*-dimethyltryptamine-*N*-oxide. *Biochemistry,* **1,** 137 (1962).

Smith, W. J. and Kirshner, N.: Enzymatic formation of noradrenaline by the banana plant. *J. Biol. Chem.,* **235,** 3589 (1960).

Smith, W. J. and Kirshner, N.: Mechanism of 3,4-dihydroxyphenylethylamine-β-hydroxylase. *J. Biol. Chem.,* **237,** 1890 (1962).

Snyder, S. H., Fischer, J. and Axelrod, J.: Evidence for the presence of monoamine oxidase in sympathetic nerve endings. *Biochem. Pharmacol.,* **14,** 363 (1965).

Snyder, S. H. and Hendley, E. D.: A simple and sensitive fluorescence assay for monoamine oxidase and diamine oxidase. *J. Pharmacol. Exp. Therap.,* **163,** 386 (1968).

Snyder, S. H. and Hendley, E. D.: Sensitive fluorometric and radiometric assays for monoamine oxidase and diamine oxidase. In "Methods in Enzymology" (H. Tabor and C. W. Tabor, *eds*), vol. 17B, p. 741. Academic Press, New York (1971).

Sommerville, A. R.: The assay of aromatic amino acid decarboxylase using radioactive substrates. *Biochem. Pharmacol.,* **13,** 1861 (1964).

Sourkes, T. L.: Inhibition of dihydroxyphenylalanine decarboxylase by derivatives of phenylalanine. *Arch. Biochem. Biophys.,* **51,** 444 (1954).

Sourkes, T. L.: DOPA decarboxylase, substrates, coenzyme, inhibitors. *Pharmacol. Rev.,* **18,** 53 (1966).

Sourkes, T. L.: Properties of the monoamine oxidase of rat liver mitochondria. In "Advances in Pharmacology" (S. Garattini and P. A. Shore, *eds*), vol. 6, Part A., Biological role of indolealkylamine derivatives., p. 61. Academic Press, New York (1968).

Sourkes, T. L. and D'Iorio, A.: Inhibitors of catecholamine metabolism. In "Metabolic Inhibitors" (R. M. Hochster and J. H. Quastel, *eds*), vol. 2, p. 79. Academic Press, New York (1963).

Sourkes, T. L., Murphy, G. F., Chavez, B. and Zielinska, M.: The action of some α-methyl and other amino acids on cerebral catecholamines. *J. Neurochem.,* **8,** 109 (1961).

Spector, S., Melmon, K., Lovenberg, W. and Sjoerdsma, A.: The presence and distribution of tyramine in mammalian tissues. *J. Pharmacol. Exp. Therap.,* **140,** 229 (1963).

Spector, S., Prockop, D., Shore, P. P. and Brodie, B. B.: Effect of iproniazid on brain levels of norepinephrine and serotonin. *Science,* **127,** 704 (1958).

Spector, S., Sjoerdsma, A. and Udenfriend, S.: Blockade of endogenous norepinephrine synthesis by alpha-methyl-tyrosine, an inhibitor of tyrosine hydroxylase. *J. Pharmacol. Exp. Therap.,* **147,** 86 (1965).

Spector, S., Sjoerdsma, A., Zaltzman-Nirenberg, P., Levitt, M. and Udenfriend, S.: Norepinephrine synthesis from tyrosine-C^{14} in isolated perfused guinea pig heart. *Science,* **139,** 1299 (1963).

Stecher, P. G., Windholz, M., Leahy, D. S., Bolton, D. M. and Eaton, L. G., *eds*: "The Merck Index," 8th Ed., Merck & Co., Inc., Rahway, N. J., U.S.A. (1968).

Steinman, A. M., Smerin, S. E. and Barchas, J. D.: Epinephrine metabolism in mammalian brain after intravenous and intraventricular administration. *Science*, **165**, 616 (1969).

Stjärne, L.: Studies of catecholamine uptake storage and release mechanisms. *Acta Physiol. Scand.*, **62**, Suppl. 228 (1964).

Stjärne, L.: Storage particles in noradrenergic tissues. *Pharmacol. Rev.*, **18**, 42 (1966 a).

Stjärne, L.: Noradrenaline biosynthesis in nerve tissue. *Acta Phisiol. Scand.*, **67**, 441 (1966 b).

Stjärne, L. and Lishajko, F.: Localization of different steps in noradrenaline synthesis to different fractions of a bovine splenic nerve homogenate. *Biochem. Pharmacol.*, **16**, 1719 (1967).

Stolz, F.: Über Adrenalin und Alkylaminoacetobrenzcatechin. *Ber. d. deutsch. Chem. Gesellsch.*, **37**, 4149 (1904).

Storm, C. B. and Kaufman, S.: The effect of variation of cofactor and substrate structure on the action of phenylalanine hydroxylase. *Biochem. Biophys. Res. Communs.*, **32**, 788 (1968).

Strömblad, B. C. R.: Observation on amine oxidase in human salivary glands. *J. Physiol.*, **147**, 639 (1959).

Strömblad, B. C. R. and Nickerson, M.: Accumulation of epinephrine and norepinephrine by some rat tissues. *J. Pharmacol. Exp. Therap.*, **134**, 154 (1961).

Studnitz, W. von: Über die Ausscheidung der 3-Methoxy-4-hydroxyphenylessigsäure (Homovanillin Säure) beim Neuroblastom und anderen neuralen Tumoren. *Klin. Wchschr.*, **40**, 163 (1962).

Suda, H., Takeuchi, T., Nagatsu, T., Matsuzaki, M., Matsumoto, I. and Umezawa, H.: Inhibition of dopamine β-hydroxylase by 5-alkylpicolinic acid and their hypotensive effects. *Chem. Pharm. Bull.*, **17**, 2377 (1969).

Sutherland, E. W. and Robison, G. A.: The role of cyclic-3',5'-AMP in responses to catecholamines and other hormones. *Pharmacol. Rev.*, **18**, 145 (1966).

Sutherland, E. W. and Rall, T. W.: The relations of adenosine-3',5'-phosphate and phosphorylase to the actions of catecholamines and other hormones. *Pharmacol. Rev.*, **12**, 265 (1960).

Szara, S., Axelrod, J. and Perlin, S.: Is adrenochrome present in the blood. *Am. J. Psychiat.*, **115**, 162 (1958).

Tabor, C. W., Tabor, H. and Rosenthal, S. M.: Purification of amine oxidase from beef plasma. *J. Biol. Chem.*, **208**, 645 (1954).

Takamine, J.: The blood-pressure-raising principle of the suprarenal glands: A preliminary report. *Therap. Gaz. s. 3.*, **16**, 221 (1901).

Takesada, M., Kakimoto, Y., Sano, I. and Kaneko, J.: 3,4-Dimethoxyphenylethylamine and other amines in the urine of schizophrenic patients. *Nature*, **199**, 203 (1963).

Taniguchi, K., Kakimoto, Y. and Armstrong, M. D.: Quantitative determination of metanephrine and normetanephrine in urine. *J. Lab. Clin. Med.*, **64**, 469 (1964).

Tautz, N. A., Voltmer, G. and Schmid, E.: Methode zur quantitativen Bestimmung von Homovanillsäure, Vanillinmandelsäure und Vanillinsäure im Urin mit dünnschicht-chromatographischer Trennung. *Klin. Wschr.*, **43**, 233 (1965).

Taylor, R. J., Stubbs, C. S. and Ellenbogen, L.: Inhibition of tyrosine hydroxylase *in vitro* and *in vivo* by 3-amino-pyrrolo[3,4c]isoxazole and derivatives. *Biochem. Pharmacol., 17,* 1779 (1968).

Taylor, R. J., Jr., Stubbs, C. S., Jr. and Ellenbogen, L.: Tyrosine hydroxylase inhibition *in vitro* and *in vivo* by chelating agents. *Biochem. Pharmacol., 18,* 587 (1969).

Taylor, R. J., Jr., Stubbs, C. S., Jr. and Ellenbogen, L.: Tyrosine hydroxylase inhibition *in vitro* and *in vivo* by deoxyfrenolicin. *Biochem. Pharmacol., 19,* 1737 (1970).

Thoenen, H., Mueller, R. A. and Axelrod, J.: Increased tyrosine hydroxylase activity after drung-induced alteration of sympathetic transmission. *Nature,* **221,** 1264 (1969).

Thoenen, H., Mueller, R. A. and Axelrod, J.: Phase difference in the induction of tyrosine hydroxylase in cell body and nerve terminals of sympathetic neurons. *Proc. Natl. Acad. Sci., 65,* 58 (1970 a).

Thoenen, H., Mueller, R. A. and Axelrod, J.: Neuronally dependent induction of adrenal phenylethanolamine-*N*-methyltransferase by 6-hydroxydopamine. *Biochem. Pharmacol., 19,* 669 (1970 b).

Tietz, A., Lindberg, M. and Kennedy, E. P.: A new pteridine-requiring enzyme system for the oxidation of glycerol ethers. *J. Biol. Chem., 239,* 4081 (1964).

Tipton, K. F.: The purification of pig brain mitochondrial monoamine oxidase. *Eur. J. Biochem., 4,* 103 (1968 a).

Tipton, K. F.: The reaction pathway of pig brain mitochondrial monoamine oxidase. *Eur. J. Biochem., 5,* 316 (1968 b).

Tipton, K. F.: A sensitive fluorometric assay for monoamine oxidase. *Anal. Biochem., 28,* 318 (1969).

Tipton, K. F.: Monoamine oxidase (pig brain mitochondria). In "Methods in Enzymology" (H. Tabor and C. W. Tabor, *eds*), vol. 17B, p. 717. Academic Press, New York (1971).

Tissot, R., Gaillard, J. M., Guggisberg, M., Ganthier, G. and de Ajuriaguerra, J.: Thérapeutique du syndrome de Parkinson par la L-DOPA "per os" associée à un inhibiteur de la decarboxylase (Ro 4-4602). *Press Méd., 77,* 619 (1969).

Tomita, E., Macha, E. and Lardy, C. A.: Enzymatic *O*-methylation of iodinated phenols and thyroid hormones. *J. Biol. Chem., 239,* 1202 (1964).

Tong, J. H., D'Iorio, A. and Benoiton, N. L.: The formation of 3,4-dihydroxy-L-phenylalanine from L-*meta*-tyrosine by rat liver and beef adrenal medulla. *Biochem. Biophys. Res. Commun., 43,* 819 (1971).

Tong, J. H., D'Iorio, A. and Benoiton, N. L.: Formation of *meta*-tyrosine from L-phenylalanine by beef adrenal medulla. A new biosynthetic route to catecholamines. *Biochem. Biophys. Res. Commun., 44,* 229 (1971).

Udenfriend, S.: Mammalian aromatic L-amino acid decarboxylase. "Proceedings of the Symposium on Chemical and Biological Aspects of Pyridoxal Catalysis, Rome, 1962," p. 267. Pergamon Press, Oxford (1962 a).

Udenfriend, S.: "Fluorescence Assay in Biology and Medicine," vol. 1, p. 129. Academic Press, New York (1962 b).

Udenfriend, S.: Factors in amino acid metabolism which can influence the central nervous system. *Am. J. Clin. Nutr., 12,* 287 (1963).

Udenfriend, S.: Biosynthesis and release of catecholamines. In "Mechanism of

Release of Biogenic Amines." Proceedings of an international Wenner-Gren symposium, Stockholm, February 1965, p. 103. Pergamon Press, London (1966 a).

Udenfriend, S.: Biosynthesis of the sympathetic neurotransmitter, norepinephrine. In "The Harvey Lectures, Series 60," p. 57. Academic Press, New York (1966 b).

Udenfriend, S.: Tyrosine hydroxylase. *Pharmacol. Rev.*, **18**, 43 (1966 c).

Udenfriend, S.: Physiological regulation of noradrenaline biosynthesis. In "Adrenergic Neurotransmission" (Ciba Foundation Study Group No. 33) (G. E. W. Wolstenholme and M. O'Connor, *eds*), p. 3. Churchill Ltd., London (1968).

Udenfriend, S.: "Fluorescence Assay in Biology and Medicine," vol. 2, p. 207. Academic Press, New York (1969).

Udenfriend, S. and Bessman S. P.: The hydroxylation of phenylalanine and antipyrine in phenylpyruvic oligophrenia. *J. Biol. Chem.*, **203**, 961 (1953).

Udenfriend, S., Clark, C. T., Axelrod, J. and Brodie, B. B.: Ascorbic acid in aromatic hydroxylation I. A model system for aromatic hydroxylation. *J. Biol. Chem.*, **208**, 731 (1954).

Udenfriend, S. and Cooper, J. R.: The enzymatic conversion of phenylalanine to tyrosine. *J. Biol. Chem.*, **194**, 503 (1952 a).

Udenfriend, S. and Cooper, J. R.: The chemical estimation of tyrosine and tyramine. *J. Biol. Chem.*, **196**, 227 (1952 b).

Udenfriend, S., Cooper, J. R., Clark, C. T. and Baer, J. E.: Rate of turnover of epinephrine in the adrenal medulla. *Science*, **117**, 663 (1953).

Udenfriend, S. and Creveling, C. R.: Localization of dopamine-β-oxidase in brain. *J. Neurochem.*, **4**, 350 (1959).

Udenfriend, S., Creveling, C. R., Ozaki, M., Daly, J. W. and Witkop, B.: Inhibitors of norepinephrine metabolism *in vivo. Arch. Biochem. Biophys.*, **84**, 249 (1959).

Udenfriend, S., Lovenberg, W. and Sjoerdsma, A.: Physiologically active amines in common fruits and vegetables. *Arch. Biochem. Biophys.*, **85**, 487 (1959).

Udenfriend, S., Weissbach, H. and Brodie, B.: Assay of serotonin and related metabolites, enzymes, and drugs. In "Methods of Biochemical Analysis" (D. Glick, *ed*), vol. 6, p. 95. Interscience Publishers Inc., New York (1958).

Udenfriend, S., Weissbach, H. and Clark, C T.: The estimation of 5-hydroxytryptamine (serotonin) in biological tissue. *J. Biol. Chem.*, **215**, 337 (1955).

Udenfriend, S., Witkop, B., Redfield, B. G. and Weissbach, H.: Studies with reversible inhibitors of monoamine oxidase: harmaline and related compounds. *Biochem. Pharmacol.*, **1**, 16 (1958).

Udenfriend, S. and Wyngaarden, J. B.: Precursors of adrenal epinephrine and norepinephrine *in vivo. Biochim. Biophys. Acta*, **20**, 48 (1956).

Udenfriend, S. and Zaltzman-Nirenberg, P.: Norepinephrine and 3,4-dihydroxyphenethylamine turnover in guinea pig brain *in vivo. Science*, **142**, 394 (1963).

Udenfriend, S., Zaltzman-Nirenberg, P. and Nagatsu, T.: Inhibitors of purified beef adrenal tyrosine hydroxylase. *Biochem. Pharmacol.*, **14**, 837 (1965).

Umezawa, H., Takeuchi, T., Iinuma, H., Suzuki, K., Ito, M., Matsuzaki, M., Nagatsu, T. and Tanabe, O.: A new microbial product, oudenone, inhibiting tyrosine hydroxylase. *J. Antibiotics*, **28**, 514 (1970).

Uretsky, N. J. and Iversen, L. L.: Effects of 6-hydroxydopamine on catechol-amine-containing neurons in the rat brain. *J. Neurochem.*, **17**, 269 (1970).

Van der Schoot, J. B., Creveling, C. R., Nagatsu, T. and Udenfriend, S.: On the mechanism of inhibition of dopamine-β-oxidase by benzyloxyamines. *J. Pharmacol. Exp. Therap.*, **141**, 74 (1963).

Van der Schoot, J. B. and Creveling, C. R.: Substrates and inhibitors of dop-amine-β-hydroxylase (DBH). In "Advances in Drug Research" (N. J. Harper and A. B. Simmonds, *eds*), vol. 2, p. 47. Academic Press, New York (1965).

Van Woert, M. H. and Bowers, M. B., Jr.: Effect of L-dopa (3,4-dihydroxyphenyl-alanine) on monoamine metabolites in Parkinson's disease. *Experientia*, **26**, 161 (1970).

Viktora, J. K., Baukal, A. and Wolff, F. W.: New automated fluorometric meth-ods for estimation of small amounts of adrenaline and noradrenaline. *Anal. Biochem.*, **23**, 513 (1968).

Viveros, O. H., Arqueros, L. and Kirshner, N.: Release of catecholamines and dopamine-β-oxidase from the adrenal medulla. *Life Sci.*, **7**, 609 (1968).

Vogel, W. H., McFarland, H. and Prince, L. N.: Decarboxylation of 3,4-dihy-droxyphenylalanine in various human adult and fetal tissue. *Biochem. Phar-macol.*, **19**, 618 (1970).

Vogel, W. H., Snyder, R. and Hara, T. A.: The enzymatic decarboxylation of DOPA in human liver homogenate. *Proc. Soc. Exp. Biol. Med.*, **134**, 477 (1970).

Vogt, M.: The concentration of sympathin in different parts of the central nerv-ous system under normal conditions and after the administration of drugs. *J. Physiol.*, **123**, 451 (1954).

Waalkes, T. P., Sjoerdsma, A., Creveling, C. R., Weissbach, H. and Udenfriend, S.: Serotonin, norepinephrine, and related compounds in bananas. *Science*, **127**, 684 (1958).

Waalkes, T. P. and Udenfriend, S.: A fluorometric method for the estimation of tyrosine in plasma and tissues. *J. Lab. Clin. Med.*, **50**, 733 (1957).

Wada, Y.: Quantitative determination of 3,4-dihydroxymandelic acid in human urine. *Tohoku J. Exp. Med.*, **79**, 389 (1963).

Walker, W. H., Kearney, E. B., Seng, R. and Singer, T. P.: Sequence and struc-ture of a cysteinyl flavin peptide from monoamine oxidase. *Biochem. Biophys. Res. Commun.*, **44**, 287 (1971).

Weil-Malherbe, H.: The fluorimetric estimation of catechol compounds by the ethylenediamine condensation method. *Pharmacol. Rev.*, **11**, 278 (1959).

Weil-Malherbe, H.: The condensation of catechols with ethylenediamine. *Bio-chim. Biophys. Acta*, **40**, 349 (1960 a).

Weil-Malherbe, H.: The fluorimetric estimation of catecholamines. In "Methods in Medical Research" (J. H. Quastel, *ed*), vol. 9, p. 130. Yearbook Medical Publishers, Chicago (1960 b).

Weil-Malherbe, H.: Simultaneous estimation of catecholamines and their meta-bolites. *Z. Klin. Chem.*, **2**, 161 (1964 a).

Weil-Malherbe, H.: Studies on the estimation of acidic metabolites of catechol-amines. *Fed. Proc.*, **23**, 491 (1964 b).

Weil-Malherbe, H.: The estimation of 3,4-dihydroxymandelic acid in urine and its excretion by man. *J. Lab. Clin. Med.*, **69**, 1025 (1967).

Weil-Malherbe, H., Axelrod, J. and Tomchick, R.: Blood-brain barrier for adrenaline. *Science,* **129,** 1226 (1959).

Weil-Malherbe, H. and Bone, A. D.: The chemical estimation of adrenaline-like substance in blood. *Biochem. J.,* **51,** 311 (1952).

Weil-Malherbe, H. and Bone, A. D.: The fluorimetric estimation of adrenaline and noradrenaline in plasma. *Biochem. J.,* **67,** 65 (1957 a).

Weil-Malherbe, H. and Bone, A. D.: The estimation of catecholamines in urine by a chemical method. *J. Clin. Path.,* **10,** 138 (1957 b).

Weil-Malherbe, H. and Bone, A. D.: Intracellular distribution of catecholamines in the brain. *Nature,* **180,** 1050 (1957 c).

Weil-Malherbe, H. and Bone, A. D.: The effect of reserpine on the intracellular distribution of catecholamines in the brain stem of the rabbit. *J. Neurochem.,* **4,** 251 (1959)

Weil-Malherbe, H. and Smith, E. R. B.: The estimation of metanephrine, normetanephrine and 3,4-dihydroxymandelic acid in urine. *Pharmacol. Rev.,* **18,** 331 (1966).

Weil-Malherbe, H., Whitby, L. G. and Axelrod, J.: The uptake of circulating (^{3}H) norepinephrine by the pituitary gland and various areas of the brain, *J. Neurochem.,* **8,** 55 (1961).

Weiner, N. and Jardetzky, O.: A study of catecholamine nucleotide complexes by nuclear magnetic resonance spectroscopy. *Arch. exp. Path. Pharmakol.,* **248,** 308 (1964).

Weiner, N. and Rabadjija, M.: The regulation of norepinephrine synthesis. Effect of puromycin on the accelerated synthesis of norepinephrine associated with nerve stimulation. *J. Pharmacol. Exp. Therap.,* **164,** 103 (1968).

Weinshilboum, R. and Axelrod, J.: Serum dopamine-beta-hydroxylase activity. *Circ. Res.,* **28,** 307 (1971).

Weissbach, H., Redfield, B. G. and Udenfriend, S.: Soluble monoamine oxidase; its properties and actions on serotonin. *J. Biol. Chem.,* **229,** 953 (1957).

Weissbach, H., Smith, T. E., Daly, J. W., Witkop, B. and Udenfriend, S.: A rapid spectrophotometric assay of monoamine oxidase based on the rate of disappearance of kynuramine. *J. Biol. Chem.,* **235,** 1160 (1960).

Welch, A. S. and Welch, B. L.: Solvent extraction method for simultaneous determination of norepinephrine, dopamine, serotonin, and 5-hydroxyindoleacetic acid in a single mouse brain. *Anal. Biochem.,* **30,** 161 (1969).

Westfall, T. C.: Effect of alpha-methyltyrosine on content and subcellular distribution of norepinephrine in rat heart and brain. *Life Sci.,* **9,** 339 (1970).

Whitby, L. G., Axelrod, J. and Weil-Malherbe, H.: The fate of H^3-norepinephrine in animals. *J. Pharmacol. Exp. Therap.,* **132,** 193 (1961).

Whiteley, J. M. and Huennekens, F. M.: 2-Amino-4-hydroxy-6-methyl-7,8-dihydropteridine as a model for dihydrofolate. *Biochemistry,* **6,** 2620 (1967).

Whittaker, V. P.: The isolation and characterization of acetylcholine-containing particles from brain. *Biochem. J.,* **72,** 694 (1959).

Whittaker, V. P.: Catecholamine storage particles in the central nervous system. *Pharmacol. Rev.,* **18,** 401 (1966).

Whittaker, V. P., Michaelson, I. A. and Kirkland, R. J. A.: The separation of synaptic vesicles from nerve ending particles (synaptosomes). *Biochem. J.,* **90,** 293 (1964).

Wilbrandt, W. and Rosenberg, T.: The concept of carrier transport and its corollaries in pharmacology. *Pharmacol. Rev.,* **13,** 109 (1961).

Wilk, S., Gitlow, S. E., Mendlowitz, M., Franklin, M. J., Carr, H. E. and Clarke, D. D.: A quantitative assay for vanillylmandelic acid (VMA) by gas-liquid chromatography. *Anal. Biochem.,* **13,** 544 (1965).

Williams, C. M., Babuscio, A. A. and Watson, R.: *In vivo* alteration of the pathways of dopamine metabolism. *Am. J. Physiol.,* **199,** 722 (1960).

Williams, C. M. and Greer, M.: Diagnosis of neuroblastoma by quantitative gas chromatographic analysis of urinary homovanillic acid and vanilmandelic acid. *Clin. Chim. Acta,* **7,** 880 (1962).

Winkler, H., Ziegler, E. and Strieder, N.: Studies on the proteins from chromaffin granules of ox, horse and pig. *Nature,* **211,** 982 (1966).

Wisser, H. and Stamm, D.: Semiautomatic method for the measurement of dopamine in urine. *Z. Klin. Chem. Klin. Biochem.,* **7,** 631 (1969).

Wisser, H. and Stamm, D.: Measurement of 4-hydroxy-3-methoxymandelic acid (vanilmandelic acid) in urine. *Z. Klin. Chem. Klin. Biochem.,* **8,** 21 (1970).

Wurtman, R. J.: The effects of endocrine, synaptic and nutritional inputs on catecholamine-containing neurons. In "Biochemistry of Brain and Behavior" (R. E. Bowman and S. P. Datta, *eds*), p. 91. Plenum Press, New York-London (1970).

Wurtman, R. J. and Axelrod, J.: Sex steroids, cardiac ^{3}H-norepinephrine, and tissue monoamine oxidase levels in the rat. *Biochem. Pharmacol.,* **12,** 1417 (1963 a).

Wurtman, R. J. and Axelrod, J.: A sensitive and specific assay for the estimation of monoamine oxidase. *Biochem. Pharmacol.,* **12,** 1439 (1963 b).

Wurtman, R. J. and Axelrod, J.: Adrenaline synthesis; Control by the pituitary gland and adrenal glucocorticoids. *Science,* **150,** 1464 (1965).

Wurtman, R. J. and Axelrod, J.: Control of enzymatic synthesis of adrenaline in the adrenal medulla by adrenal cortical steroids. *J. Biol. Chem.,* **241,** 2301 (1966).

Wurtman, R. J., Noble, E. P. and Axelrod, J.: Inhibition of enzymatic synthesis of epinephrine by low doses of glucocorticoids. *Endocrinology,* **80,** 825 (1967).

Wurzburger, R. J. and Musacchio, J. M.: Subcellular distribution and aggregation of bovine adrenal tyrosine hydroxylase. *J. Pharmacol. Exp. Therap.,* **177,** 155 (1971).

Yagi, K. and Nagatsu, T.: Condensation products of ethylenediamine with catechol derivatives. *J. Biochem. (Tokyo),* **48,** 439 (1960).

Yagi, K., Nagatsu, T. and Nagatsu, I.: Condensation product of ethylenediamine with noradrenaline or 3,4-dihydroxymandelic acid. *Nature,* **186,** 310 (1960).

Yagi, K., Nagatsu, T. and Nagatsu-Ishibashi, I.: Condensation reaction of DOPA with ethylenediamine. *J. Biochem. (Tokyo),* **48,** 617 (1960).

Yamada, H. and Yasunobu, K. T.: Monoamine oxidase. I. Purification, crystallization, and properties of plasma monoamine oxidase. *J. Biol. Chem,* **237,** 1511 (1962).

Yamada, H. and Yasunobu, K. T.: Monoamine oxidase. IV. Nature of the second prosthetic group of plasma monoamine oxidase. *J. Biol. Chem.,* **238,** 2669 (1963).

Yamamoto, I., Oka, M. and Iwata, H.: *In vitro* activation of monoamine oxidase in rat tissue homogenates by 4(or 5)-diazoimidazole-5(or 4)-carboxamide.

Biochem. Pharmacol., **19**, 1831 (1970).

Yasunobu, K. T. and Gomes, B.: Mitochondrialamine oxidase (monoamine oxidase) (beef liver). In "Methods in Enzymology" (H. Tabor and C. W. Tabor, *eds*), vol. 17B, p. 789. Academic Press, New York (1971).

Yasunobu, K. T., Igaue, I. and Gomes, B.: The purification and properties of beef liver mitochondrial monoamine oxidase. In "Advances in Pharmacology" (S. Garattini and P. A. Shore, *eds*), vol. 6, Part A, Biological role of indole-alkylamine derivatives, p. 43. Academic Press, New York (1968).

Yoshinaga, K., Itoh, C., Ishida, N., Sato, T. and Wada, Y.: Quantitative determination of metadrenaline and normetadrenaline in normal human urine. *Nature,* **191**, 599 (1961).

Youdim, M. B. H., Collins, G. G. S. and Sandler, M.: Multiple forms of rat brain monoamine oxidase. *Nature,* **223**, 626 (1969).

Youdim, M. B. H. and Collins, G. G. S.: Dissociation and reassociation of rat liver mitochondrial monoamine oxidase. *Biochem. J.,* **117**, 37P(1970).

Youdim, M. B. H. and Collins, G. G. S.: The dissociation and reassociation of rat liver mitochondrial monoamine oxidase. *Europ. J. Biochem.,* **18**, 73 (1971).

Youdim, M. B. H. and Sandler, M.: Isoenzymes of soluble monoamine oxidase from human placenta and rat-liver mitochondria. *Biochem. J.,* **105**, 43P(1967).

Youdim, M. B. H. and Sandler, M.: Activation of monoamine oxidase and inhibition of aldehyde dehydrogenase by reserpine. *Eur. J. Pharmacol.,* **4**, 105 (1968).

Youdim, M. B. H. and Sourkes, T. L.: Properties of purified, soluble monoamine oxidase. *Can. J. Biochem.,* **44**, 1397 (1966).

Zaimis, E., Berk, L. and Callingham, B. A.: Morphological, biochemical and functional changes in the sympathetic nervous system of rats treated with NGF-antiserum. *Nature,* **206**, 1220 (1965).

Zeller, E. A. and Barsky, J.: *In vivo* inhibition of liver and brain monoamine oxidase by 1-isonicotinyl-2-isopropylhydrazine. *Proc. Soc. Exp. Biol. Med.,* **81**, 459 (1952).

Zeller, E. A., Barsky, J. and Berman, E. R.: Amine oxidase; inhibition of monoamine oxidase by 1-isonicotinyl-2-isoprophylhydrazine. *J. Biol. Chem.,* **214**, 267 (1955).

Zeller, E. A., Barsky, J., Fouts, J. R., Kirchheimer, W. F. and Van Orden, L. S.: Influence of isonicotinic acid hydrazide (INH) and 1-isonicotinyl-2-isopropyl-hydrazide (IIH) on bacterial and mammalian enzymes. *Experientia,* **8**, 349 (1952).

Zhelyaskov, D. K., Levitt, M. and Udenfriend, S.: Tryptophan derivatives as inhibitors of tyrosine hydroxylase *in vivo* and *in vitro*. *Mol. Pharmacol.,* **4**, 445 (1968).

Zilversmit, D. B.: The design and analysis of isotope experiments. *Am. J. Med.,* **29**, 832 (1960).

Zöllner, N. and Wolfram, G.: TLC in clinical diagnosis. In "Thin-layer Chromatography" (E. Stahl, *ed*), p. 578. Springer-Verlag, Heidelberg (1969).

SUPPLEMENT REFERENCES

Christenson, J. G.: Studies on aromatic L-amino acid decarboxylase. Thesis, The City University of New York (1972).

Ellenbogen, L., Markley, E. and Taylor, R. J.: Inhibition of histidine decarboxylase by benzyl and aliphatic aminooxyamines. *Biochem. Pharmacol.,* **18**, 683 (1969).

Foldes, A., Jeffrey, P. L., Preston, B. N. and Austin, L.: Dopamine β-hydroxylase of bovine adrenal medulla. A rapid purification procedure. *Biochem. J.,* **126**, 1209 (1972).

Friedman, P. A., Lloyd, T. and Kaufman, S.: Production of antibodies to rat liver phenylalanine hydroxylase, cross-reactivity with other pterin-dependent hydroxylases. *Mol. Pharmacol.,* **8**, 501 (1972).

Fuxe, K., Goldstein, M., Hödfelt, T. and Joh, T.H.: Cellular localization of dopamine-β-hydroxylase and phenylethanolamine-N-methyltransferase as revealed by immunohistochemistry. *Progress in Brain Research*, **34**, 127 (1971).

Geffen, L. B., Livett, B. G. and Rush, R. A.: Immunohistochemical localization of protein components of catecholamine storage vesicles. *J. Physiol.,* **204**, 593 (1969).

Goldstein, M., Fuxe, K., Hökfelt, T. and Joh, T. H.: Immunohistochemical studies on phenylethanolamine-N-methyltransferase, dopa-decarboxylase and dopamine-β-hydroxylase. *Experientia*, **27**, 951 (1971).

Hartman, B. K., Yasunobu, K. T. and Udenfriend, S.: Immunological identity of the multiple forms of beef liver mitochondrial monoamine oxidase. *Arch. Biochem. Biophys.,* **147**, 797 (1971).

Hartman, B. K., Zide, D. and Udenfriend, S.: The use of dopamine-β-hydroxylase as a marker for the central noradrenergic nervous system in rat brain. *Proc. Natl. Acad. Sci. U. S. A.,* **69**, 2722 (1972).

Hidaka, H. Hartman, B. and Udenfriend, S.: Comparison of mitochondrial monoamine oxidases from bovine brain and liver using antibody to purified liver monoamine oxidase. *Arch. Biochem. Biophys.,* **147**, 805 (1971).

Kuzuya, H. and Nagatsu, T.: Properties of dopamine β-hydroxylase in soluble and particulate fractions of bovine adrenal medulla. *Biochem. Pharmacol.,* **21**, 737 (1972).

Kuzuya, H. and Nagatsu, T.: Intracellular distribution of endogenous inhibitors of dopamine β-hydroxylase in bovine adrenal medulla. *Biochem. Pharmacol.,* **21**, 740 (1972).

Laduron, P.: N-Methylation of dopamine to epinine in brain tissue using N-methyltetrahydrofolic acid as the methyl donor. *Nature New Biology,* **238**, 212 (1972).

Mizutani, K., Nagatsu, T., Asashima, M. and Kinoshita, S.: Inhibition of tyrosine hydroxylase by naphthoquinone pigments of echinoids. *Biochem. Pharmacol.,* **21**, 2463 (1972).

Nagatsu, I., Sudo, Y. and Nagatsu, T.: Tyrosine hydroxylation in the banana plant. *Enzymologia,* **43**, 25 (1972).

Nagatsu, T., Kato, T., Kuzuya, H., Umezawa, H., Matsuzaki, M. and Takeuchi, T.: Serum dopamine-β-hydroxylase in spontaneously hypertensive rats. *Experientia,* **28**, 905 (1972).

Nagatsu, T., Mizutani, K., Nagatsu, I., Umezawa, H., Matsuzaki, M. and Takeuchi, T.: Enzymes of catecholamine biosynthesis and metabolism in spontaneously hyperten-

352

sive rats and hypotensive effects of the specific inhibitors from microbial origin. In "Spontaneous Hypertension-Its Pathogenesis and Complications" (K. Okamoto, *ed.*), p. 31. Igaku Shoin, Tokyo (1972).

Nakashima, Y., Suzue, R., Sanada, H. and Kawada, S.: Effect of ascorbic acid on tyrosine hydroxylase activity *in vivo*. *Arch. Biochem. Biophys.*, **152**, 515 (1972).

Oreland, L.: Purification and properties of pig liver mitochondrial monoamine oxidase. *Arch. Biochem. Biophys.*, **146**, 410 (1971).

Rhoads, R. E. and Udenfriend, S.: Decarboxylation of α-ketoglutarate coupled to collagen proline hydroxylase. *Proc. Nat. Acad. Sci. U. S. A.*, **60**, 1473 (1968).

Rush, R. and Geffen, L.: Radioimmunoassay and clearance of circulating dopamine-β-hydroxylase. *Circ. Res.*, **31**, 444 (1972).

Udenfriend, S., Stein, S., Böhlen, P., Dairman, W., Leimgruber, W. and Weigele, M.: Fluorescamine: a reagent for assay of amino acids, peptides, proteins and other primary amines in the picomole range. *Science*, **178**, 871 (1972).

Walsh, D. A., Perkins, J. P. and Krebs, E. G.: An adenosine 3′,5′-monophosphate-dependent protein kinase from rabbit skeletal muscle. *J. Biol. Chem.*, **243**, 3763 (1968).

Waymire, J. C., Bjur, R. and Weiner, N.: Assay of tyrosine hydroxylase by coupled decarboxylation of Dopa formed from 1-^{14}C-L-tyrosine. *Anal. Biochem.*, **43**, 588 (1971).

Weigele, M., Blount, J. F., Tengi, J. P., Czajkowski, R. C. and Leimgruber, W.: The fluorogenic ninhydrin reaction. Structure of the fluorescent principle. *J. Am. Chem. Soc.*, **94**, 4052 (1972).

Weinshilboum, R. M., Thoa, N. B., Johnson, D. G., Kopin, I. J. and Axelrod, J.: Proportional release of norepinephrine and dopamine-β-hydroxylase from sympathetic nerves. *Science*, **174**, 1349 (1971).

INDEX

1976

)k may be kept

TEEN DAYS